Pharmaceutical Analysis

(Volume 2)

Pharmaceutical Analysis

(Volume 2)

THIRD EDITION

Dr Anees Ahmad Siddiqui
Head, Department of Pharmaceutical Chemistry
Jamia Hamdard University
Hamdard Nagar, New Delhi-110062

Dr Seemi Siddiqui
Vice Principal
International Institute of Pharmaceutical Sciences,
Sonepat, Haryana

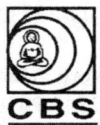

CBS PUBLISHERS & DISTRIBUTORS PVT. LTD.

NEW DELHI • BENGALURU • CHENNAI • KOCHI • MUMBAI • PUNE

ISBN : 978-81-239-2491-5

First Edition : 2006
Reprint : 2007
Second Edition : 2009
Reprint : 2011
Third Edition : 2014

Copyright © Authors & Publisher

All rights reserved. No part of this book may be reproduced or transmitted in any form or by any means, electronic or mechanical, including photocopying, recording, or any information storage and retrieval system without permission, in writing, from the publisher.

Published by Satish Kumar Jain and produced by V.K. Jain for
CBS Publishers & Distributors Pvt. Ltd.,
4819/XI Prahlad Street, 24 Ansari Road, Daryaganj,
New Delhi - 110002, India.
e-mail: cbspubs@vsnl.com, cbspubs@airtelmail.in
Website: www.cbspd.com

- *Bengaluru:* Seema House, 2975, 17th Cross, K.R. Road,
  Bansankari 2nd Stage, Bengaluru - 560070
  - Ph.: +91-80-26771678/79 • Fax: +91-80-26771680
  - E-mail: cbsbng@gmail.com, bangalore@cbspd.com
- *Pune:* Bhuruk Prestige, Sr. No. 52/12/2+1+3/2,
  Narhe, Haveli (Near Katraj-Dehu Road By-pass), Pune - 411041
  - Ph.: +91-20-64704058/59, 020-32392277 • E-mail: pune@cbspd.com
- *Kochi:* 36/14, Kalluvilakam, Lissie Hospital Road,
  Kochi - 682018, Kerala • Ph.: +91-484-4059061-65
  • Fax: +91-484-4059065 • E-mail: cochin@cbspd.com
- *Chennai:* 20, West Park Road, Shenoy Nagar, Chennai - 600030
  Ph.: +91-44-26260666, 26208620 • Fax: +91-44-42032115
  • E-mail: chennai@cbspd.com
- *Mumbai:* 83-C, Ist Floor, Dr. E. Moses Road, Worli, Mumbai-400 018,
  Maharashtra   Ph.: +91-9833017933, 022-24902340/24902341
  • E-mail: mumbai@cbspd.com

Printed at :
J.S. Offset Printers, Delhi

Preface to the Third Edition

The Volume-II of the book titled **'Pharmaceutical Analysis'** is concerned with the analysis by instrumental methods. These methods are in practice for the quality control of pharmaceutical raw materials & finished products and food stuffs.

Our previous two editions on this subject were quite appreciated and recommended by our fellow colleagues. Hence, it is worth take out third edition which is updated with the inclusion of recent developments.

Each chapter is corrected from some prevailing typographic mistakes and updated. The validation process is included as separate chapter because it is required almost in every field of analysis. The UV-Visible spectroscopy is given the status of separate chapter. The ^{13}C-NMR and 2D-NMR spectroscopy are updated as per recent developments with some examples. The numerical exercises are added for better understanding of the concepts. The new figures and tables are also included for clear understanding of the subjects.

We hope, the third edition will be more demanding for the students as well as to the teachers.

The authors are thankful to their fellow colleagues for their useful suggestion in bringing out this edition.

The authors are thankful to Mr. Satish Kumar Arya and Mr. Rajiv Tonk, for checking the manuscript.

We are thankful to the authors of articles from where informations are gathered for compiling this volume.

We are also thankful to Shri S.K. Jain and Mr V.K. Jain of M/s CBS Publishers & Distributors Pvt. Ltd. for their encouragement to bring this edition.

New Delhi

Dr. Anees Ahmad Siddiqui
Seemi Siddiqui

Preface to the First Edition

Pharmaceutical analysis is an important subject for the quality control of raw material, drugs, food stuffs and pharmaceuticals. This is due to the fact that drugs, pharmaceuticals and food stuffs of maximum purity are essential for the safeguard of the health of human beings.

The purity and stability of the drugs are checked with the help of various physical, chemical and instrumental techniques. These techniques have been developing/modifying day by day with the aim to increase the sensitivity, selectivity and accuracy of the method. The new techniques have replaced the old ones in the various Pharmacopeias.

To justify the rapid development and applications of various analytical techniques, the present book is written in easy understandable language in two volumes. The Volume-I, useful for B.Pharmacy IInd year has already been compiled. The present Volume-II, useful for final year B.Pharmacy will provide the understanding of the subject to undergraduate as well as to postgraduate students specially in the field of instrumental analysis.

We are grateful to Mr. R. Rajesh, Mojahidul Islam, S. Rizwan Ahmad and Aftab for their help in compilation of the volume-I.

We express our indebtness to those authors of articles, books and Pharmacopeias from which informations are gathered for writing this book.

We appreciate the co-operation of Mr. S.K. Jain and Vinod Kumar Jain of M/s. CBS Publishers & Distributors, Delhi for publishing this volume.

We will be grateful to all teachers and students to be kind enough to give constructive suggestions for improvement of this book in the future.

New Delhi
2006

Dr. Anees A Siddiqui
Seemi Siddiqui

Contents

Preface to the Third Edition v
Preface to the First Edition vi
1. Introduction 1
2. Mass Spectrometry 8
3. UV-Visible Spectroscopy 49
4. Infrared Spectroscopy 78
5. NMR Spectroscopy 111
6. Atomic Absorption Spectroscopy 141
7. Fluorimetry 162
8. Flame Photometry 175
9. Turbidimetric and Nephelometric Titrations 186
10. Potentiometric Titration 192
11. Conductometric Titration 208
12. Polarography 220
13. Amperometric Titrations 232
14. Polarimetry 240
15. X-ray Absorption, Diffraction and Fluorescence Spectroscopy 246
16. Refractometry 277
17. Thermoanalytical Methods 286
18. Electron Spin Resonance (ESR) Spectroscopy 310
19. Introduction to Validation Process 318
    Question Bank 327
    Index 339

CHAPTER 1

Introduction

In quantitative chemical analysis, a sample is prepared and then analyzed to identify or to determine the concentration of one (or more) of its components. The Fig. 1.1 gives a general overview of this process.

There are a very large number of techniques used in chemical analysis. It can be very useful to classify the measurement process according to a variety of criteria:

- by the type of analytical technique – *classical* or *instrumental tecniques*;
- by the nature of the measurement data generated – *single-channel* or *multi-channel techniques*; and
- by the quantitation method (by which the analyte concentration will be illustrated to describe the characteristics of a variety of analytical techniques.

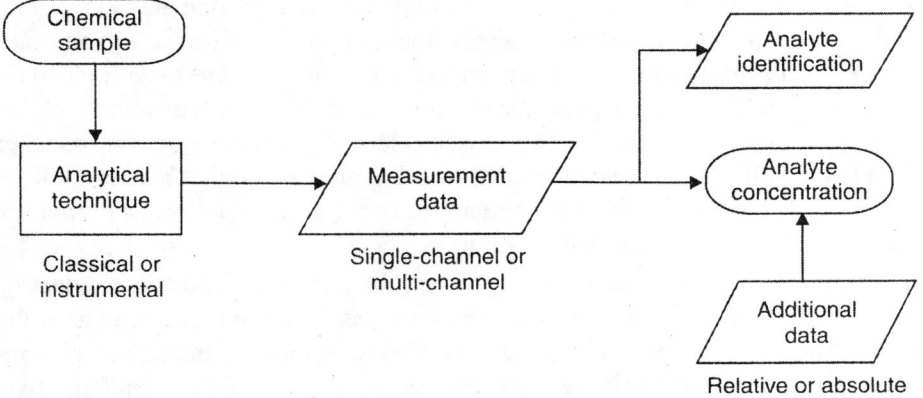

Fig. 1.1. Schematic showing measurement steps involved in quantitative chemical analysis of a sample. There are three ways of classifying the process, based on the technique (classical vs instrumental), the measurement data (single-channel vs multi-channel), or on whether additional data is needed to estimate the analyte concentration (relative vs absolute).

CLASSICAL VS INSTRUMENTAL TECHNIQUES

In *classical* analysis, the signal depends on the chemical properties of the sample: a reagent reacts completely with the analyte, and the relationship between the measured signal and the analyte concentration is determined by chemical stoichiometry. In *instrumental analysis*, some physical property of the sample is measured, such as the electrical potential difference between two electrodes immersed in a solution of the sample, or the ability of the sample to absorb light. Classical methods are most useful for accurate and precise measurements of analyte concentrations at the 0.1% level or higher. On the other hand, some specialized instrumental techniques are capable of detecting individual atoms or molecules in a sample. Analysis at the ppm (μg/ml) and even ppb (ng/ml) level is routine.

The advantages of instrumental methods over classical methods include:
  (i) The ability to perform *trace analysis*, as mentioned here.
  (ii) Generally, large numbers of samples may be analyzed very quickly.
  (iii) Many instrumental methods can be automated.
  (iv) Most instrumental methods are multi-channel techniques (we will discuss these shortly).
  (v) Less skill and training is usually required to perform instrumental analysis than classical analysis.

Because of these advantages, instrumental methods of analysis have revolutionized the field of analytical chemistry, as well as many other scientific fields. However, they have not entirely supplanted classical analytical methods, due to the fact that the latter are generally more accurate and precise, and more suitable for the analysis of the major constituents of a drug sample. In addition, the cost of many analytical instruments can be quite high.

Instrumental analysis can be further classified according to the principles by which the measurement signal is generated. A few of the methods are listed below:

1. **Electrochemical methods** of analysis, in which the analyte participates in a redox reaction or other process. In potentiometric analysis, the analyte is part of a galvanic cell, which generates a voltage due to a drive to thermodynamic equilibrium. The magnitude of the voltage generated by the galvanic cell depends on the concentration of analyte in the sample solution. In voltammetric analysis, the analyte is part of an electrolytic cell. Current flows when voltage is applied to the cell due to the participation of the analyte in a redox reaction; the conditions of the electrolytic cell are such that the magnitude of the current is directly proportional to the concentration of analyte in the sample solution.

2. **Spectrochemical methods** of analysis, in which the analyte interacts with electromagnetic radiation. Most of the methods in this category are based on the measurement of the amount of light absorbed by a sample; such *absorption-based techniques* include atomic absorption, molecular absorption, and NMR methods. The rest of the methods are generally based on the measurement of light emitted or scattered by a sample; these *emission based techniques* include atomic emission, molecular fluorescence, and Raman scatter methods.

3. **The technique of mass spectroscopy** is a powerful method for analysis in which the analyte is ionized and subsequently detected. Although in common usage, the term "spectroscopy" is

not really appropriate to describe this method since electromagnetic radiation is not usually involved in mass spectroscopy. Perhaps the most of the quantitative analysis involving the mass spectrometry is done by GC-MS or LC-MS technique. In these techniques, mass spectrometer is used as detector. A more recent innovation is the use of an inductively coupled plasma (ICP) as an ion source for a mass spectrometer; this combination (ICP-MS) is a powerful tool for elemental analysis.
4. **Scattering methods:** Nephelometry, turbidimetry, etc. are best examples for this class. These are based on scattering features of sample.
5. **Thermal methods:** The technique of thermal analysis actually comprises of a series of methods, which detect the changes in the physical and mechanical properties of the given substance by the application of heat or thermal energy. The physical properties include mass, temperature, enthalpy, dimension, dynamic characteristics, etc. It finds its application in finding the purity, integrity, crystallinity and thermal stability, of the chemical substances under study.
6. **Optical methods:** These include the refractometry and polarimetry. The former measures the refractive index due to refraction of light and the later measure the optical rotation, caused due to rotation of plane polarized light.
7. **Radiometric methods:** It involves the measurement of activity in the radioactive analyte or artificially induced radioactive analyte (discussed in Volume I).
8. **Chromatographic methods:** The technique through which the chemical components present in complex mixtures are separated, identified and determined is termed as chromatography. This technique is widely used like spectroscopy and is a very powerful tool not only for analytical methods but also for preparative methods (discussed in Volume I).

Finally, we should note that a number of methods that are based on stoichiometry, and so must be considered "classical", still have a significant "instrumental" aspect to their nature. In particular, the techniques of *electrogravimetry*, and *potentiostatic* and *amperostatic coulometry* are relatively sophisticated classical methods that have a significant instrument component. Let us not forget that instrumental methods can be used for endpoint detection in titrimetric analysis even though potentiostatic titrimetry uses an instrumental method of endpoint detection, it is still considered a classical method.

SINGLE-CHANNEL VS MULTI-CHANNEL TECHNIQUES

This way of classification is based on method of generation of measurement data. Another useful distinction between analytical techniques is based on the information content of the data generated by the analysis:

- *Single-channel techniques* will generate but a single number for each analysis of the sample. Examples include gravimetric and potentiometric analysis. In the former, the signal is a single mass measurement (e.g. mass of the precipitate) and in the latter method, the signal is a single voltage value.
- *Multi-channel techniques* will generate a series of numbers for a single analysis. Multi-channel techniques are characterized by the ability to obtain measurements while changing some independently controllable parameter. For example, in a molecular absorption method, an

absorption *spectrum* may be generated, in which the absorbance of a sample is monitored as a function of the wavelength of the light transmitted through the sample. Measurement of the sample thus produces a series of absorbance values.

Any multi-channel technique can thus produce a plot of some type when analyzing a single sample, where the signal is observed as a function of some other variable: absorbance as a function of wavelength (in molecular absorbance spectroscopy), electrode potential as a function of added titrant volume (potentiometric titrimetry), diffusion current as a function of applied potential (voltammetry), etc. Multi-channel methods provide a lot more data and informations than single-channel technique.

Multi-channel methods have two important advantages over their single-channel counterparts:
(i) They provide the ability to perform *multicomponent analysis*. In other words, the concentrations of more than one analyte in a single sample may be determined.
(ii) Multi-channel methods can detect, and sometimes correct for, the presence of a number of types of interferences in the sample. If uncorrected, the presence of the inter-ference will result in biased estimates of analyte concentration.

Multi-channel measurements simply give more information than a single-channel signal. For example, imagine that measurement of one of the calibration standards gives the data pictured in Fig. 1.2(a).

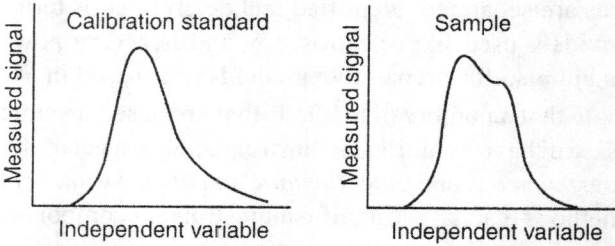

Fig. 1.2. Illustration of how multi-channel data allow for the detection of interferences. Comparison of the multi-channel signal of the (a) the calibration standard, and (b) the sample reveals that there is interference in the latter.

Plots of the measurements of the other calibration standards (assuming they are not contaminated) should give the same general shape, although the magnitude of the signal will of course depend on the analyte concentration.

Now imagine that you obtain multi-channel measurements of a sample, recording the following data shown in Fig. 1.2(b). It is immediately obvious that the shape has changed due to some interference. A likely explanation is that some component of the sample matrix is also contributing to the measured signal, so that the result is the sum of the two (or perhaps more than two) sample components. Another possibility is that the sample matrix alters the response of the analyte, giving rise to an altered peak shape.

More than just identifying the presence of an interfering substance, multi-channel data often allows the analyst to correct for its presence. For example, if it is suspected that the altered peak in Fig. 1.2(b) is due to an additional component, then a channel can be chosen for quantitation where the interfering substance does not contribute. The left side of the peak looks unaltered, so perhaps the data in one of these channels can be used to estimate analyte concentration. An important point, although multi-channel methods are capable of collecting measurements on multiple channels (e.g. different wavelengths), it is possible to use them in "single-channel" mode. In other words, to decrease measurement time, the analyst has the option of measuring the response on only a single channel (e.g., the wavelength corresponding to the peak response). If the nature of the sample or standard is well known, this may be perfectly acceptable. However, the analyst must realize that a lot of information is being thrown away – the advantages of multi-channel data described above (multicomponent analysis and detection/correction of interferences) will be lost. As a general guideline, it is always a good idea to collect the multi-channel response of at least one of the calibration standards to see what the analyte response looks like, and then to collect the multi-channel response of at least one of the samples to ensure that no interferences are present.

One last item: There is another way of classifying analytical techniques according to the measurement data produced. Rather than single- and multi-channel techniques, we may speak of the order of the analytical technique. The order is equal to the number of independent parameters that are controlled as the data is collected for each sample. Thus, single-channel techniques would be *zeroth order methods*, since only a single data point is collected. If absorbance is measured as a function of wavelength, as in molecular absorption spectroscopy, the technique is labelled *first order*. Examples of second order techniques include the following:

- gas chromatography with mass spectrometric detection (the two inependent parameters are retention time and ion mass/charge ratio);
- liquid chromatography with UV-visible spectrophotometric detection (signal is determined as a function of retention time and wavelength); and
- molecular fluorescence (signal measured as a function of both excitation wavelength and emission wavelength).

As discussed, techniques with first-order data are able to identify, and in many cases correct, for the presence of interferes. Due to their ability to provide data with higher information content, second-order techniques are even more powerful than first-order methods; further discussion of the additional capabilities of these methods is beyond the scope of this course.

RELATIVE VS ABSOLUTE TECHNIQUES

Another way of classifying analytical techniques is according to the method by which the analyte concentration is calculated from the data:

- in absolute analytical techniques, the analyte concentration can be calculated directly from measurement of the sample. No additional measurements are required (other than a measurement of sample mass or volume).
- in relative analytical techniques, the measurement of the sample must be compared to measurements of additional samples that are prepared with the use of analyte *standards* (e.g., solutions of known analyte concentration).

The Fig. 1.3 illustrates the difference between the two types of methods.

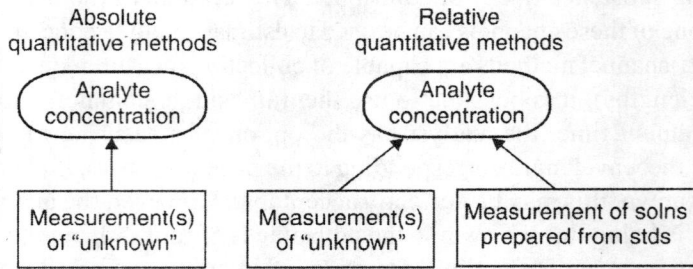

Fig. 1.3. The difference between absolute and relative techniques is that the latter requires additional measurements in order to obtain an estimate of the analyte concentration.

SUMMARY: CHARACTERIZATION OF ANALYTICAL TECHNIQUES

There are a large number of techniques used for quantitative chemical analysis. As we have discussed, any analytical technique may be classified according to a variety of criteria, revealing something of its characteristics. Table 1.1 summarizes the techniques discussed in this course.

Table 1.1. Principle of various instrumental methods

Method	*Basic principle*
1. **Electroanalytical methods**	Concerned with change in electrical properties of the system
(i) Potentiometry	Measures the change in electrode potential during a chemical reaction of the system
(ii) Conductometry	Measure the change in electrical conductivity during a chemical reaction
(iii) Polarography	Measure the current at various applied potential indicating the polarisation at indicator electrode
(iv) Amperometry	Measure the change (or decrease) in current at a fixed potential during addition of titrant
2. **Spectroscopic methods**	
(i) Absorption spectroscopy (ultraviolet, visible and infrared)	Measure the absorbance of percent transmittance during the interaction of monochromatic radiation (of particular wavelength) by the same
(ii) Fluorimetry	Measure the intensity of fluorescence caused by emission of electromagnetic radiation due to absorption of UV radiation
(iii) Flame photometry	Measure the intensity of emitted light of particular wavelength emitted by particular element
(iv) Turbidity	Measure the turbidity of a system by passing light beam in a turbid media
(v) Nephelometry	Measure the opalescence of the medium by reflection of light by a colloidal solution
(vi) Atomic absorption spectrometry	Measure the intensity of absorption when atoms absorb the monochromatic radiation

(Contd.)

Method	Basic principle
(vii) X-ray spectroscopy	Measure the position and intensity of spectral lines during emission of X-ray spectrum by atoms under influence of X-rays
(viii) NMR spectroscopy	Observe the position and intensity lines in NMR spectrum when proton interact with electromagnetic radiation in radiofrequency region
3. **Scattering methods**	
(i) Turbidimetry	Measure the turbidity of a system by passing light beam in a turbid media
(ii) Nephelometry	Measures the opalescence of the medium by reflection of light by a colloidal solution
4. **Optical methods**	
(i) Refractometry	Measure the refractive index by causing refraction of light by matter
(ii) Polarimetry	Measure the optical rotation by caus-ing the rotation of plane polarized light
5. **Mass spectrometry**	Observe the position and intensity of signals in mass spectrum by causing the ionisation of molecules
6. **Thermal methods**	Measure the physical parameters of the system as a function of temperature. It includes thermogravimetry, differential thermal analysis, differential scanning calorimetry etc.
7. **Radiometric methods**	Measure the radioactivity either present naturally or induced artificially
8. **Chromatographic methods**	
(i) Higher Performance Liquid Chromatography (HPLC)	To separate and analyse complex mixtures or solutions which include liquids and solids of both organic and inorganic origins
(ii) Gas Chromatography (GC)	To separate and analyse mixtures of volatile organic compounds

CHAPTER 2

Mass Spectrometry

INTRODUCTION

Mass Spectrometry is one of the most sensitive analytical techniques, used for the structural elucidation of chemical compounds. Basically in mass spectrometry, molecule is broken down into the fragments; these fragments are separated on the basis of their mass/charge ratio. Each fragment of particular mass gives its response as peak on reaching to the detector. The response of all the fragment ions is finally recorded in the form of the mass spectrum. The *mass spectrum* (Fig. 2.1) is a graphical representation of mass of fragments versus relative intensity/relative abundance. The highest peak (response) at m/e 56 is recorded as 100% (base peak) and the other peaks are recorded with respect to the base peak. From the fragments, the structure of original compound is predicted. It is similar to the routine fact, for example, when the letter is torned out and we want to read this

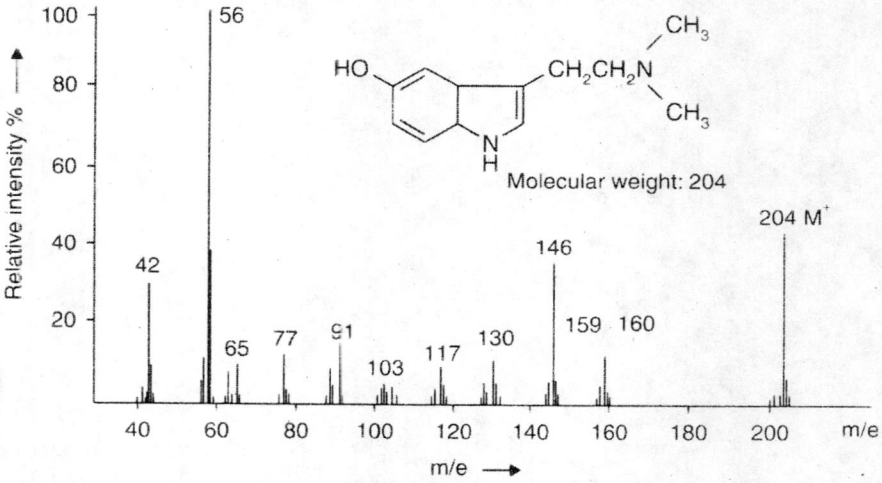

Fig. 2.1. Example of mass spectrum.

letter. This original content of letter can only be read out by reuniting a piece of torned letter in a possible original shape.

Mass Spectrometry measures molecular masses while all other spectroscopic method such as ultraviolet (UV) spectroscopy, infrared (IR) spectroscopy, and nuclear magnetic resonance (NMR) spectroscopy, measure frequency. Mass spectrometry in its present form can be used to identify unknown compounds, to quantify known materials and to elucidate the structural and chemical properties of the molecules. This can be accomplished with very small quantities, usually less than picogram amounts, even in chemically complex environment. Mass Spectrometry provides valuable information to a wide range of professionals including physicians, law enforcement officials, chemists, astrologers, process control engineers and biologists.

Some of the most important analyses where mass spectrometry can be quite a useful tool are listed below :

- To detect dioxins in contaminated fish. *The dioxins are produced as a waste product by industrial plants and waste incineration. These may cause hormonal changes, cancer and other severe disorder.*
- To determine the composition of molecular species found in space.
- To detect and identify the illegal use of steroids by athletes.
- To detect the adulteration of honey with corn syrup.
- To locate oil deposits by measuring petroleum precursors in rock.
- To monitor fermentation process in the biotechnology industry.
- To determine gene damage from environmental causes.
- To establish elemental composition of semiconductor material.
- For real time breathe monitoring of patients by anesthesiologists during surgery.
- To identify the structure of biomolecules, such as carbohydrates and nucleic acids.
- To sequence biopolymers such as proteins and oligosaccharides.
- To determine how drugs are metabolised by the body.
- To perform forensic analysis for confirmation and quantitation of drugs of abuse.
- To analyze environmental pollutants.
- To determine the age and origin of specimens in geo-chemistry and archaeology.
- To identify the quantity components of complex organic mixtures.

INSTRUMENTATION

Mass spectrometer in generalised may consist of following fundamental components, namely :
1. Ionisation source
2. Analyser
3. Detector
4. Vacuum system

Ionisation source ⟶ Mass analyser ⟶ Detector ⟶ Recorder

The sample under investigation is introduced into *ionisation source* of the instrument. In the ionisation source, the sample molecules are ionised, because ions are easier to manipulate than neutral molecules. These ions are forced to enter into the analyser region of the mass analyser where they are separated according to their mass (m) to charge (e) ratios. As most of the ions are singly charged, so it can be said that ions are separated on the basis of their mass. The separated ions are detected and this signal sent to a data system where m/e ratios are stored together with their relative abundance for presentation in the format of a *mass spectrum*.

1. IONISATION SOURCE

Ionisation of sample occurs in the Ionisation chamber. The minimum energy required to ionize an atom or molecule is referred to as its **"Ionisation potential"**. This energy may be supplied in a number of ways depending on the physical and chemical nature of sample.

The appearance of mass spectrum for a given molecular species is highly dependent upon the method used for ion formation. The ionisation sources are divided into two major categories. The first one are *gas phase sources* in which the sample is volatilized, following which the gaseous components are ionized in various ways. The volatilization may be carried out externally (batch inlet system) or internally from a heated probe. The second category of sources is *desorption sources* in which bulk sample vaporization is dispensed with. As a consequence, this technique is always the use of a sample probe or sample holder. Here, energy in a variety of forms is imparted to the solid or liquid sample, causing ionisation and a direct transfer of ions from the condensed phase into gaseous ionic state. It can be used for non-volatile and thermally fragile molecules such as those commonly encountered in biochemistry. Probes are also used where the quantity of the sample is limited because less sample is wasted than with the batch system. Thus, mass spectrum can often be obtained with as little as few nanograms of sample.

Ion sources are sometimes categorized as *hard* or *soft*. The most pioneer type hard source is electron impact source. *Hard sources* impart large energies to the sample molecule and so ions formed are in highly excited vibrational and rotational states. A good deal of fragmentation accompanies relaxation of these ions and complex mass spectra result due to appearance of more number of peaks (as a result of formation of more ions). In contrast, *soft sources*, such as Chemical ionisation and desorption sources, cause relatively little ion excitation. Thus, little fragmentation occurs and spectra are simple. The Fig. 2.2 shows the mass spectra of ionised by hard and soft sources respectively. The hard ionization source spectrum shows large number of peaks due to entensive fragmentation. In contrast, soft source shows less peaks due to less fragmentation. Both types of spectra are useful. The simple spectra from soft sources allow the ready determination of the *molecular weight* of the analyte. The more complex spectral patterns from hard sources often give the structural information of the analyte. Various types of ionisation source are as follows:

A. Gaseous sources

In gaseous sources, sample is inserted in the ionisation chamber in vapour form. These are as follows:

Electron impact ionisation

Here, the sample molecules are bombard with energetic electrons. Electron impact bombarding electrons are produced by thermionic emission from an electrically heated (several thousand degree)

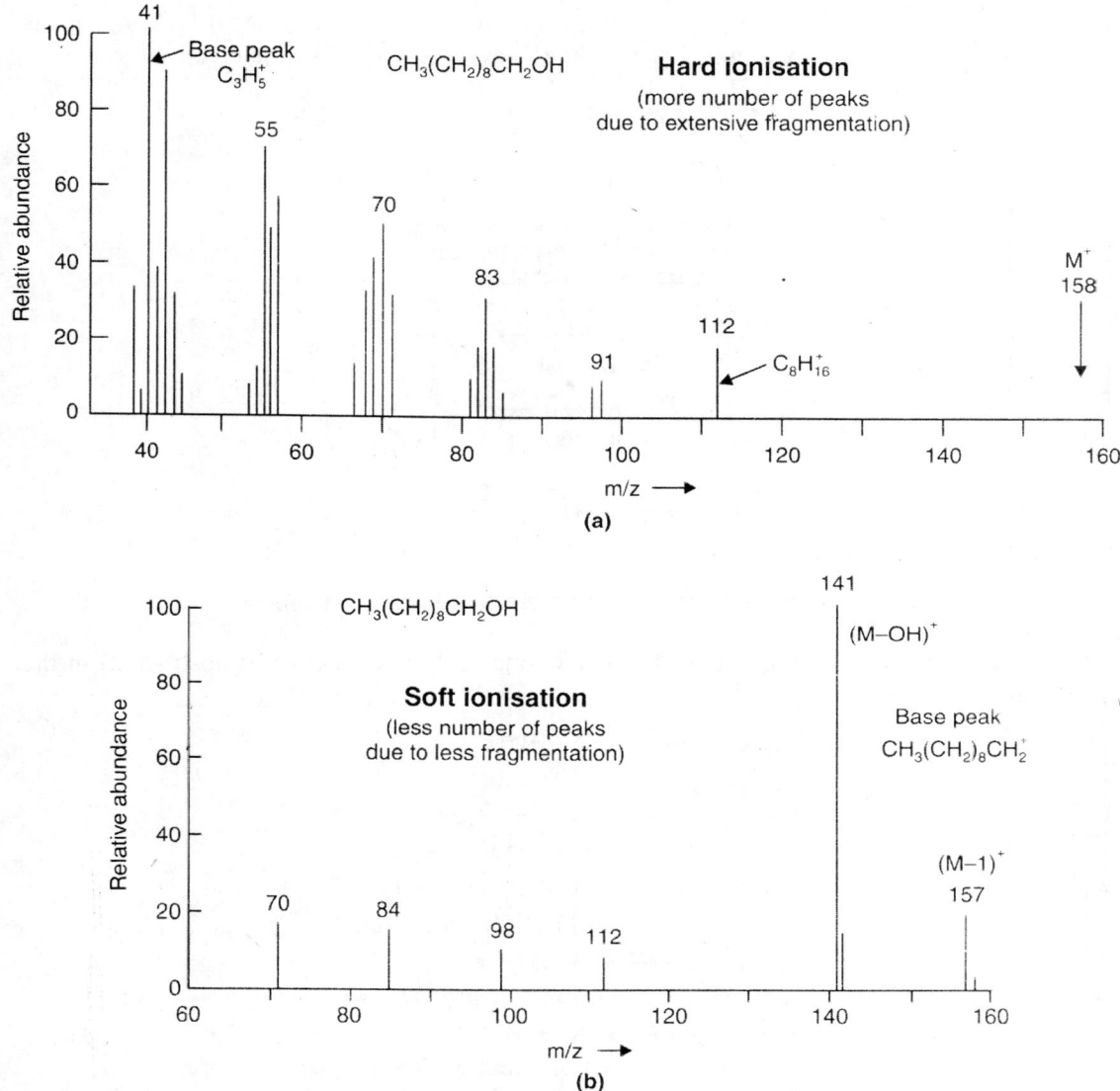

Fig. 2.2. Mass spectrum of Decanol using (a) Hard ionisation source; (b) Soft ionisation source.

rhenium or tungston filament. These electrons are collimated by an electric field. The sample pressure is of order 10^{-5} to 10^{-6} torr. The vapour of the sample to be analysed is introduced at right angles to the electron beam (Fig. 2.3). Energy transfer take place between the bombarding electrons and the neutral molecules. When the transferred energy is equal to the ionisation potential of the molecule, it loses an electron and ionizes. For most elements, the ionisation potential is in the range of 5 to 15 eV. It varies from 8 to 12 eV for organic compounds. When more energy is transferred to the molecule by the bombarding electron, a hypothetical molecule, molecule A–B can undergo the various type of electron impact induced reactions, fragmentation of the molecule takes place as shown below. Generally, the spectrum is run at 70 eV (average energy of the electron beam).

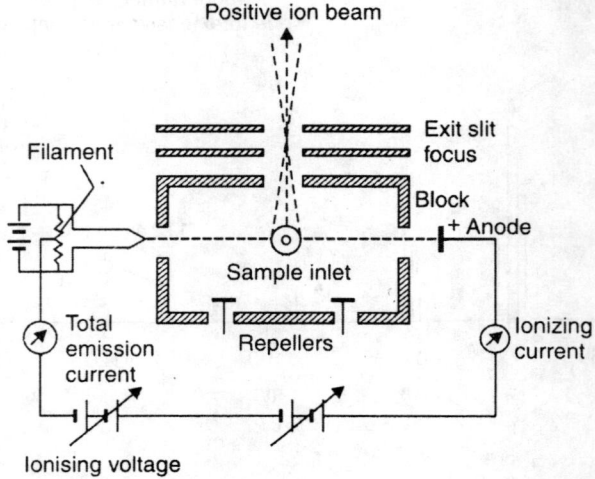

Fig. 2.3. Schematic diagram of an electron impact ion source.

The primary product is singly charged positive ions (only one electron is abstracted) in the electron impact method.

$$A - B + e \longrightarrow A - B^*$$
(Excitation)

$$A - B + e \longrightarrow A - B^{+\bullet} + 2e$$
(Single Ionisation)

$$A - B + e \longrightarrow A - B^{n+} + (n + 1)e$$
(Multiple Ionisation)

$$A - B + e \longrightarrow A^+ B^- + e$$
(Ion pair production)

$$A - B + e \longrightarrow A^+ + B + 2e$$
(Dissociative Ionisation)

$$A - B + e \longrightarrow A - B^-$$
(Electron capture)

Due to high energy, ions of lower mass (occasionally greater), called daughter ions are formed.

Chemical Ionisation

It is a useful technique for organic compounds. A reaction gas (e.g. hydrocarbon CH_4, isobutane, ammonia, nitric oxide, tetramethylsilane) is introduced into the ionisation chamber of mass spectrometer at a pressure of 1 torr. Primary Ionisation of the reaction gas is effected by electron impact (50 to 70 eV). Because of the high pressure, these primary ions undergo ion-molecule reaction with the neutral molecules of the reaction gas and with the sample molecules which are present at relatively low concentration (~1%). If the reaction gas is methane, it react with high energy electron to give primary ions e.g., CH_4^+, CH_3^+ and CH_2^+. These ions react rapidly with additional methane molecules as follows :

$$CH_4^+ + CH_4 \longrightarrow CH_5^+ + CH_3^{\cdot}$$
$$CH_3^+ + CH_4 \longrightarrow C_2H_5^+ + H_2$$

Generally, collisions between the sample molecule (XH) and highly reactive CH_5^+ or $C_2H_5^+$ involve proton or hydride transfer.

$$CH_5^+ + XH \longrightarrow XH_2^+ + CH_4 \quad \text{(Proton transfer)}$$
$$C_2H_5^+ + XH \longrightarrow XH_2^+ + C_2H_4 \quad \text{(Proton transfer)}$$
$$C_2H_5^+ + XH \longrightarrow X^+ + C_2H_6 \quad \text{(Hydride transfer)}$$

Proton transfer give the $(M + 1)^+$ ion whereas the hydride transfer produces $(M - 1)^+$ ion leak. Mass spectra resulting from chemical Ionisation is simple one and supplement to electron impact.

Field Ionisation

In this, ions are formed under the influence of high electric field (10^8 V/cm). Such fields are produced by applying high voltages (10 to 20 kV) to specially formed emitters consisting of numerous fine tips having diameters of less than 1 μm. In this, sample is allowed to diffuse in the ionization chamber. The molecular ion peak is a significant ion peak in this technique. Fragmentation process is minimum, so spectra is not complex due to presence of less number of peaks in the mass spectrum.

B. Desorption sources

In the previous one, ionising agents act on gaseous samples. Such methods are not applicable to nonvolatile substances. A number of desorption type ionisation methods have been developed. As a consequence, mass spectra for delicate biochemical species having molecular weight of greater than 10^3 dalton have been reported.

Desorption methods dispense with volatilization. Instead, energy in various forms is transferred into the solid or liquid sample in such a way to cause direct formation of gaseous ions.

Field desorption

In this, electrode is mounted on a probe that can be removed from the sample compartment. The sample solution is applied on this electrode and then the probe is reinserted into sample compartment, Ionisation again take place by application of *high potential* to this electrode. It also gives more simpler spectra.

Thermal ionisation (surface Ionisation)

Sample is applied to a filament wire or ribbon and inserted into the ion source. A part of the substance on the hot filament is vaporized in the vacuum of the mass spectrometer. Some of the atoms or molecules evaporate directly as ions. The method is used to analyse substances of low Ionisation potential. The method is highly sensitive.

Fast atom bombardment (FAB)

Samples in a condensed state often in glycerol matrix, are ionised by bombardment with energetic (several eV) xenon or argon atoms. Both positive (with low ionisation potential organic molecule) and negative analyte ion (high electronegativity molecule) are sputtered from the surface of the sample. This treatment provide very rapid sample heating which reduces sample fragmentation.

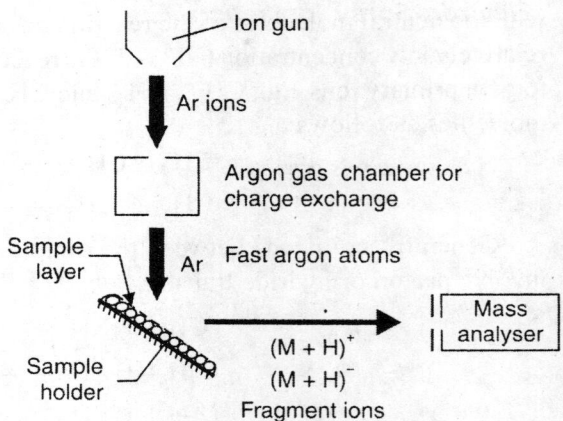

Fig. 2.4. Principle of FAB ionisation method.

A beam of fast atoms is obtained by passing accelerated argon or xenon ions from an ion source or gun through a chamber containing argon or xenon atoms at a pressure of *about* 10^{-5} *torr* (Fig. 2.4). The speeding ions undergo a *resonant electron exchange reaction* with atoms without substantial loss of translational energy. With FAB technology, molecular weight over 10,000 have been determined and detailed structural information has been obtained for compounds but the mass spectrum also contain peaks due to matrix.

Photoionisation

Ionisation of molecules can be accomplished by a beam of UV light of sufficiently shortwave length. Many Ionisation processes occur at 10 eV or more. This corresponds to 1200 Å or less. Ionisation occurs by collision between photons and neutral molecules.

$$A + h\nu \longrightarrow A^+ + e$$

where

ν is the frequency of light wave

h = planck constant

Laser desorption

Laser beam is also used for causing Ionisation

Matrix assisted laser desorption Ionisation (MALDI)

It is based on the bombardment of sample molecules in matrix with a laser light to bring out the ionisation (Fig. 2.5). The sample is pre-mixed with highly absorbing matrix compound (nicotinic acid, sinapinic acid derivatives, α-cyano-4-hydroxy cinnamic acid, 2,5-dihydroxy-benzoic acid derivatives) for the most consistent and reliable results. The laser is fired and the energy arriving at the sample/matrix surface optimised. The matrix transforms the laser energy into excitation energy for the sample for causing ionisation. In this way, energy transfer is efficient and also the analyte molecules are spared excessive direct energy that may otherwise cause decomposition.

Electron Spray Ionisation (ESI)

It is one of the atmospheric pressure Ionisation (API) technique and well suited for the analysis of polar molecules.

The sample is dissolved in polar volatile solvent and pumped through a narrow, stainless steel capillary (75–150 μm) at a flow rate of 1 μl/minute to form droplets (Fig. 2.6). The droplet carry the charge when exit the capillary and as the solvent vaporizes, the droplet disappears leaving highly charged sample molecules. A high voltage of 3 or 4 kV is applied to the tip of the capillary, which is situated within the ionisation source of mass spectrometer and as a consequence of this strong electric field, the sample emerging from the tip is dispersed into an aerosol of highly charged droplets. This process is aided by a co-axially introduced nebulising gas flow around the outside of the capillary. For this technique, sample must be soluble in low boiling solvents (acetonitrile, $CHCl_3$ etc.) and stable at a very low concentration, i.e. 10^{-2} mole/L.

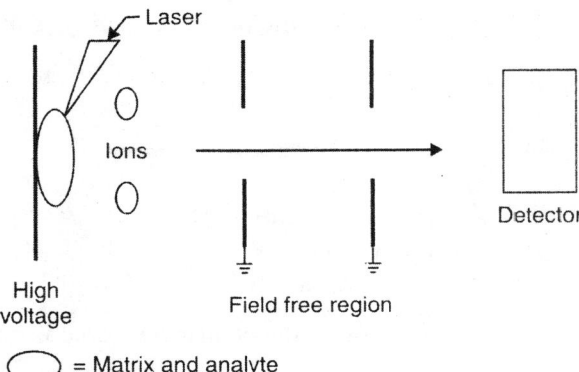

Fig. 2.5. Simplified schematic of MALDI-TOF mass spectrometry.

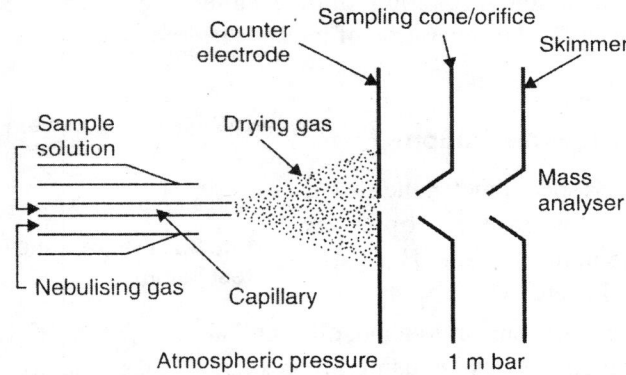

Fig. 2.6. Schematic representation of electrospray ionisation source.

2. MASS ANALYSER

Ions produced in the ionisation chamber are accelerated by the application of acceleration potential (2 to 8 kV). These ions enter in the mass analyser which differentiate them on the basis of mass to charge ratio by magnetic and electric field. There are two main functions of a mass analyser (i) resolve the ion beam into its component ions and (ii) to maximise the resolved ions intensities (dispersive focussing).

In electrical field, the potential energy is balanced by kinetic energy:

$$eV = \frac{1}{2}mv^2 \qquad ....(eq.\ 2.1)$$

where
- e = electric charge
- V = acceleration potential
- m = mass of an ion
- v = velocity of an ion

In magnetic field, the centripetal force is balanced by centrifugal force.

$$Hev = \frac{mv^2}{R} \qquad ....(eq.\ 2.2)$$

where
- H is strength of magnetic field
- R is the radius of curvature which ions take place on entering in the magnetic field

Rearranging the eq. 2.2 and substituting the value of v in the eq. 2.2

$$\frac{m}{e} = \frac{H^2 R^2}{2V} \qquad ....(eq.\ 2.3)$$

The eq. 2.3 is the fundamental equation for the magnetic deflection type of mass spectrometer. Either 'H' or 'V' is varied for the separation of ions of different mass but for the very fast scanning V is varied.

High resolution and low resolution

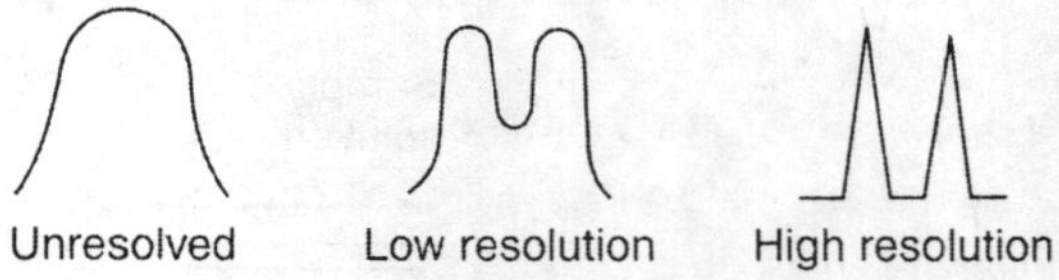

In the low resolution mass spectrometer, the atomic weight of the most abundant isotopes are determined as a whole number, means $^1H = 1$; $^{16}O = 16$; $^{12}C = 12$; $^{14}N = 14$, etc.

Fig. 2.7. Diagram showing three states of peaks resolution.

Low resolution mass spectrometers cannot differentiates the CO, N_2, C_2H_4 as all will be recorded as whole number of which mass is 28, using low resolution mass spectrometer, the peaks are not resolved (Fig. 2.7).

From a physical point of view, only the atomic weight of most abundant isotope of carbon is equal to 12 exactly. The other atoms are not equal to whole numbers and their actual atomic weight can be determined to the sixth decimal place.

For example,

$^1H = 1.007825$ $^{16}O = 15.994915$

$^{12}C = 12.000000$ $^{19}F = 18.998405$

$^{14}N = 14.003074$ $^{32}S = 31.972074$

From these values, it can be observed that CO, C_2H_4 and N_2 show a significant difference in their actual masses.

$$CO = 27.994914, N_2 = 28.006158, C_2H_4 = 28.031299.$$

The mass spectrometer with good resolving power can differentiate them. Resolving power can be calculated as :

$$\text{Resolving power (RP)} = \frac{m_1}{m_2 - m_1} = \frac{m_1}{\Delta m}$$

where m_1 and m_2 are the masses of two sample molecule.

For example, to separate the nitrogen and ethylene :

$$RP = \frac{28.006158}{28.031299 - 28.006158} = 1110$$

Hence, mass spectrometer possessing RP = 1,110 can differentiate the masses of nitrogen and ethylene. The different mass spectrometer can be classified on the basis of mass analyzers which are as follows:

Single focussing mass spectrometer

The ions produced in the source are accelerated by a variable potential difference applied to plates 'b'. The ions entered in the magnetic field through slit 'c'. Magnetic field bend the trajectories of ions into circular path of radii that depend on the mass to charge ratio of ions. Ions of larger m/e deflected more and so follow larger radius path than ions of smaller m/e values. After the beam has been deflected through 180°, the ions are focussed through slit e and impinge on collector 'f'. By changing the ion through variation of the magnetic field strength ions of different nominal mass to charge ratio can be focussed on collector. It is a directional focussing so the instrument is defined as a 'direction' or 'single' focussing mass spectrometer (Fig. 2.8).

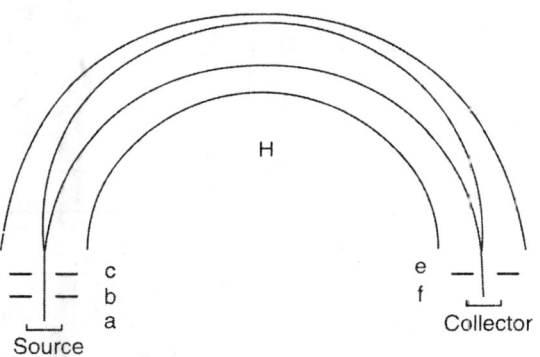

Fig. 2.8. Single focussing mass analyser.

The mass spectrum is obtained when ions of different mass arrive at collector, one after the other. The time of arrival will be proportional to the square root of the m/e ratio. They have lower mass ranges.

Double focussing mass spectrometer

It uses a combination of magnetic and electrical fields to sort and focus ions. It is directional as well as velocity focussing (Fig. 2.9). Trajectory of ions is not only a function of the m/e ratio but also of the kinetic energy. Ions are differentiated on the basis of their kinetic energy by applying electrical field before the beam of ion enters in the magnetic field. The electrostatic analyser consist of tube of a fixed radius under constant electric field (Fig. 2.9). Only ions the kinetic energy of which correspond to the radius of curvature are able to pass into the magnetic field. The mass ranges are higher (2000-5000) in comparison to single focussing mass spectrometer.

The quadrupole mass analyser

The operative principle of the quadrupole mass spectrometer is given by the *Mathieu* equations which describe the trajectory of a particle moving through the lines of force of two fields at continuous current modulated by a radio frequency.

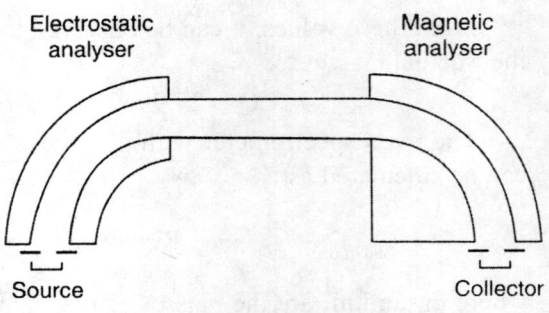

Fig. 2.9. Double focussing mass analyser.

The quadrupole mass analyser has four metal bars, fixed at the angles of square and ceremically isolated, connected alternatively to form two couples to which are applied DC and RF potential with charges of opposite sign (Fig. 2.10).

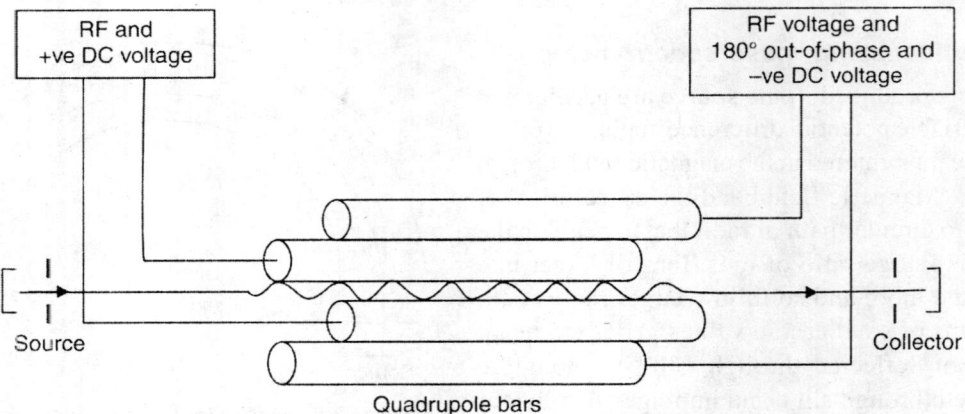

Fig. 2.10. Quadrupole mass analyser.

The accelerated particles enter the analyser and begins to oscillate in a complex manner according to their m/e and applied RF/DC ratio. For every value of these ratio, only one mass is able to pass completely through the filter and impinge on the collector. The other ions of the other m/e value strikes the pole and discharged. Therefore, by varying the RF/DC ratio, it is possible to select a single value of m/e able to give a signal and by continuous variation from minimum to maximum, the whole spectrum can be recorded.

Time of flight (ToF) analyser

The accelerated particles passes into a field free drift tube about a meter in length (Fig. 2.11). Because all ions entering the tube was supplied with same kinetic energies, their velocity in the tube must vary invariably with their masses, with the lighter particles arriving at the detector earlier than the heavier ones. Typical flight times are 1 to 30 µs. Resolution power is less than 1000 and also have low mass ranges.

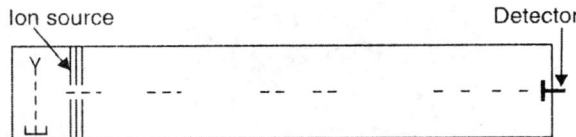

Fig. 2.11. A time of flight mass analyser.

Ion trap analysers

An analytic ion from an electron impact or chemical ionisation source is entered in specially designed chamber. Ions with a appropriate m/e value circulate in the orbit. As the *radio frequency voltage* is increased, the orbits of heavier ions become stabilised while those of lighter ions become destabilised (trapped) goes to the detector (leave the chamber).

3. DETECTORS USED IN MASS SPECTROMETRY

There are three methods of ion detection:

(i) *The electron multiplier*: The ions strikes on the photoemissive surface, present on the cathode to release the electron. The electrons are attracted toward the anode to generate the current which is measured. The cathode and several dynodes have Cu/Be surfaces (Fig. 2.12) from which burst of electrons are emitted when struck by energetic ion or electrons. These electrons move towards the anode, causing the generation of electric current. The intensity of current is proportional to number of electrons (number of ions reach to detector). The strength of current is measured and recorded.

(ii) Photographic plates coated with a *silver bromide emulsion* are sensitive to energetic ions. All these ions are allowed to fall on the photographic plates, to cause impression. This detector is well suited for wide range of m/e values.

(iii) *Scintillation type detector*: Crystalline phosphor dispersed on thin aluminium sheet that is mounted on photomultiplier tube. The ions strike the scintillator to emit out the light which is detected by phosomultiplier tube.

Sample handling system

(i) Heated inlet system

In this, the sample is vapourized externally and then slowly allowed to diffuse through a molecular leak into the ionisation chamber. Solids and liquids with sufficient vapour pressure at any temperature below 350°C in vacuum are introduced through a *glass heated* inlet system. Volatile liquids are introduced by the freeze out technique. The sample in the sample holder is frozen with dry ice or liquid nitrogen. After evacuation, the tube is warmed to room temperature or higher to evaporate the sample into reservoir. Compounds of low volatility such as sugar, amino acid are converted to more volatile derivatives (ester, ether or amine) to be used by this system.

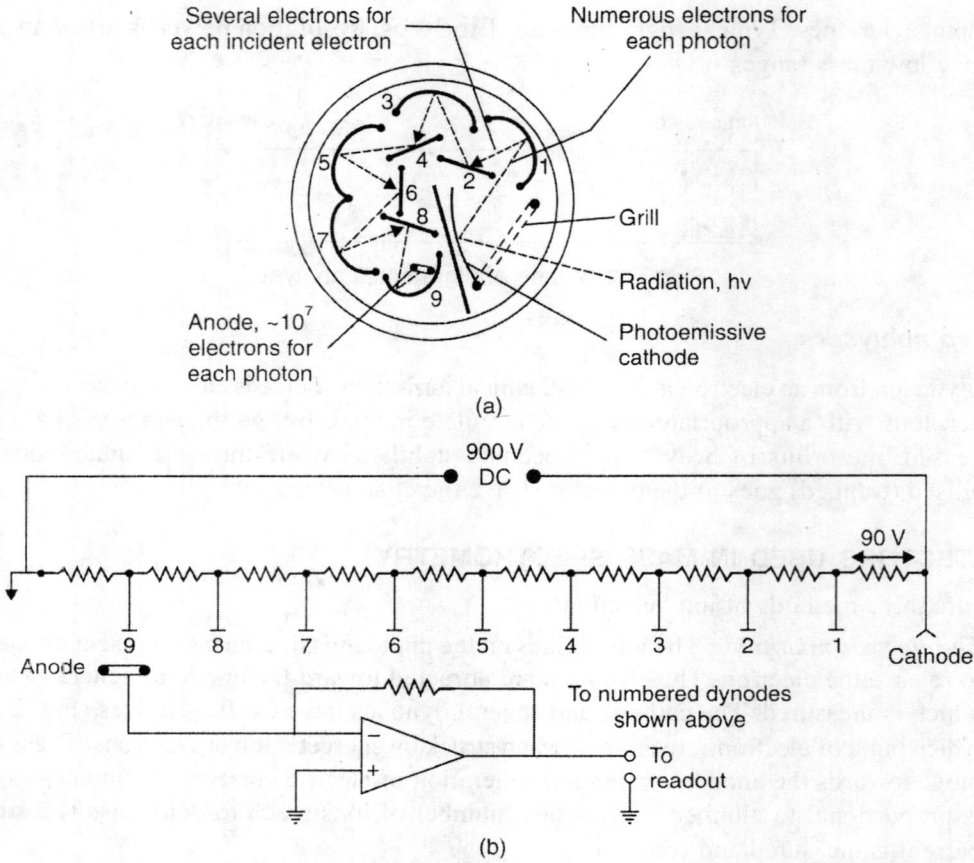

Fig. 2.12. Photomultiplier tube: (a) cross section of the tube; (b) electrical circuit.

(ii) Direct inlet system

Solids and liquids of very low vapour pressure are directly introduced into the ionization chamber and slowly vaporized in the electron bombardment region. In this case, only a fraction of milligram or less quantity of the sample is sufficient to record a spectrum.

4. VACUUM SYSTEM

The vacuum system 10^{-7} to 10^{-8} torr is required to avoid sputtering of ion. This is produced with mechanical attached with diffusion pump.

Tandem or Multistage Mass Spectrometry

An ion produced by fast atom bombardment (FAB) will indicate the molecular weight of the sample but often may not fragment much, if at all, thus giving little structural information. By coupling together two mass spectrometers, separated by a collision cell, further information can be obtained. The first analyzer is used to select, the ion of interest. This ion is then passed into the collision cell, which usually will have been pressurized with an inert gas such as argon, collision of the ion with the atoms in the cell can induce dissociation of the ion. This is known as *collision induced dissociation* (CID). The original ion is referred to as the 'precursor' ion and the dissociated ions are known as 'product' ions. These products are then analysed in second mass spectrometer thus generating a product ion mass spectrum of the original precursor ion.

Isotope Ratio Mass Spectrometry

It is useful in a wide range of applications, for example metabolic studies using isotopically enriched elements as tracers; climate studies using measurements of temperature dependent oxygen and carbon isotope ratios in foraminifers; rock age dating using radiogenic isotopes of elements such as lead or strontium. In isotopic ratio mass spectrometry, element isotope ratios are determined very accurately and precisely. Typically, single focussing magnetic sector mass spectrometers with fixed multiple detectors (one per isotope) are used. Complex compounds are reduced to simple molecules prior to measurement, for example, organic compounds are combusted to CO_2, H_2O and Na.

Elemental Mass Spectrometry

This technique is used mostly for inorganic material, the elemental composition of a sample is determined rather than the structural identities of its chemical constituents. It provides quantitative information about the concentration of these elements.

TYPES OF IONS

The ions which forms in mass spectrometer are molecular ions, isotopic ions, fragment ions, rearrangement ions, multiple charge ions, metastable ions, negative ions and ions formed by ion-molecule interaction.

(i) Molecular ions ($M^{+\cdot}$)

The ion formed by loss of one electron from molecule is called 'molecular ion' or the 'parent ion'. For example,

$$CH_4 + e^- \longrightarrow CH_4^{+\cdot} + 2e^-$$
Methane → Molecular ion

$$^{12}CH_3CO^{12}CH_3 + e^- \longrightarrow CH_3CO-CH_3^{+\cdot} + 2e^-$$
Acetone → Molecular ion

The corresponding peak in the mass spectrum is called 'molecular ion peak' or the parent ion peak. The formation of molecular ion require minimum energy. It is the precursor of all the other fragment ions in the mass spectrum. The nominal mass of such an ion corresponds to the molecular weight of the compound. The mass number obtained by this method is the exact molecular weight and not an approximate value as obtained by classical chemical methods such as cryoscopy and ebullioscopy. The relative intensity of the molecular ion depend on its stability with respect to the decomposition products and it thus indicates the type of compounds under examination. For example, the aromatic compounds give rise to intense molecular peak because of π electron in the system.

Cyclic molecules also give intense molecular ion peak because of the fact, two bonds must be broken before they fragment. For example, cyclohexanol gives the intense molecular ion peak. In general, every structural characteristic that favours the delocalisation of the electronic charge leads to increase in stability and thus to a particularly intense peak.

(ii) Isotopic ions

The molecular ion contains the most abundant isotopes of the constituent elements. The parent peak is always accompanied by other peaks of higher mass, appeared due to ions which contain the heavier isotopes. For example, benzene shows an intense peak at m/e 78 for the most abundant ion $^{12}C_6\ ^1H_6$ and another peak at m/e 79 due to the heavier isotopes ion $^{13}C\ ^1H_6$ and in part, to the ion $^{12}C_6\ ^1H_5\ ^2H$. The intensity of peak due to later ion is very less due to isotopic abundance of hydrogen (only 0.015%) in nature. The intensity of peak at m/e 79 is 6.6% with respect to molecular peak (m/e 78) because for every 100 atoms of ^{12}C, 1.1 atom of ^{13}C is present. The isotopic abundance (% of the most frequently occurring elements are shown in Table 2.1.

Table 2.1. Natural abundance of various isotopes

^1H = 99.985	^2H = 0.015	
^{12}C = 98.89	^{13}C = 1.108	
^{14}N = 99.64	^{15}N = 0.36	
^{16}O = 99.96	^{17}O = 0.04	^{18}O = 0.20
^{32}S = 95.06	^{33}S = 0.66	^{34}S = 4.20 $\quad$ ^{36}S = 0.14
^{35}Cl = 75.4	^{37}Cl = 24.6	
^{39}Br = 50.57	^{81}Br = 49.43	

The isotopic ion peaks are useful for detecting of the presence of Cl, Br and sulphur atoms. For, organic molecule containing one chlorine atom shows the $M^{+\bullet}$ and $M^{+\bullet} + 2$ peak with an intensity ratio of 3 : 1. The molecular ion and isotopic ion peaks together are helpful in determination of molecular formula.

Determination of molecular formula by mass spectrometer

(i) Formula from high resolution mass spectrometer

Formula can often be derived from the exact mass of the molecular ion peak. High resolution instrument capable of detecting mass differences of few thousands of a mass unit.

For example:

Purine $C_5H_4N_4$ (m = 120.044)

Benzimidine $C_7H_8N_2$ (m = 120.069)

Ethyl toluene C_9H_{12} (m = 120.096)

Acetophenone C_7H_8O (m = 120.058)

If the measured mass of molecular ion peak is 120.070 ($\pm$ 0.005), then all except $C_7H_8N_2$ are excluded as possible formula.

(ii) Formula from isotope ratios

Low resolution instrument can discriminate between ions differing in mass by whole mass number. It can also yield useful information about the formula of a compound provided only that the molecular ion peak is sufficiently intense ion peak that its height and the height of the ($M^{+\bullet}$ + 1) and ($M^{+\bullet}$ + 2) isotope can be determined accurately. For example,

$C_6H_4N_2O_4$ (dinitrobenzene)

$C_{12}H_{24}$ (Olefin)

Both has molecular weight ~ 168 but calculation of $M^{+\bullet}$ + 1/$M^{+\bullet}$ ratio give the possibility of appropriate molecular formula.

$C_6H_4N_2O_4$
- ^{13}C 6 × 1.08 = 6.48%
- ^{2}H 4 × 0.015 = 0.060%
- ^{15}N 2 × 0.37 = 0.74%
- ^{17}O 4 × 0.04 = 0.16%

$C_{12}H_{24}$
- ^{13}C 12 × 1.08 = 12.96%
- ^{2}H 24 × 0.015 = 0.36%

$$\frac{M^{+\bullet}+1}{M^{+\bullet}} = 7.44\%$$

$$\frac{M^{+\bullet}+1}{M^{+\bullet}} = 13.32\%$$

In an approximate but rapid manner, ratios $M^{+\bullet}$ + 1/$M^{+\bullet}$ and $M^{+\bullet}$ + 2/$M^{+\bullet}$ can be determined in the following ways :

$$\frac{M^{+\bullet}+1}{M^{+\bullet}} = (1.1\% \times \text{No. of carbon atom}) + 0.36\% \times \text{No. of nitrogen atoms}$$

$$\frac{M^{+\bullet}+2}{M^{+\bullet}} = \frac{(1.1\% \times \text{No. of carbon atom})^2}{200} + 0.2\% \times \text{No. of nitrogen atoms}$$

(iii) Formula from Beynon table

Generally, position of the molecular ion and isotopic ion peak along with their intensities are mentioned in mass spectral data. For example, in a compound following mass spectral data are recorded:

150 ($M^{+\bullet}$)	100%
151 ($M^{+\bullet}$ + 1)	9.9%
152 ($M^{+\bullet}$ + 2)	0.9%

To know the molecular formula of this compound, we select all the compounds the Baynon table of molecular weight – 150 possessing the nearly same M^+ + 1 and M^+ + 2 peak intensities:

		$M^{+\bullet}+1$	$M^{+\bullet}+2$			$M^{+\bullet}+1$	$M^{+\bullet}+2$
(i)	$C_7H_{10}N_4$	9.25	0.38	(v)	$C_9H_{10}O_2$	9.96	0.84
(ii)	$C_8H_8NO_2$	9.23	0.78	(vi)	$C_9H_{12}NO$	10.34	0.68
(iii)	$C_8H_{10}N_2O$	9.61	0.61	(vii)	$C_9H_{14}N_2$	10.71	0.52
(iv)	$C_8H_{12}N_3$	9.98	0.45				

There are seven molecular formula at the molecular weight – 150 possessing same or nearly same $M^{+\bullet}+1$ and $M^{+\bullet}+2$ (intensities peak). According to nitrogen rule, molecular formulas, (ii), (iv) and (vi) are rule out (compound possessing even numbered molecular weight should possess even number nitrogen or no nitrogen atoms). Then, it is observed that molecular formula $C_9H_{10}O_2$ (V) possess the more close $M^{+\bullet}+1$ (9.96) and $M^+ + 2$ (0.84) values. Hence, it is the possible molecular formula of the compound which should be further verified from the IR, NMR and mass fragmentation pattern.

(iv) Fragment ions

Due to high energy, many inter atomic bonds are broken, producing fragments of lower mass.

$$CH_4 + e^- \longrightarrow CH_4^{+\bullet} + 2e$$
$$\text{(Molecular ion)}$$
$$\downarrow$$
$$CH_3^+ + H^\bullet$$
$$\text{(fragment ion)}$$

$$CH_3-COCH_3 + e^- \longrightarrow CH_3-CO-CH_3^{+\bullet}$$
$$\text{(Molecular ion)}$$
$$\downarrow$$
$$CH_3-C \equiv O^+ + CH_3$$
$$\text{(Fragment ion)}$$

(v) Rearrangement ions

The ions formed by rearrangement process are those whose origin cannot be explained by the simple rupture of a bond in the molecule. The classical example is "Mclafferty rearrangement". This mechanism is confined to compounds such as aldehydes, ketones, acids amides and ester which contain a suitable hydrogen atom on the γ-carbon atom with respect to carbonyl group.

Butyl methyl ketone   (Molecular ions)

The resulting positive ion is established by three resonating structures. The stability of the fragment is a driving force for this type of rearrangement. In butylpentanoate, on McLafferty rearrangement on the acidic side generates a m/e = 116 ion. Subsequent rearrangement on the alcohol side generates m/e 60 and 56 ions.

The rearrangement ions can be predicted by observing the m/e value. The formation of even mass or odd mass fragment ions take place via simple cleavage from the odd mass or even mass molecular ion respectively. But if the rearrangement process is taking place then even mass or odd mass molecular ion gives even mass or odd mass fragment ion respectively.

(vi) Multiple charged ions

The removals of two or more electrons from a molecule without fragmentation is possible in case of organic compounds with aromatic rings and conjugated systems. Double and triple charged ions are formed by removal of two or more electrons respectively and they appear at ½ and 1/3 of the actual mass respectively.

(vii) Metastable ions

The presence of metastable ion is indicated by broad diffuse peaks, called "metastable peak", that do not usually appear at whole mass numbers.

If the average life time of ion (m_1) is $>5 \times 10^{-6}$ secs, the ion become accelerated, deviated and recorded as m_1. If the average life time of ion m_1 $<5 \times 10^{-6}$ secs, it fragment before acceleration to give a new ion of mass m_2.

If the ion decomposed in the zone between the source and analyser, there will be an ion with the acceleration of m_1 that becomes deviated as m_2. The ion m_2 appears in the spectrum at m^*. The value of mx will be equal to $(m_2)^2/m_1$. For example, toluene shows intense peak at m/e 91($C_7H_7^+$) and m/e 65 ($C_5H_5^+$) and diffuse peak at 46.4 (= $65^2/91$). It indicates that at least some of the ions at m/e 65 arise through ejection of C_2H_2 (26 mass unit) from the ions at m/e 91. Such a decomposition is called "metastable transition". The Fig. 2.13 is an example of metastable transition in anthraquinone.

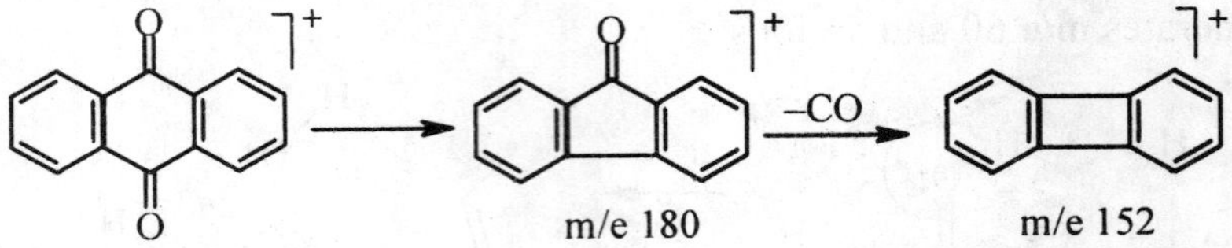

Fig. 2.13. Metastable ions.

(viii) Negative ions

Negative ions formed in the ion source are less abundant than positive ions by a factor of 10^{-4}. These are formed from a neutral molecule by three mechanisms :

(i) Poduction of a couple of ions
$$AB + e \longrightarrow A^+ + B^- + e$$

(ii) Capture of an electron with dissociation
$$AB + e^- \longrightarrow A + B^-$$

(iii) Capture of electron
$$AB + e^- \longrightarrow AB^-$$

(ix) Ions formed by ion-molecule interaction

The percentage of molecules of a compound ionized to the vapour in ionisation chamber is very low. Therefore, there is possibility of collision between molecular ion and neutral molecule. In such a collision, the molecular ion can subtract an atom from the neutral molecule, forming a heavier ion. The simplest example is the protonation of the molecular ion, resulting in the formation of M + 1 peak. This peak can be differentiated from the isotopic peak with the help of high resolution data. This reaction occur when the sample pressure is high.

APPLICATION OF MASS SPECTROMETRY

The fundamental equation of a mass spectrometer is:

$$\frac{m}{e} = \frac{m^2 R^2}{2V} \qquad \text{....(i)}$$

This equation expresses the relationship between the mass to charge ratio (m/e) of an ion, the magnetic field (H), the radius of the trajectories of the ions (R) and the applied accelerating voltage (V).

$$m = \frac{k}{V}$$

where $k = \frac{1}{2} H^2 R^2$

The mass of the ion focussed on the collector of the mass spectrometer is therefore, inversely proportional to the applied accelerating voltage and this relationship suggests that the different ions can be focussed by varying the acceleration potential at constant magnetic field. By releasing appropriate values of the voltage, the desired ions (single ion detection) can be focussed. By suitably varying the accelerating voltage between certain fixed mass numbers, the ion corresponding to these prescribed values can be focussed, successively (multiple ion detection).

Some of the compounds like hallucinogens are active in the order of micrograms, quantities and therefore, their identification from tissues or biological liquids requires the use of a very sensitive method, such as mass spectrometry. It can be detected by either single or multiple ions detection technique.

Single ion detection

Only one ion is focussed (generally an intense one). This technique can be used either by coupling with gas chromatograph or by using high resolution mass spectrometer.

In the first method, mass spectrometer is combined with gas chromatograph. Here, mass spectrometer is used as a selective gas chromatograph detector. This technique can increase the sensitivity of detection by a factor of between 1,000 and 10,000 with respect to normal gas chromatographic detectors like electron capture, flame ionisation or thermal conductivity detector.

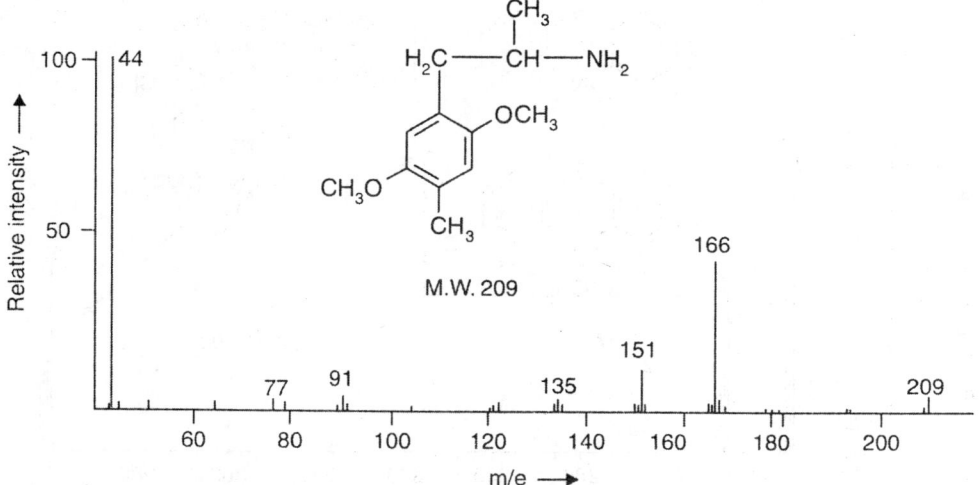

Fig. 2.14. Mass spectrum of 2,5-dimethoxy-4-methyl-amphetamine.

28 Pharmaceutical Analysis

An example of this application is the determination of 2,5-dimethoxy 4-methyl amphetamine. Its mass spectrum show prominent peak at m/e 166. Hence, acceleration potential corresponding to this mass is focussed and mass spectrum is recorded. Mass fragmentogram is a graph of total ion current versus time.

By this method, it can be detected in quantities as low as 100 pg. DDT, in trace amounts as low as 10 pg. has been similarly determined.

In second method (high resolution mass spectrometry), it is possible to differentiate the ions that have the same nominal m/e ratio but have different elemental composition. This method can be applied for determination of p-tyramine, a precursor of catechol-amines, isolated from brain extract. The sample is introduced directly into the ion source and a doublet is observed at the nominal mass 108. The high resolution mass spectrometer is focussed on m/e 108.0575, an ionic fragment corresponding to lipid-hydrocarbon that have a peak at m/e 108.0939.

Multiple ion detection

When the mass spectrometer is employed as a multiple ion detector, it focuses on two or three ionic fragments within a 10–30% range of the magnetic scan of the instrument or on upto eight fragments over the whole field using a quadrupole mass spectrometer. For example, the mass spectrum of desmethyl chloropromazine trifluoro-acetate shows three prominent peaks at m/e 232, 234 and 246. The component separated by gas chromatograph (Fig. 2.15) is focussed on the three peaks at m/e 232, 234 and 246.

Desmethyl chloropromazine trifluoro acetate

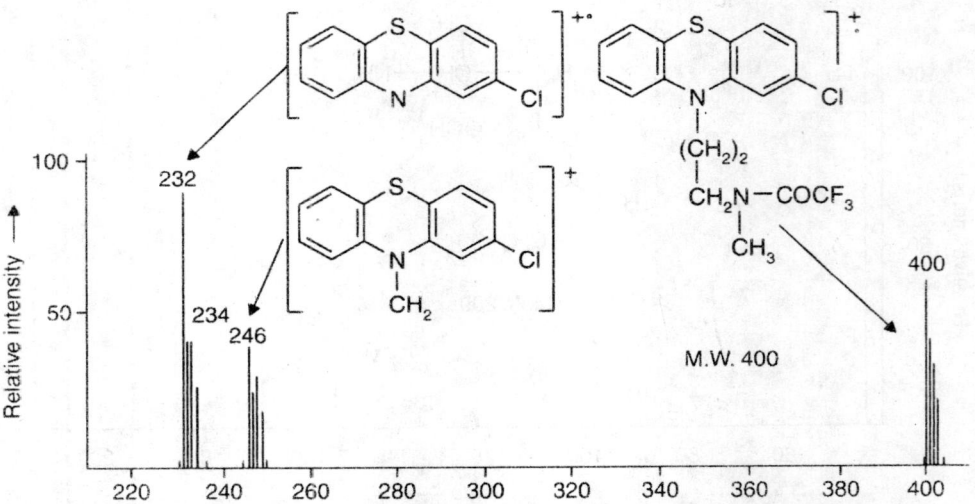

Fig. 2.15. Partial mass spectrum of desmethyl chlorpromazine trifluoro acetate.

Quantitative mass spectrometry

This method is analogous to those illustrated above using the single ion detection method but has the additional advantage of greater specificity. This result is obtained by focussing on more than one characteristic ionic fragment of a molecule and this ensures the identity of compound displayed. One of the channels on the AVA (accelerating voltage alternator) can also be used to detect the intensity of a fragmentation derived from internal standard.

This method is useful in the quantitative determination of imipramine. The spectrometer is focussed on fragment at m/e 235. The quantitative estimation is given by the relative peak areas of the ion fragment. The quantity is directly read out from calibration curve, obtained from standard. This method is useful to estimate the compound in the presence of complex mixtures as in extracts from biological fluids without interference.

For quantitative estimation, calibration curve is plotted with the help of internal standard, then from this calibration curve, quantity of unknown sample is determined.

Imipramine

HYPHENATED TECHNIQUES

1. GC-MS

Here, gas chromatography (GC) and mass spectrometry (Fig. 2.16) are combined together. GC can separate volatile and semivolatile compounds with great resolution, but it cannot identify them. MS can provide detailed structural information on most compounds such that they can be exactly

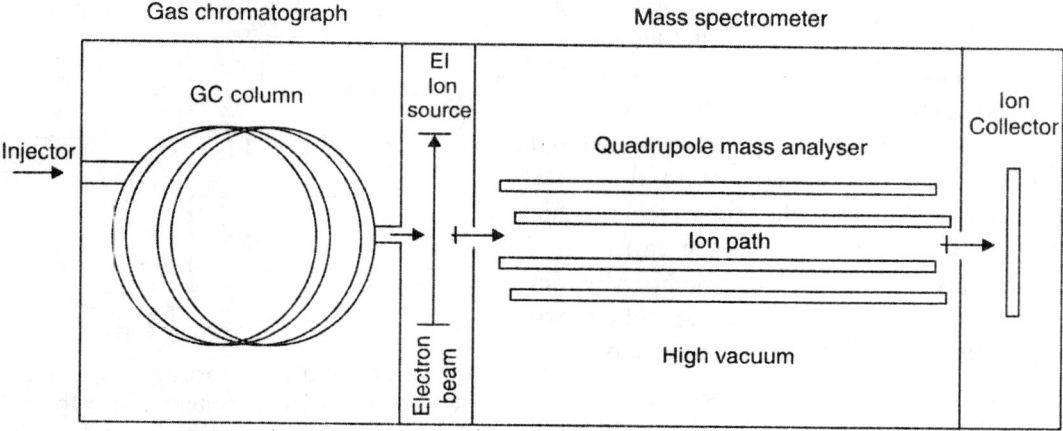

Fig. 2.16. Schematic diagram of GC-MS.

identified, but it cannot readily separate them. It means, mass spectrometer act as detector when it is combined with Gas Chromatography. This combination of the two techniques was suggested shortly after the development of GC in the mid-1950s. Gas chromatography and mass spectrometry are, in many ways, highly compatible techniques. In both techniques, the sample is in the vapor phase, and both techniques deal with about the same amount of sample (typically less than 1 ng). Unfortunately, there is a major incompatibility between the two techniques. The compound exiting the gas chromatograph is a tree component in the GC's carrier gas at a pressure of about 760 torr, but the mass spectrometer operates at a vacuum of about 10^{-6} to 10^{-5} torr. This is a difference in pressure of 8 to 9 orders of magnitude, a considerable problem.

The pressure incompatibility problem between GC and MS is solved in several ways. The earliest approach, dating from the late 1950s, simply split a small fraction of the gas chromatographic effluent into the mass spectrometer. Depending on the pumping speed of the mass spectrometer, about 1 to 5% of the GC effluent is split off into the mass spectrometer, venting the remaining 95 to 99% of the analytes into the atmosphere. It is soon recognized that this is not the best way to maintain the high sensitivity of the two techniques, and so improved GC-MS interfaces are designed. These interfaces reduced the pressure of the GC effluent from about 760 torr to 10^{-6} to 10^{-5} torr, but at the same time, they allow to pass all (or most) of the analyte molecules from the GC into the mass spectrometer. These interfaces are no longer just GC carrier gas splitters, but carrier gas separators; that is, they separated the carrier gas from the organic analytes and actually increased the concentration of the organic compounds in the carrier gas stream.

The most important commercial GC carrier gas separator is called the *jet separator*; see Fig. 2.17). This device takes advantage of the differences in diffusibility between the carrier gas and the organic compound. The carrier gas is almost always a small molecule such as helium or hydrogen with a high diffusion coefficient, whereas the organic molecules have much lower diffusion coefficients. In operation, the GC effluent (the carrier gas with the organic analytes) is sprayed through a small nozzle, indicated as d_1 in Fig. 2.17, into a partially evacuated chamber (about 10^{-12} torr). Because of its high diffusion coefficient, the helium is sprayed over a wide solid angle, whereas the heavier organic molecules are sprayed over a much narrower angle and tend to go straight across the vacuum region. By collecting the middle section of this solid angle with a skimmer (marked d_3 in Fig. 2.17) and passing it to the mass spectrometer, the higher-molecular-weight organic compounds are separated from the carrier gas, which is removed by the vacuum pump. Most jet separators are made from glass by drawing down a glass capillary, sealing it into a vacuum envelope, and cutting out the middle spacing (marked d_2 in Fig. 2.17). It is important that the spray orifice and the skimmer be perfectly aligned.

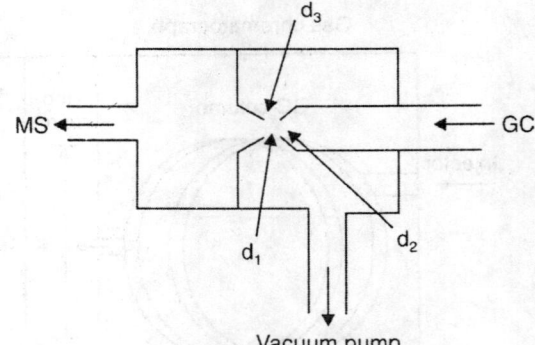

Fig. 2.17. The jet separator, a device for interfacing a packed column GC with an MS. The three distances are typically d_1, 100 μm; d_2, 300 μm; and d_3, 240 μm.

Mass spectrometry provides us uniquely valuable information about molecular weight (via mass to charge (m/e) ratio); molecular structural information and quantitative data, all at high sensitivity. However, it is best to apply separation techniques to complex mixtures before mass spectrometry is undertaken. High performance liquid chromatography (LC) is excellent for separating mixtures but generally poor at identification of compounds. The combination of these two techniques (LC/MS) thus provides an extraordinarily powerful analytica tool. LC/MS is a hyphenated technique, combining the separation power of HPLC, with the detection power of mass spectrometry. Most instruments now use atmospheric pressure ionization (API) technique where solvent elimination and ionization steps are combined in the source and take place at atmospheric pressure. When electron impact ionization (EI) is the choice, the solvent elimination and ionization steps are separate. The interface is a particle beam type, which separates the sample from the solvent, and allows the introduction of the sample in the form of dry particles into the high vacuum region. Electron impact is of interest for molecules which do not ionize with API technique, or when an electron impact spectrum is necessary, since it provides spectral information independent of the sample introduction technique (GC or LC, or direct introduction) and instrument supplier.

FACTORS INFLUENCING THE FRAGMENTATION

The mass spectrum of a molecule shows the numerous peaks, some of them are intense whereas others are weak or scarcely visible. The formation of ions depend on the (i) preferential breakage of some bonds in comparison to others, and (ii) on the stability of some fragments because of their structure. In conclusion, the formation of ions depend on three factors :

1. The relative strength of the bonds.
2. The stability of the fragmentation products. These may be neutral molecule, radicals and positive ions.
3. The relative spatial arrangements of the atoms or groups.

1. Relative strength of the bonds

The energies of the most common bonds of an organic molecule are shown in Table 2.2. The weakest bond (C-I, C-Br, C-Cl) are preferentially broken in comparison to other. Similarly, breakage of single bond require less energy in preference to double or triple bond.

Table 2.2. Energy profile of some bonds present in organic compounds (kCal/mole)

Bond	Energy	Bond	Energy	Bond	Energy
C–H	97.8	C=N	147	C–F	116
C–C	82.6	C–O	85.5	C–Cl	81
C=C	145.1	C=O	179	C–Br	68
C≡C	199.6	C–S	65	C–I	51
C–N	72.8	C=S	128	O–H	110.6

2. Stability of the fragments

Fragment ions are established by following undermentioned process.

(a) Inductive effect

In the mass spectra of n–butyl and t–butyl alcohol, the ions $C_4H_9^+$

$$CH_3CH_2CH_2CH_2 - \overset{+\bullet}{O}H \longrightarrow CH_3CH_2CH_2CH_2^+ + {}^\bullet OH$$

$$\begin{array}{c} H_3C \\ H_3C-C-\overset{+\bullet}{O}H \\ H_3C \end{array} \longrightarrow \begin{array}{c} H_3C \\ H_3C-C^+ + {}^\bullet OH \\ H_3C \end{array}$$

are formed in both cases but more abundant in the case of t-butanol because tertiary ion is stabilized by the inductive effect of the alkyl groups attached to carbon atom, carrying the positive charge. To some extent, it is also stabilized by hyperconjugation effect, that is delocalisation of the electron of σ C–H bond to form a π bond with an adjacent carbon atom having an empty orbital.

$$\begin{array}{c} H \\ | \\ -C-C+ \\ | \quad | \end{array} \longrightarrow \begin{array}{c} H^+ \\ | \\ -C=C- \\ | \quad | \end{array}$$

Similarly, in isopentane, the fragmentation occurs at different bond position and the various ions have the following order of stability. Out of these, the ion resulting from the breakage of bond at C-2 position will be most stabilised.

$$\underset{\text{Isopentane (Molecular ion)}}{CH_3-CH_2-\overset{\overset{CH_3}{|}}{CH}-CH_3}\Big]^{+\bullet} \longrightarrow CH_3-CH_2-\overset{\overset{CH_3}{|}}{\overset{}{CH}} > \overset{\overset{CH_3}{|}}{\overset{}{CH}}-CH_3 > CH_3-CH_2^+ > CH_3^+$$

The inductive effect also has an influence on the breaking of a bond. In a compound R–X in which X can be Cl, Br, O, S or N, the electronegativity of hetero atom lowers the electron density of the R–X bond. Formation of an alkyl ion occurs according to below mentioned reaction :

$$R-Cl \longrightarrow R^+ + {}^\bullet Cl$$

$$R-O-R \longrightarrow R^+ + {}^\bullet OR$$

The order of electron attraction is Cl > Br, O, S > I > N, C, H.

The unsaturated functional groups, such as carbonyl group, have a similar effect.

$$R-\overset{\overset{O}{\|}}{C}-R \longrightarrow R-CO^\bullet + R^+$$

(b) Neighbouring electron participation

The carbonyl compounds, such as ketones, aldehydes, esters, amides and the corresponding sulphur derivatives, give rise to ions of $\ce{>C+ = \ddot{X}}$ stabilised in the canonical form, $-C \equiv X^+$.

$$\underset{\displaystyle CH_3-\overset{\overset{\displaystyle O^{+\bullet}}{\|}}{C}-CH_3}{} \longrightarrow CH_3-C \equiv O^+ + \overset{\bullet}{C}H_3$$

The canonical form is stabilised by heteroatom that possess at least a couple of electrons not used in bonding.

Similarly, alcohols, ethers, thiols, thioethers and amines shows the presence of ion which are stabilised by heteroatom.

$$R-\underset{\underset{\displaystyle \overset{+}{:}OH}{|}}{CH}-R^1 \longrightarrow R^{\bullet} + \underset{\underset{\displaystyle OH}{\|}}{CH}-R^1$$

$$\searrow \underset{\underset{\displaystyle R-\overset{\|}{C}+{}^{\bullet}R^1}{}}{\overset{+}{OH}}$$

$$R-CH_2-\overset{+\bullet}{\underset{\displaystyle ..}{O}}-CH_2-R^1 \longrightarrow R-CH_2-\overset{+}{O}=CH_2 + {}^{\bullet}R^1$$
$$R^{\bullet} + CH_2=\underset{+}{O}-CH_2-R^1$$

$$R-\underset{\underset{\displaystyle \overset{+}{\cdot}NH_2}{|}}{CH}-R^1 \longrightarrow R-\underset{\underset{\displaystyle +NH_2}{\|}}{C}+{}^{\bullet}R^1$$

$$\downarrow$$

$$R^{\bullet} + \underset{\underset{\displaystyle +NH_2}{\|}}{CH}-R^1$$

The capacity of a heteroatom to stabilize an adjacent positive charge is very high for nitrogen atom and decrease gradually, passing through S, O and the halogen for which is very low.

(c) Resonance effect

Allylic cleavage is a favoured fragmentation mode in unsaturated compound. The resonance stabilization of an allyl cation leads to increased probability of fragmentation of carbon-carbon bond β to a double bonds.

$$\overset{|}{\underset{|}{C}}-\overset{|}{\underset{|}{\overset{\alpha}{C}}}-\overset{|}{\underset{|}{\overset{\beta}{C}}}-\overset{|}{\underset{|}{C}} \longrightarrow \overset{|}{\underset{|}{\overset{+}{C}}}-\overset{|}{\underset{|}{\overset{\bullet}{C}}}-\overset{|}{\underset{|}{C}}-\overset{|}{\underset{|}{C}} \longrightarrow \overset{|}{\underset{|}{\overset{+}{C}}}-C=\overset{|}{\underset{|}{C}} + \overset{\bullet}{\underset{|}{C}}- \longleftrightarrow \overset{|}{\underset{|}{C}}=\overset{|}{\underset{|}{C}}-\overset{|}{\underset{|}{\overset{+}{C}}}$$

The β cleavage is one of the most characteristic fragmentation of aromatic hydrocarbons with an alkyl side chain. The ion that is formed is represented by tropylium structure because all the carbon atoms are equivalent.

The β cleavage is also characteristic for five membered aromatic heterocycles with an alkyl side chain in the α or β position.

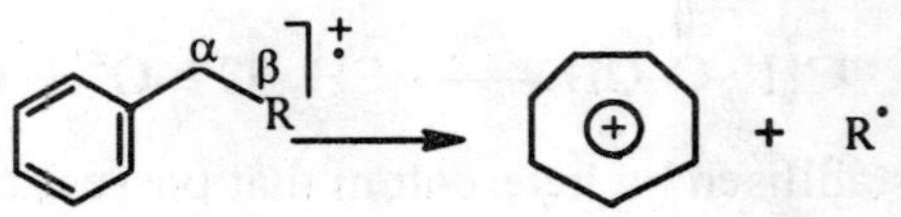

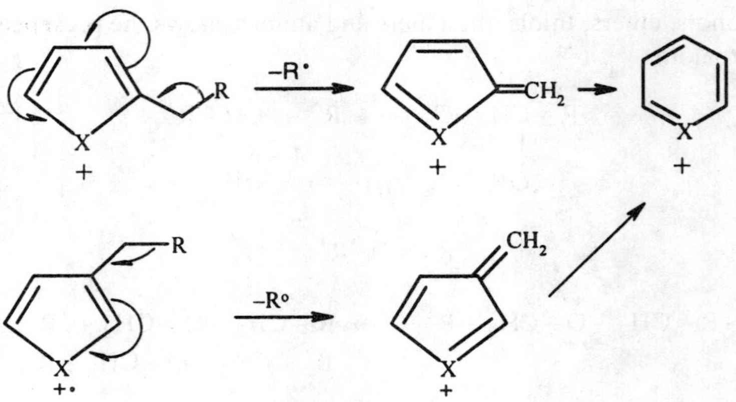

3. Multicenter fragmentations and steric factors

The fragmentation so far observed involve the cleavage of only one bond. In a complex molecule, the interaction of various functional groups can give a complicated fragmentation pattern that involves the rupture of more than one bond. This is called a multi-center fragmentation. In this, there may be hydrogen atom migration with the expulsion of neutral fragment (elimination and Mclafferty rearrangement) and the reaction of internal rearrangement of bonds (Retro diels-alder).

(a) Elimination reaction

This elimination process can be represented by following scheme:

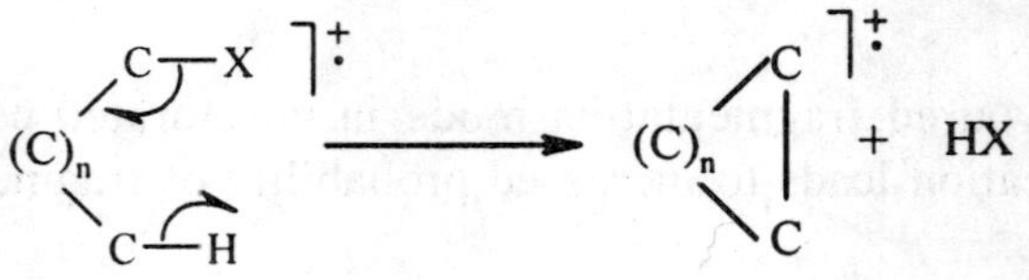

where X = Cl, Br, I, OH, OR, OCOR, NH_2, NR_2, SH.

For example, alcohol shows the M–H_2O peak due to elimination reaction.

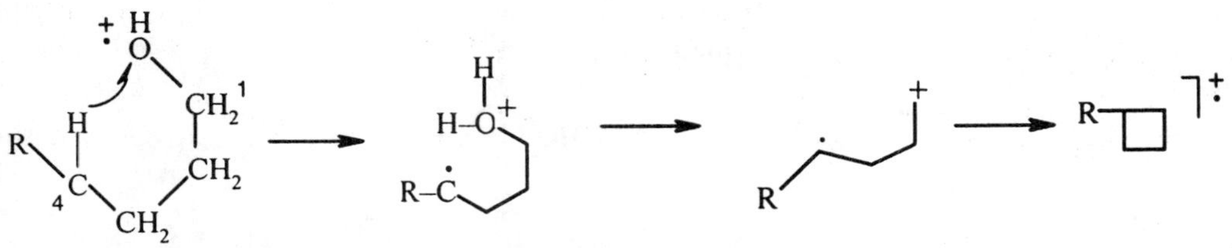

Similarly, there is elimination of hydrogen chloride in alkyl chloride.

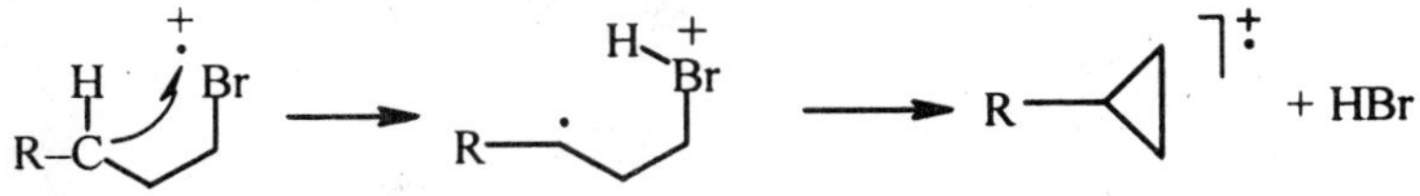

(b) Ortho effect

Ortho disubstituted aromatic system or cis olefins can give rise to the specific migration of a hydrogen atom onto an atom or group that is eliminated in a form of neutral molecule. For example, in o-methyl acetophenone, there is migration of 'H' atom to release the methyl alcohol.

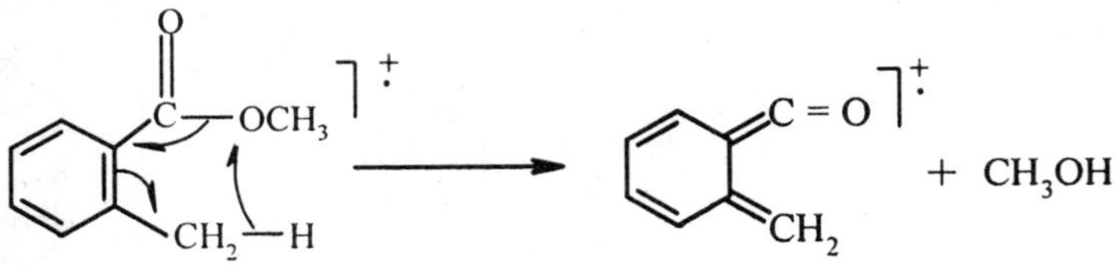

o-methyl acetophenone

Similarly, o-methyl benzyl alcohol shows the ortho effect to form the water molecule.

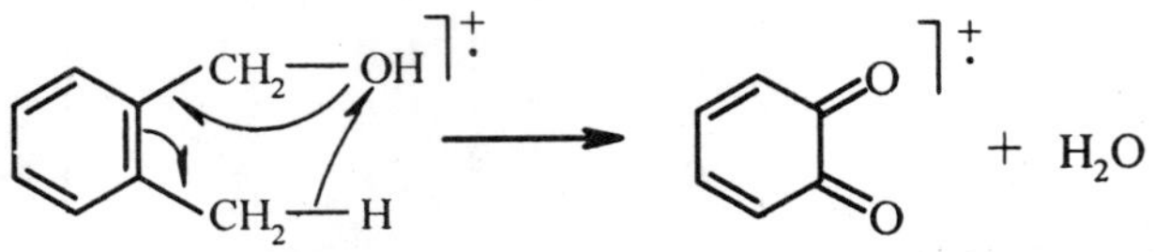

o-methyl benzyl alcohol

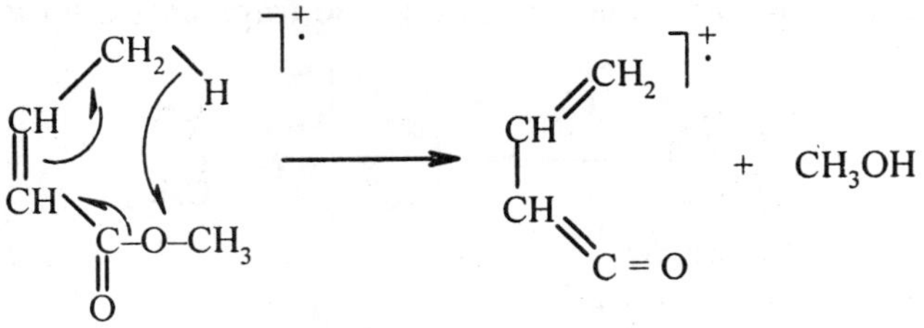

It is useful to distinguish between cis and trans compounds and o, m and p-isomers.

(c) Maclafferty rearrangement (MR)

This fragmentation mode is characteristic of ketones, aldehydes, acids, esters, olefins, alkyl benzene, oximes and hydrazones.

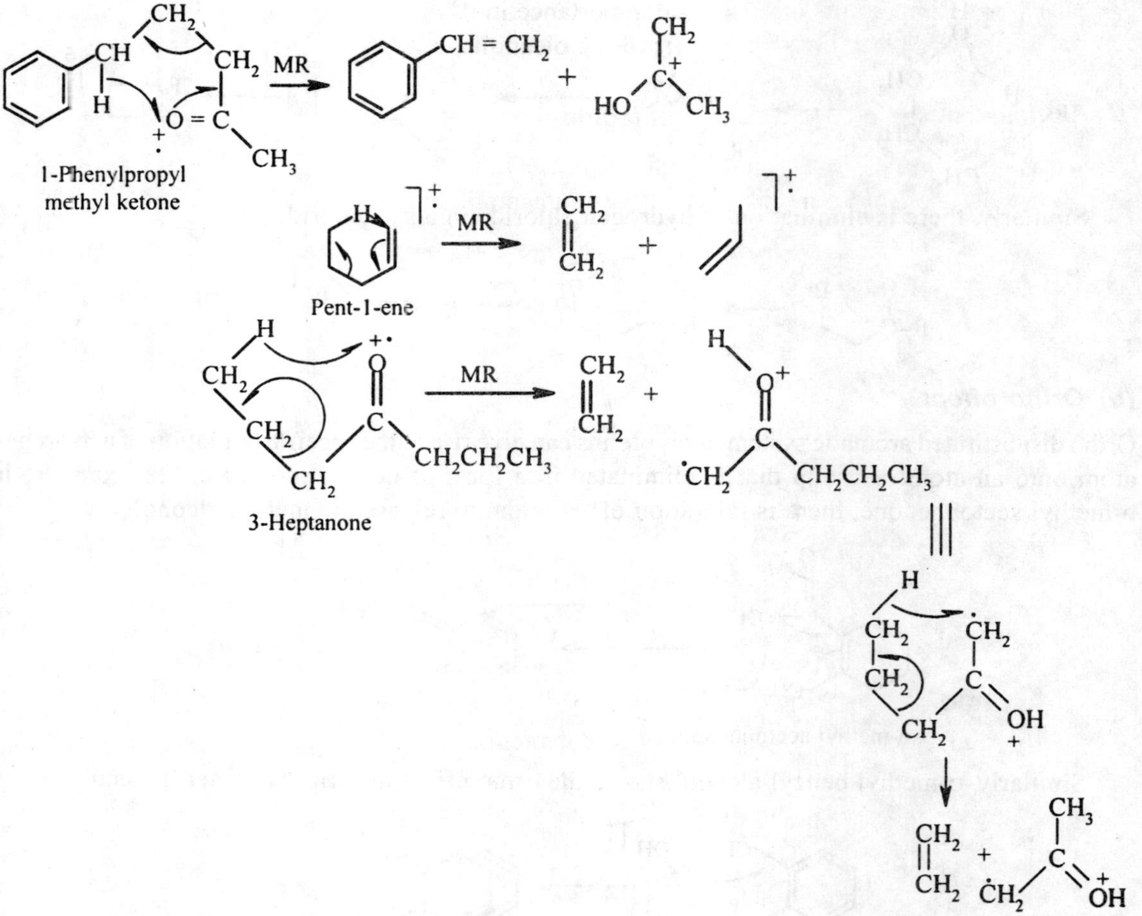
1-Phenylpropyl methyl ketone
MR
Pent-1-ene
MR
3-Heptanone
MR

(d) Retro diels-alder reaction

This multi centre fragmentation is very common in mass spectrum of cyclic olefins. Usually, a positively charged, diene fragment and a neutral olefinic fragments are formed.

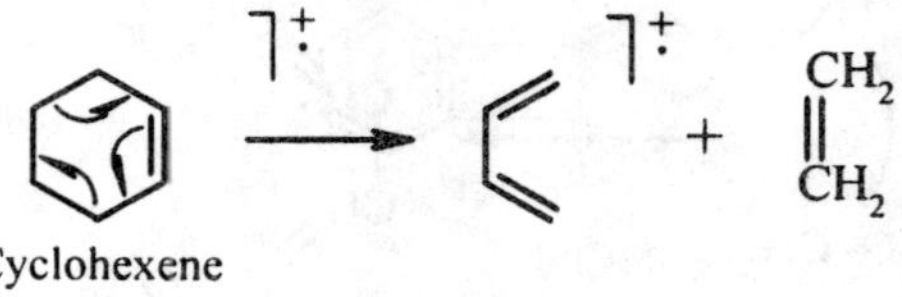
Cyclohexene

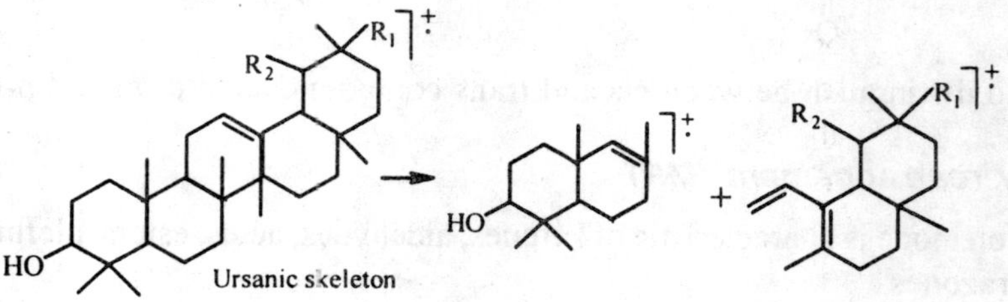
Ursanic skeleton

This type of reaction is considerable importance in the structural determination of numerous compounds, such as tetraline, triterpenes of the oleanolic or ursolic skeleton.

(e) Expulsion of a stable neutral molecule

Expulsion of neutral molecules like CO, CO_2, N_2, SO_2, $CH_2 = CO$, $CH_2 = CH_2$ and $CH \equiv CH$ has a considerable importance in the course of a fragmentation.

$$R-\overset{+}{O}\cdots H + O=C=CH_2 \quad \text{(Acetate)} \longrightarrow R-\overset{+\cdot}{O}-H + O=C=CH_2$$

The mass spectrum of phthalic anhydride shows the elimination first of CO_2 and then of CO to give an ion at m/e 76, designated as benzene.

$$\text{phthalic anhydride} \xrightarrow{+e} \xrightarrow{-CO_2} [C_7H_4O]^{+\cdot} \xrightarrow{-CO} [C_6H_4]^{+\cdot} \quad m/e\ 76$$

Anthraquinone losses two molecules of carbon monooxide to give a compound $C_{12}H_{10}$ to which is attributed the diphenyl structure.

GENERAL RULES OF FRAGMENTATION

A number of general rules for predicting prominent peaks in electron impact spectra can be written and rationalized by using standard concepts of physical organic chemistry :

1. The relative height of the molecular ion peak is greatest for the straight-chain compound and decreases as the degree of branching increases (See Rule 3).
2. The relative height of the molecular ion peak usually decreases with increasing molecular weight in a homologous series. Fatty esters appear to be an exception.

3. Cleavage is favored at alkyl substituted carbons; the more substituted, the more likely is cleavage. This is a consequence of the increased stability of a tertiary carbocation over a secondary, which in turn is more stable than a primary.

$$\text{R–}\overset{|}{\underset{|}{C}}\text{–} \longrightarrow \text{R}^{\bullet} + \overset{|}{\underset{|}{C}}^{+}$$

Cation stability order:

$$R_3C^+ > R_2CH^+ > RCH_2^+ > CH_3^+$$

Generally, the largest substituent at a branch is eliminated most readily as a radical, presumably because a long-chain radical can achieve some stability by delocalization of the lone electron.

4. **Stevenson's rule:** The most probable fragmentation is the one that leaves the positive charge on the fragment with the lowest ionization energy. For example, in the molecule (AB), either A^+ or B^+ possessing positive charge may form during fragmentation.

$$AB^+ \diagup\!\!\!\diagdown \begin{array}{l} A^+ + B^{\bullet} \\ A^{\bullet} + B^+ \end{array}$$

Whichever species (A or B) that has the lowest electron affinity will be the cationic fragmentation species. It means fragmentation pattern that leads to the formation of stable ions, is favoured over the formation of less stable ions.

Stevenson's rule also leads to the corollary, that when two radicals are possible, the largest alkyl radical will be lost preferentially. Therefore, the ease in fragmentation increases:

$$H_3C^+ < RCH_2^+ < R_3^+ < H_2C=CHCH_2^+$$
$$\sim HC\equiv CCH_2^+ < C_6H_5CH_2^+$$

5. Double bonds, cyclic structures, and especially aromatic (or heteroaromatic) rings stabilize the molecular ion, and thus increase the probability of its appearance.
6. Double bonds favour allylic cleavage and give the resonance-stabilized allylic carbonium ion.

$$CH_2^{+\bullet} : CH-CH_2-R \xrightarrow{-R^{\bullet}} {}^+CH_2-CH=CH_2$$
$$\updownarrow$$
$$CH_2=CH-CH_2^+$$

7. Saturated rings tend to lose side chains at the a-bond. This is merely a special case of branching (Rule 3). The positive charge tends to stay with the ring fragment. Unsaturated rings can undergo a *retro*-Diels-Alder reaction:

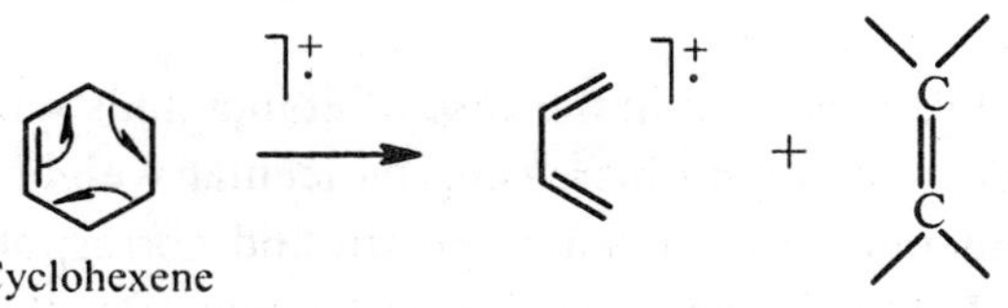

Cyclohexene

8. In alkyl-substituted aromatic compounds, cleavage is very probable at the bond beta to the ring, giving the resonance-stabilized benzyl ion or, more likely, the tropylium ion:

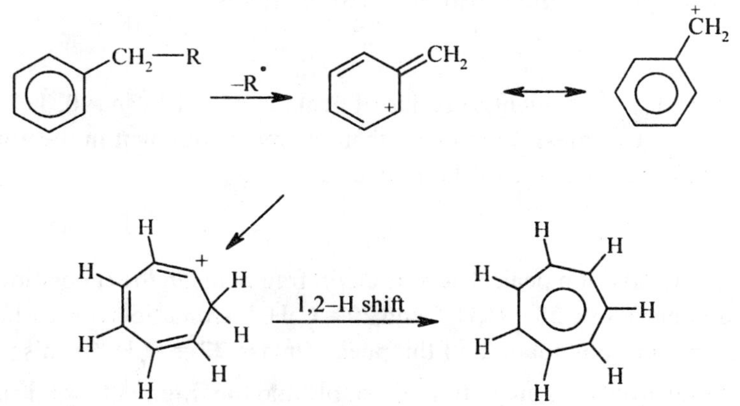

1,2–H shift

9. C–C bonds next to a heteroatom (Y) are frequently cleaved, leaving the charge on the fragment containing the heteroatom whose nonbonding electrons provide resonance stabilization.

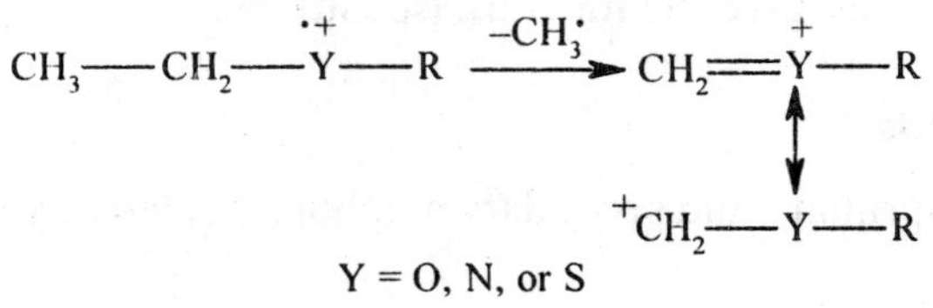

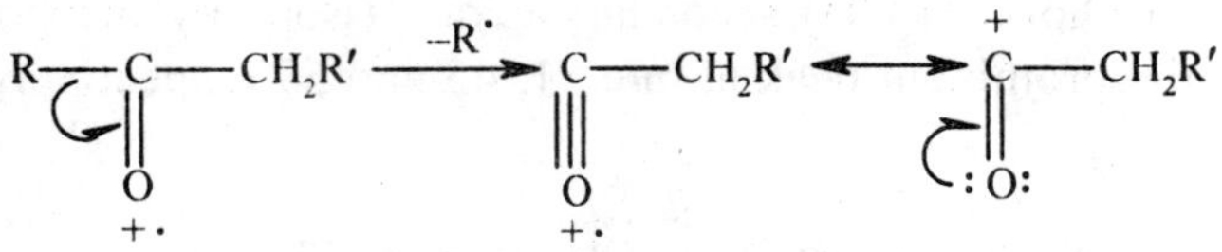

$Y = O, N,$ or S

10. Cleavage is often associated with elimination of small stable neutral molecules, such as carbon monoxide, olefins, water, ammonia, hydrogen sulphide, hydrogen cyanide, mercaptans, ketene, or alcohols.

COMMON FRAGMENTATION PATTERN OF SOME CLASSES OF ORGANIC COMPOUNDS

Hydrocarbons

Aliphatic

The molecular peak is always present in the case of compounds with linear chains. The intensity of molecular ion peak decreases with increasing molecular weight. Two series of fragmentation homologues are preponderant in their mass spectra and correspond to the empirical formulae $C_nH_{2n+1}^+$ and $C_nH_{2n-1}^+$. The peaks corresponding to the loss of methyl group $(M-15)^+$ is of reduced intensity unless there is a branched methyl group.

The peaks at m/e $43 = C_3H_7^+$ and $57 = C_4H_9^+$ are abundant. In the case of branched hydrocarbons, the fragmentation takes place at the substituted carbon atoms.

Olefins

The molecular peak $C_nH_{2n}^+$ is evident. A series of peak, at $41 + 14n$ ($n = 0, 1, 2, ...$) is observed, corresponding to a series two mass units lower than the most abundant in the aliphatic series. The base peak occurs by allylic cleavage of the molecule.

Saturated cyclic

It shows an intense molecular ion peak. The side chain fragments in the α position and the cleavage of the ring give fragments at m/e $28 = C_2H_4^+$ and $29 = C_2H_5^+$ Aromatic hydrocarbon. The molecular ion peak is, in general very abundant, and the peak at mass $77 = C_6H_5^+$ is also evident.

The condensed ring aromatics are extremely stable and the fragmentation is much reduced and generally non-consistent. In the alkyl aromatics, the base peak is that of mass $91 = C_7H_7^+$, as the tropylium ion. If, however, the carbon in the α position, with respect to the ring, is substituted, the base peak becomes $91 + 14$ n. The positional isomers on the ring (o, m and p-) are difficult to differentiate in as much as they give identical transpositions.

Hydroxylated compounds

The molecular ion peak of primary and secondary alcohols is relatively small. It is undetectable in tertiary alcohol.

The molecular ion decomposes by α cleavage with a tendency to lose a radical of large dimension. The primary alcohol (CH_3OH), secondary alcohol (isopropyl alcohol) and tertiary alcohol (t-butyl alcohol) show the prominent peak at m/e 31, 45 and 59 respectively.

$$\overset{H}{\underset{|}{C}}H_2\overset{+\cdot}{O}H \xrightarrow{H^\cdot} \overset{+}{C}H_2\text{--}\overset{..}{O}H \longleftrightarrow CH_2 = \overset{+}{O}H$$
$$\text{m/e } 31$$

$$\underset{CH_3}{\overset{CH_3}{>}}CH\text{--}\overset{\cdot+}{O}H \xrightarrow{CH_3^\cdot} CH_3\text{--}\overset{+}{C}H\text{--}\overset{..}{O}H \longleftrightarrow CH_3\text{--}CH = \overset{+}{O}H$$
$$\text{m/e } 45$$

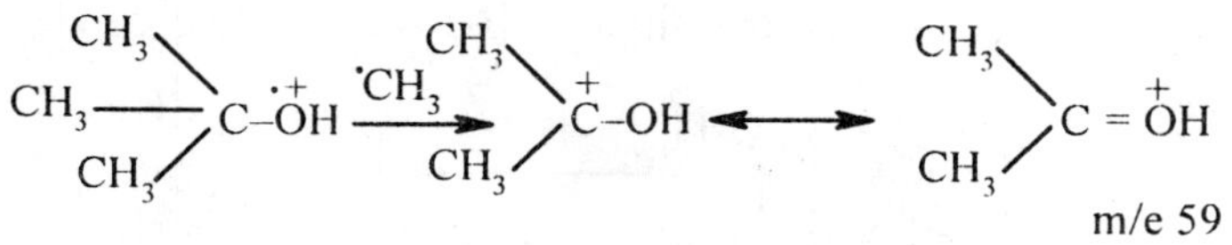

The peak (M-18)⁺ occurs by loss of water molecule from the molecular ion in alcohol containing 4 or more carbon atoms :

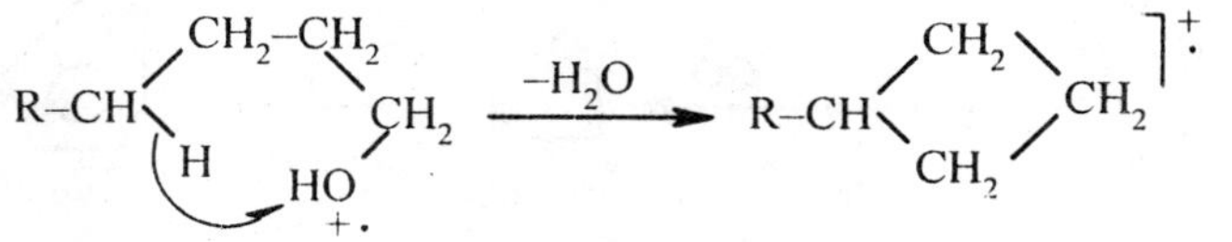

α-cleavage occur in unsaturated alcohol. In allyl alcohol, formation of the (M–H) ion is favoured due to high stability of the resulting ion.

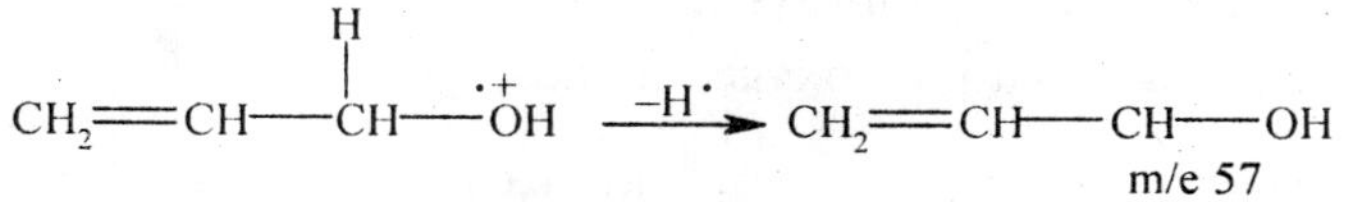

The McLafferty rearrangement has also been reported in these compounds.

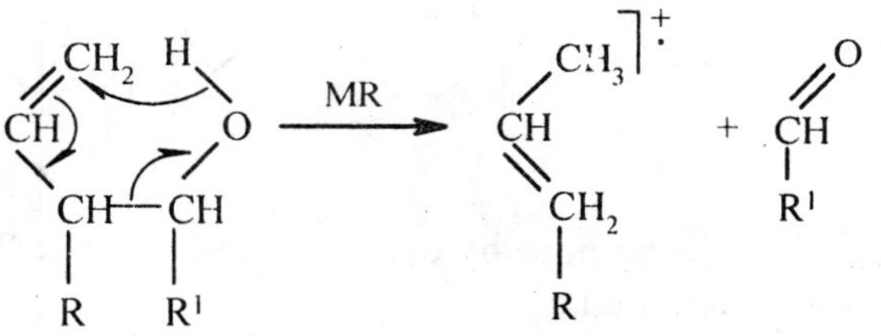

The cyclic alcohol e.g. cyclohexanol show peak at m/e 57 due to cleavage of ring.

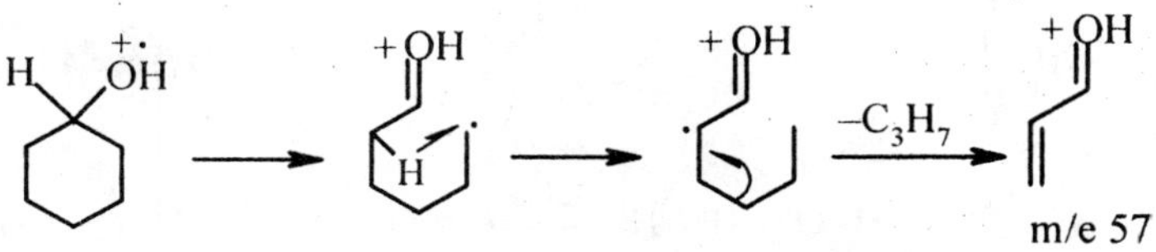

Benzyl alcohol show the ion peak caused by liberation of carbon monoxide molecule.

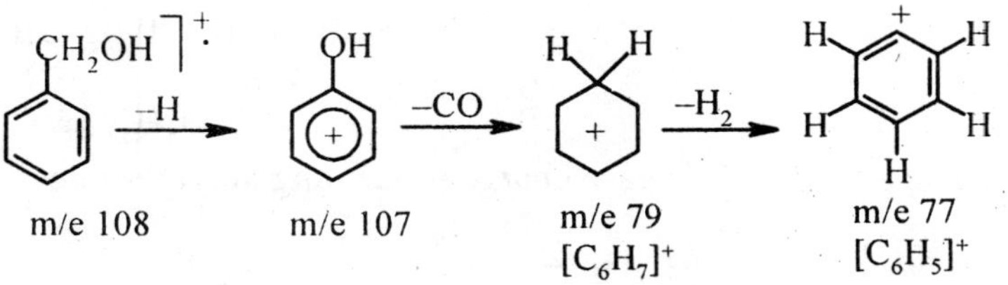

Ortho-substituted benzyl alcohol give a distinct M-18 due to loss of H_2O (ortho effect).

In phenol, peak resulting from loss of CO is usually found.

m/e 66 → m/e 65

ETHERS

Aliphatic ether

There are two major fragmentation pathways :

(i) Cleavage of C–C bond next to the oxygen atom.

$$RCH_2-CH_2-\overset{+\cdot}{CH}-\overset{\cdot\cdot}{O}-CH_2-CH_3 \xrightarrow{-RCH_2CH_2^\cdot} \underset{CH_3}{\overset{|}{CH}}=\overset{+\cdot}{O}-CH_2-CH_3$$

$$\underset{CH_3}{\overset{|}{\overset{+}{CH}}}=\overset{\cdot\cdot}{O}-CH_2-CH_3 \quad m/e\ 73$$

This fragment may further decompose by the following process. This pathway is important when α-carbon atom is substituted.

$$\underset{\underset{m/e\ 73}{CH_3\ H-CH_2}}{\overset{+\cdot}{\overset{|}{CH}}=O-CH_2} \xrightarrow{CH_2=CH_2} \underset{CH_3}{\overset{|}{\overset{+\cdot}{CH}}=OH} \longleftrightarrow \underset{CH_3\ m/e\ 45}{\overset{+}{\overset{|}{CH}}-\overset{\cdot\cdot}{OH}}$$

$$RCH_2-CH_2-\overset{+\cdot}{\underset{|}{CH}}-\overset{\cdot\cdot}{O}-CH_2CH_3 \xrightarrow{CH_3^\cdot} RCH_2-CH_2-\underset{CH_3}{\overset{|}{CH}}-\overset{+}{\underset{\cdot\cdot}{O}}=CH_2$$

$$RCH_2-CH_2-\underset{CH_3\ m/e\ 73}{\overset{|}{CH}}-\overset{\cdot\cdot}{\overset{+}{O}}-CH_2$$

(ii) C–O bond cleavage occurs to release charge possessing alkyl fragment.

$$CH_3-\overset{+\cdot}{\underset{\cdot\cdot}{O}}-C_2H_5 \longrightarrow CH_3-\overset{\cdot\cdot}{\underset{\cdot\cdot}{O}}- + C_2H_5^+$$

Aromatic ether

The molecular peak is intense. Generally base peak is obtained by β cleavage with respect to the ring.

$$[C_6H_5-O-CH_2-CH_2-H]^{+\cdot} \longrightarrow C_6H_5-\overset{+\cdot}{OH} + CH_2=CH_2$$

There are also other concurrent reactions.

$$[C_6H_5-O-CH_2]^{+\cdot} \xrightarrow{-CH_3^{\cdot}} C_6H_5-\overset{+}{O} \xrightarrow{-CO} \left[\bigcirc\right]^{+}$$

$$\downarrow -CH_2=O$$

$$C_6H_6^{+\cdot}$$

Carbonyl compounds

Aliphatic ketones

They show intense molecular ion peak. There is cleavage of carbon–carbon bond adjacent to oxygen atom to release alkyl group with greater probability of losing the heavier group. The charge is mainly located on the fragments bearing oxygen atom.

$$\underset{R_2}{\overset{R_1}{>}}C=O \;{}^{+\cdot} \xrightarrow{-R_1^{\cdot}} R_2-C\equiv \overset{+}{O} \longleftrightarrow R_2-\overset{+}{C}=\ddot{O}$$
$$\xrightarrow{-R_2^{\cdot}} R_1-C\equiv \overset{+}{O} \longleftrightarrow R_1-\overset{+}{C}=O$$

McLafferty rearrangement occur if one of the allyl group possess γ-hydrogen.

$$\left[R-\overset{O}{\underset{}{C}}\overset{H}{\underset{CH_2-CH_2}{\diagdown}}CHR_1\right]^{+\cdot} \longrightarrow R-\overset{OH}{\underset{CH_2}{\overset{\|}{C}}} {}^{+\cdot} + CH_2=CHR_1$$

Aromatic ketones

There is an intense molecular ion peak. In general, a base peak is obtained by fragmentation α to carbonyl group.

$$C_6H_5-\overset{\overset{+}{O}}{\underset{}{\overset{\|}{C}}}-R \xrightarrow{-R^{\cdot}} C_6H_5-C\equiv \overset{+}{O}$$

When the alkyl chain contain 3 carbon atom or more, McLafferty rearrangement may occur.

Aliphatic aldehydes

The molecular peak M^+ and $(M-1)^+$ are intense, the latter following alpha cleavage.

$$R-\underset{H}{\underset{|}{C}}=O \overset{\cdot +}{} \longrightarrow \begin{cases} R-C\equiv O^+ \\ R-C\equiv O^+ \end{cases}$$

Peak at m/e 29 also appears due to presence of $H-C\equiv O^+$ formed by α cleavage.

β cleavage, for linear aldehydes of more than three carbon atoms also occurs, with a base peak of m/e 44 following a McLafferty rearrangement.

$$\begin{array}{c} HC=O \quad H \\ | \quad \quad | \\ H_2C \quad \quad CH-R \\ \diagdown CH_2 \diagup \end{array} \xrightarrow{MR} \begin{array}{c} OH \\ | \\ HC \\ \| \\ CH_2 \end{array} + H_2C=CHR$$

m/e 44

If the carbon atom in position 2 is substituted, peaks occur at masses 44 + 14n.

Aromatic aldehydes

The peak M^+ and $(M-1)^+$ are intense. There is a tendency to form the benzoylic cation (m/e 105).

$$Ph-CHO^+ \xrightarrow{H^\cdot} Ph-C\equiv O^+$$

Carboxylic acid

Aliphatic acid

The direct loss of hydroxyl (M-17) and carboxyl radical (M-45) by α cleavage occur from the molecular ion in short chain acid. McLafferty rearrangement leads to the formation of characteristic peak at m/e 60.

$$\begin{array}{c} H \\ \diagdown \\ CH_2 \quad O^+ \\ | \quad \| \\ CH_2 \quad C \\ \diagdown CH_2 \diagup \quad \diagdown OH \end{array} \xrightarrow{MR} CH_2=\underset{}{\overset{\overset{\cdot +}{O}H}{C}}-OH + CH_2=CH_2$$

In the spectra of long chain acids, oxygen containing fragments at m/e 45, 59, 87, ... and alkyl fragments at m/e 29, 43, 57, 71, 85, ... are observed. Following α cleavage with respect to carboxyl group, two series of fragments are formed depending on the localisation of the charge.

$$[R-CO{\mid}OR_1]^+ \longrightarrow R-C=O^+ + {}^{\bullet}OR, \text{ giving a series of } 29 + 14\ n.$$

$$R{\mid}CO-OR_1 \longrightarrow R^{\bullet} + {}^+O\equiv C-OR_1, \text{ giving a series of } 59 + 14\ n.$$

With β cleavage, following a Mclafferty rearrangement, the methyl ester give a base peak at m/e 74 ($CH_2=C-OMe$), ethyl ester a peak at m/e 88.
$$\qquad\qquad\qquad\qquad\quad |$$
$$\qquad\qquad\qquad\qquad +OH$$

Aromatic acid

The molecular ion peak in aromatic acid is more intense in comparison to aliphatic acids. Loss of hydroxyl and carboxyl radical by α-cleavage is generally observed. Loss of H_2O (M-18) is also observed if hydrogen bearing ortho group is present.

In the case of methyl ester, M-31 (M–OCH_3) is the base peak, and M-59 (M–$COOCH_3$) is also intense.

Esters

Aliphatic acids

The molecular ion peak is irrelevant. Following α cleavage, with respect to carbonyl group, two series of fragments are formed depending on the localization of the charge.

Amines

Aliphatic amines

The molecular ion peak of an aliphatic amines is usually quite weak and in long chain or highly branched amines, is undetectable. The base peak usually appears due to C–C cleavage next to nitrogen atom giving rise to $CH_2=\overset{+}{N}H_2$ fragment.

$$CH_3-CH_2-\overset{+\bullet}{N}H_2 \longrightarrow CH_2=\overset{+}{N}H_2 + {}^{\bullet}CH_3$$

This cleavage also accounts for base peak in tertiary and secondary amines that are not branched at α-carbon. Loss of largest fragment from α-C atom is preferred.

All amines show peak at mass 30 + 14n due to hydrogen atom migration.

Aromatic amines

The molecular ion peak of aromatic monoamine is intense. For example, loss of one H atoms of aniline gives a moderately intense M-1 peak, loss of neutral molecule of HCN followed by loss of hydrogen atom gives a prominent peaks at m/e 66 and 65 respectively.

Amides

Apthalic amide

Molecular ion peak is irrelevant. In low molecular weight amide, α fragmentation is predominant.

$$R-C(=O)-NH_2 \xrightarrow{-R^\bullet} \overset{+}{O}\equiv C-NH_2 \longrightarrow O=C=\overset{+}{NH_2}$$

If R contain three or more carbon atoms, loses an H atom, cleavage in the β position by McLafferty rearrangement gives a prominent peak at m/e 59.

$$R-C(H)(=O)(NH_2) \longrightarrow CH_2=C(OH)(NH_2) + R-CH=CH_2$$
$$m/e\ 59$$

The long chain amides also break in the γ position (m/e 72) and when followed by H transposition give an ion at m/e 73. There are peaks at M-16 (–NH$_2$) obtained by α cleavage with respect to the carbonyl.

Nitro compounds

Intense peak is derived by elimination of NO$_2$. The loss of NO occurs frequently due to isomerization of the nitro group.

$$[C_6H_5-NO_2]^{+\cdot} \rightarrow [C_6H_5-ONO]^{+\cdot} \xrightarrow{-NO} [C_6H_5O]^{+\cdot} \xrightarrow{-CO} C_5H_5^+$$

At the same time, there is an intense peak at m/e 30 (NO$^+$).

Halogenated derivatives

The halogen having a great affinity for electrons, do not show a tendency to carry the positive charge.

The aliphatic compounds lose the halogen or the hydrohalide. Similarly, the loss of halogen is preferred in the aromatic derivatives.

The compounds are easily recognised in the mass spectrum by the isotopic peaks of the bromo and chloro derivatives.

Aliphatic chloride

The molecular ion peak is generally visible in the lower monochloride. Cleavage of straight chain monochloride at –C–C bond adjacent to the chlorine atoms accounts for a small peak at m/e 49 and at m/e 51 due to heavier isotope.

$$R-CH_2-Cl \xrightarrow{-R^\cdot} CH_2=Cl^+ \leftrightarrow \overset{+}{C}H_2-\ddot{Cl}$$
$$m/e\ 49/51$$

Cleavage of C–Cl bond leads to small Cl$^+$ peak and to a R$^+$ peak.

Straight chain chlorides contain 6 carbon atoms give $C_3H_6Cl^+$, $C_4H_8Cl^+$ and $C_5H_{10}Cl^+$ ions. Among all these ions, $C_4H_8Cl^+$ ion dominates due to formation of cyclic structure.

Aromatic chloride

The molecular ion peak is more intense. The M–Cl peak is large for all compounds in which chlorine is attached directly to the ring.

CHAPTER 3

UV-Visible Spectroscopy

Spectroscopy is a branch of science that involves the study of interaction of electromagnetic radiations with atoms or molecules. Spectroscopy is of two types:
- Emission Spectroscopy
- Absorption Spectroscopy

When an atom is excited thermally or electrically, its electrons are promoted from their ground energy state to a higher energy state. The lifetime of the electron in this metastable state is short and in their return to a lower excited or ground level, the absorbed energy is released as light.

Emission spectroscopy is the measure of this emitted light and the spectroscopic analysis of this emitted light gives the emission spectrum. An emission spectrum thus obtained, gives the information about the light source under study. This phenomenon is primarily caused by the excitation of atoms by the thermal or electrical means; absorbed energy causes the promotion of electrons from ground state to state higher energy where they are short lived and so return to the ground state by emitting the radiations. In some cases, the excited state may have appreciable lifetime such that emission of light continues even after excitation has seized. Such a phenomenon is called **phosphorescence**. Flame photometry, fluorimetry, etc. are the examples of emission spectroscopy.

Absorption spectroscopy is the measure of the energy absorbed by an excited atom or molecule and the spectroscopic analysis of the absorbed energy gives the absorption spectrum. It also represents the energy absorbed relative to the energy of given frequency of electromagnetic radiation. IR, UV and NMR spectroscopy are the examples of absorption spectroscopy but the mechanism of absorption of energy is different in UV, infrared and nuclear magnetic resonance regions.

ELECTROMAGNETIC RADIATION

In absorption spectroscopy, radiant energy is given in the form of electromagnetic radiation which transfers energy as photons (bundles of energy) when it interacts with matter. The energy of photon is proportional to the frequency of electromagnetic radiation that has an electric and magnetic component. Only electric component is involved in the transfer of energy in the wave's interaction with matter.

The **wavelength,** λ of the wave is the linear distance in 'cm' travelled by one complete wave (Fig. 3.1).

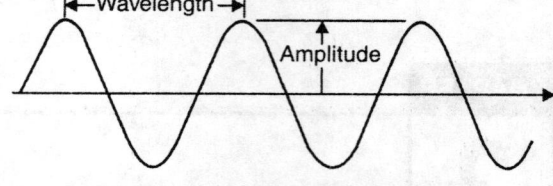

Fig. 3.1. Electromagnetic wave.

The intensity of a wave is characterized by its radiant power. The number of wave cycle passing a fixed point per unit time is termed as frequency of electromagnetic wave. The energy of electromagnetic wave is given by the relationship :

$$E = h\nu \qquad ....\text{(eq. 3.1)}$$

h is plank's constant (6.62×10^{-27} erg/sec)
ν = frequency

The characteristics of an electromagnetic wave is represented by the frequency or wavelength or wave number.

Frequency of a wave is related to wavelength by the equation

$\nu = \dfrac{c}{\lambda}$ (c is velocity of light in air and this value is 3.0×10^{10} cm/sec.). On substituting this value in eq. 3.1

$$E = h \cdot \dfrac{c}{\lambda} \qquad ....\text{(eq. 3.2)}$$

Wavenumber is the reciprocal of wavelength. The wavelength is most commonly indicated in Angstron 'A' (= 10^{-8} cm), mμ (=10^{-7} cm) and μ (=10^{-4} cm).

$$\nu = \dfrac{1}{\lambda}$$

The electromagnetic spectral series ranges from cosmic rays to radio waves as given in Fig. 3.2.

ABSORPTION OF RADIANT ENERGY

The total energy in a molecule is the sum of energies associated with the translational, rotational, vibrational and electronic energy of the molecule.

Translational energy is associated with the motion (velocity) of the molecule.
Rotational energy is associated with the overall rotation of molecule.
Vibrational energy is associated with the movement of atoms within the molecule.
Electronic energy is associated with the motion of electron around the molecule.

Therefore, total energy is sum of Translational, rotational, vibrational and electronic energy (eq. 3.3)

$$E = E_{trans} + E_{vib} + E_{rot} + E_{elect} \qquad ....\text{(eq. 3.3)}$$

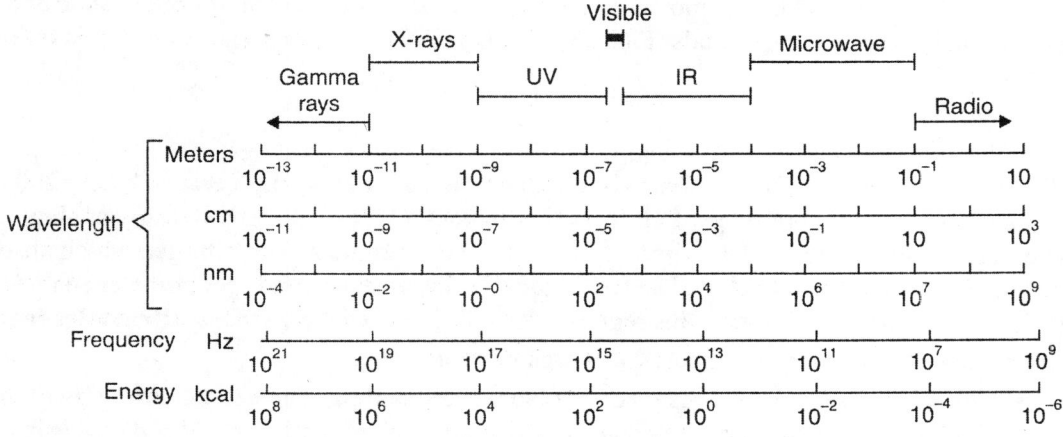

Fig. 3.2. Electromagnetic spectrum.

The sum of vibrational, rotational and electronic energy component may assume certain values for a given molecule. This permitted level of E_{vib}, E_{rot} and E_{elect} is related to the structure means no two kinds of molecule possess identical combination of vibrational, rotational and electronic energy on interaction with electromagnetic radiation.

When energy of certain wavelength or frequency is incident on a molecule discrete amount of energy (energy required for particular transition) is absorbed and the molecule jump from lower energy level (E_1) to higher energy level (E_2) and the difference in the energy is equivalent to hν.

$$E_2 - E_1 = h\nu \qquad ....(eq.\ 3.4)$$

This energy jump from one level to another is known as *transition*. This absorption of energy is represented as absorption spectrum. It consists of graph of extent of light absorption against the frequency or wavelength. As allowed (permitted) transitions are different for molecules of different structure, absorption spectrum is also different. The excited molecules emit the absorbed energy as heat or electromagnetic radiation.

TRANSITION

The energy required for the transition from a state of lower energy (E_1) to state of higher energy (E_2) is directly related to the frequency of electromagnetic radiation. That is, for a given excitation process a molecule absorbs only one discrete amount of energy and hence absorbs radiation of only one frequency. If this is the case with all molecule of a substance, one would observe a series of absorption lines. However, a group of molecule exists in a number of different vibrational and rotational states. Each state is differing from another by a relatively small amount of energy.

ABSORPTION OF UV AND VISIBLE RADIATION

The absorption of photons in the UV-Visible region of electromagnetic radiation occurs because of electronic transition in a molecule from the ground state to higher energy state. These higher energy states are described by the molecular orbitals that are vacant in the unexcited state and are commonly called antibonding orbitals (Fig. 3.3). The UV-Visible region is characterized as follows:

Far UV: 100–200 nm
UV: 200–380 nm
Visible: 380–780 nm

The ultraviolet region (200–380 nm) is commonly used for analysis. Because below 200 nm, there is a problem due to presence of air in the instrument. Oxygen absorbs strongly at about 200 nm and below. This range can be utilized by flushing the instrument with nitrogen which absorbs strongly at about 150 nm and below. The technique of using an evacuated spectrometer enables the range below 200 nm to be studied. This region is frequently called the **vacuum ultraviolet region**.

Four kinds of electrons are important in organic molecules.

- *Closed shell electrons*: These are not involved in bonding. The excitation energy of these electrons is very high and they don't contribute to absorption in the UV and visible region. It means $\sigma \rightarrow \sigma^*$ transition don't contribute in UV absorption.
- *Sigma electrons* (electron in covalent single bonds): These also consist of high excitation energy; absorption may be seen exceptionally in far UV region, e.g., cyclopropane shows the absorption at the wavelength at 190 nm.
- *Non bonding* paired outer shell electron such as those oxygen, sulphur and halogens (n electrons) can lead to absorption in UV region. $n \rightarrow \sigma^*$ near 200 nm (end absorption), $n \rightarrow \pi^*$ (low energy transition).
- π *electrons* (in double or triple bond) are much responsible for much of the absorption in the UV and visible region.

The possible six types of electron jumps (transitions) that light might causes are given in Fig. 3.3. In each possible case, an electron is excited from a full orbital into an empty anti orbital. Each jump needs energy for transition. The big jump obviously more energy than a small one.

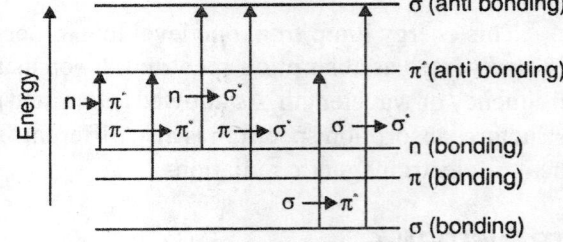

Fig. 3.3. Energy levels of various electronic transition.

There are three important transitions in UV region that are as follows:

- From π orbitals to π^* antibonding orbitals
- From nonbonding orbitals to π^* antibonding orbitals
- From nonbonding orbitals to σ^* antibonding orbitals

Other jumps (transitions) shown in Fig. 3.3 absorbs UV light of wavelength less than 200 nm.

CHARGE-TRANSFER COMPLEX

Many a times, a given compound that is transparent in the UV region starts absorbing after interacting with another species. This happens if the species has an electron donor group and the interacting species has an electron acceptor group. When two species bind to each other, the resulting species becomes intensely colored. This is due to formation of complex between the two species. Such a complex is called charge transfer complex. For example, the blood red color of the complex ion, thiocyanate iron (III) ion, $(FeSCN)^{2+}$ is due to form formation of charge transfer complex.

UV Spectrum

An UV absorption spectrum is a plot of energy absorbed (A) (intensity) and wavelength (λ) of an absorbing molecule. A characteristic spectrum of Isoprene is shown in Fig. 3.4.

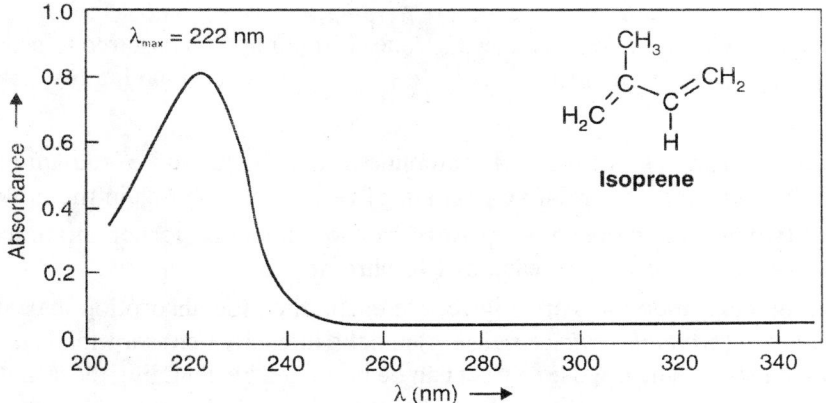

Fig. 3.4. UV spectrum of Isoprene.

From the above discussion, it is clear that the only molecular moieties which likely to absorb light in the 200 to 800 nm region have the π-electron functions and hetero atoms having non-bonding valence shell electron pairs. Such light absorbing groups are referred to as **chromophores**. A list of some simple chromophores and their characteristics light absorption is provided in the Table 3.1.

Table 3.1. Examples of Chromophore along with their transitions

Chromophore	Example	Excitation	λ_{max} nm	ε	Solvent
C=C	Ethene	$\pi \to \pi^*$	171	15,000	Hexane
C≡C	1-Hexyne	$\pi \to \pi^*$	180	10,000	Hexane
C=O	Acetaldehyde	$n \to \pi^*$	290	15	Hexane
		$\pi \to \pi^*$	180	10,000	Hexane
N=O	Nitromethane	$n \to \pi^*$	275	17	Ethanol
		$\pi \to \pi^*$	200	5,000	Ethanol
C–Br	Methyl bromide	$n \to \sigma^*$	205	200	Hexane
C–I	Methyl iodide	$n \to \sigma^*$	255	360	Hexane

The oxygen non-bonding electrons in alcohols and ethers do not give rise to absorption above 160 nm. Consequently, pure alcohol and ether solvents may be used for spectroscopic studies. The absorption maximum (λ max) of a molecule is due to chromophoric group in its structure. Chromophore is the covalently bonded unsaturated functional group e.g. –C=O in acetone, phenyl ring in toluene, $CONH_2$, CN, –N=N–, etc.

Types of Chromophores

There are two types of chromophores:

(i) Independent chromophore: Single chromophore is sufficient to impart color to the compound e.g. azo group.

(ii) Dependent chromophore: When more than one chromophore is required to produce color e.g. acetone having one ketonic group is colorless whereas diacetyl having two ketonic groups is yellow in color.

Many molecules contain 2 or more chromophores. The interaction of radiant energy with the molecule then depends upon the relative position of two chromophores in the molecules:

(a) When two chromophores are separated by more than one carbon atom, total absorption is the sum of absorption of each of two chromophores.

(b) When two chromophores are adjacent to each other, the absorption max shifts to longer wavelength (*bathochromic or red shift*) and the intensity of absorption is increased (*hyper chromic effect*). The opposite effect can be produced by changing the structure of organic structure. A shift to the shorter wavelength (blue shift) and a reduction of intensity (hypochromic or blue effect) is obtained. When two chromophoric groups are conjugated, the high intensity transition ($\pi \rightarrow \pi^*$) absorption band is shifted to longer wavelength (generally 15–45 nm) with respect to unconjugted chromophore.

Some saturated functional group OH, NH_2, Cl etc. when attached to the chromophore affects both intensity and wave length, they are called **auxochrome**. For example, C_6H_6 shows the maximum absorption at the wavelength of 255 nm but aniline that contain auxochrome group (NH_2) shows its λ_{max} at 280 nm. All the auxochromic groups contain non bonding which are responsible for this effect. They are likely to interact with the chromophonic group for causing the shift of λ_{max}.

A chromophore producing two peaks

A chromophore such as the carbon-oxygen double bond in acetone, for example, obviously has π electrons as a part of the double bond, but also has lone pairs on the oxygen atom. It means, two types of the important transition ($\pi-\pi^*$ and $n \rightarrow \pi^*$) are possible as shown in Fig. 3.5.

The non bonding orbital has a higher energy than a π-bonding orbital. That means that the jump from an oxygen lone pair into a pi anti-bonding orbital needs less energy. That means it absorbs light of a lower frequency and therefore a higher wavelength.

Acetone (Fig. 3.5) can therefore absorb light of two different wavelengths:

- the π bonding to π^* anti-bonding absorption peaks at 195 nm.
- the non-bonding to π^* anti-bonding absorption peaks at 274 nm.

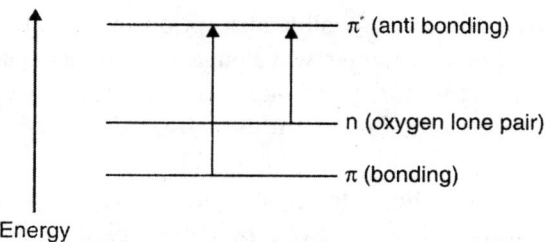

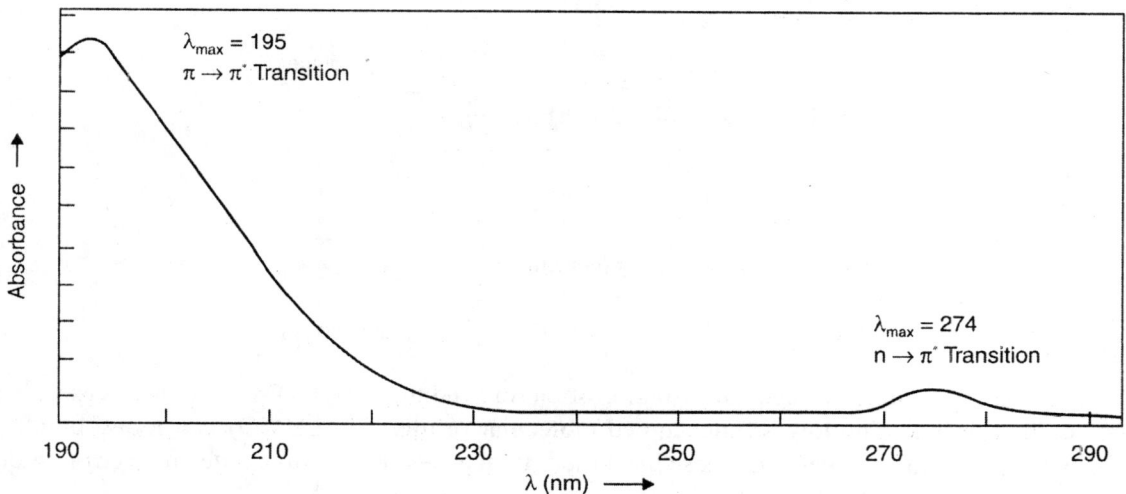

Fig. 3.5. UV spectrum of acetone showing the π→π* and n→π* transitions.

The π→π* transitions are generally intense while the n→π* transitions are weak.

Both of these absorptions are in the ultra-violet, but most spectrometers won't pick up the one at 195 nm because they work in the range from 200–800 nm.

Importance of conjugation in UV absorption

Consider these three molecules:

$$CH_2=CH_2 \qquad CH_2=CH-CH=CH_2 \qquad CH_2=CH-CH=CH-CH=CH_2$$
$$\text{Ethene} \qquad \text{Buta-1,3-diene} \qquad \text{Hexa-1,3,5-triene}$$

Ethene contains a simple isolated carbon-carbon double bond, but the other two have conjugated double bonds. In these cases, there is delocalisation of the π bonding orbitals over the whole molecule. Now observe at the wavelengths of the light which each of these molecules absorbs.

Molecule	λ_{max} (nm)
Ethene	171
Buta-1,3-diene	217
Hexa-1,3,5-triene	258

All of the molecules give similar UV-visible absorption spectra, the only difference being that the absorptions move to longer and longer wavelengths as the amount of delocalisation in the molecule increases. It indicates the shifting of maximum absorption (λ_{max}) to longer wavelengths as the amount of delocalisation increases. Therefore, absorption needs less energy as the amount of delocalisation increases.

Compare ethene with buta-1,3-diene. In ethene, there is one π bonding orbital and one π anti-bonding orbital. In buta-1,3-diene, there are two π bonding orbitals and two π anti-bonding orbitals as shown below.

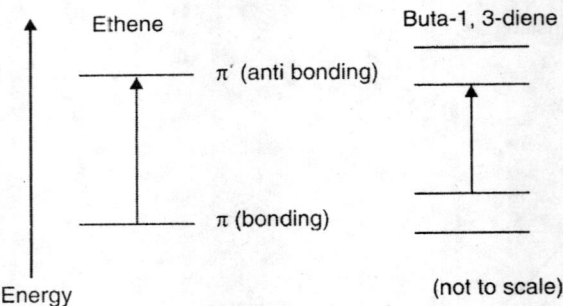

The highest occupied molecular orbital is often referred to as the HOMO - in these cases, it is a π bonding orbital. The lowest unoccupied molecular orbital (the LUMO) is a π anti-bonding orbital. Note that the gap between these has fallen. It takes less energy to excite an electron in the buta-1,3-diene than with ethene.

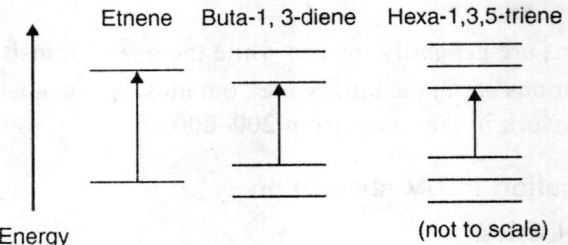

Why beta-carotene is orange colored?

β-carotene has the sort of delocalisation on a much greater scale with 11 carbon-carbon double bonds conjugated together. The structure of β-carotene shows the presence of double and single bonds shown in alternate position.

UV-Visible Spectroscopy

The more delocalisation there is, the smaller the gap between the highest energy π-bonding orbital and the lowest energy π-anti-bonding orbital. To promote an electron therefore takes less energy in β-carotene so β-carotene absorbs throughout the ultra-violet region into the violet - but particularly strongly in the visible region between about 400 and 500 nm with a peak about 470 nm (Table 3.2).

Table 3.2. Colors in visible spectrum

Color region	Wavelength (nm)
Violet	400–420
Indigo	420–440
Blue	440–490
Green	490–570
Yellow	570–585
Orange	585–620
Red	620–780

Why indicators change the color?

Phenolphthalein

It is colorless in acidic conditions and magenta (bright pink) colored in an alkaline solution. How is this color change related to changes in λ_{max} of the molecule?

The structures of the two differently colored forms are:

Colorless form → (Add alkali / Add acid) → Magenta colored form

In alkaline medium, conjugation increases which in turn increases the delocalisation of π electrons. Hence, due to increased delocalisation, λ_{max} is shifted to longer wavelength to impart bright pink color.

Methyl orange

It is yellow in alkaline solutions and red in acidic ones. The structure in alkaline solution is:

Methyl orange (yellow form)

In acid solution, a hydrogen ion is (perhaps unexpectedly) picked up on one of the nitrogens in the nitrogen-nitrogen double bond and acquire positive charge.

The positive charge on the nitrogen is delocalised (spread around over the structure) - especially out towards the right-hand end of the molecule ad we have written it. The normally drawn structure for the red form of methyl orange is given below.

Methyl orange (red form)

The yellow has an absorption peak at about 440 nm. The red form has an absorption peak at about 520 nm (shifted to longer wavelength). That means that there must be more delocalisation in the red form than in the yellow one.

Effect of solvent on UV absorption

Highly pure, non-polar solvents such as saturated hydrocarbons do **not interact** with solute molecules either in the ground or excited state and the absorption spectrum of a compound in these solvents is similar to the one in a pure gaseous state. However, polar solvents such as water, alcohols etc. may stabilize or destabilize the molecular orbitals of a molecule either in the ground state or in excited state and the spectrum of a compound in these polar solvents may significantly vary from the one recorded in a hydrocarbon solvent.

(i) $\pi \rightarrow \pi^*$ Transitions

In case of $\pi \rightarrow \pi^*$ transitions, the excited states are more polar than the ground state and the dipole-dipole interactions with solvent molecules lower the energy of the excited state more than that of the ground state. Therefore a polar solvent decreases the energy of $\pi \rightarrow \pi^*$ transition and absorption maximum appears ~10–20 nm red shifted in going from hexane to ethanol solvent.

(ii) $n \rightarrow \pi^*$ Transitions

In case of $n \rightarrow \pi^*$ transitions, the polar solvents form hydrogen bonds with the ground state of polar molecules more readily than with their excited states. Therefore, in polar solvents the **energies of electronic transitions** are increased. For example, the absorption maximum of acetone in hexane appears at 279 nm which in water is shifted to 264 nm, with a blue shift of 15 nm (Fig. 3.6). The use of polar solvent also influence the $\pi \rightarrow \pi^*$ transition but shadowed by the blue light resulting from solvation of lone pair.

Due to the solvent effects, solvents having double or triple bonds or heavy atoms (e.g. S,

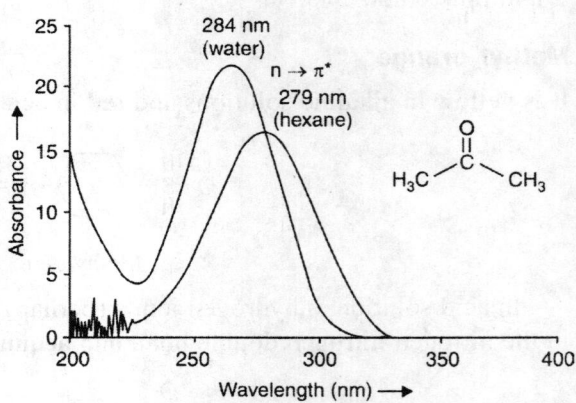

Fig. 3.6. UV-spectra of acetone in hexane and in water.

Br, and I) are generally avoided. Typical solvents, used in UV spectroscopy are water, ethanol, hexane and cyclohexane.

Effect of Hydrogen bonding on UV spectrum

The n→σ* transitions are very sensitive to hydrogen bonding. Alcohols as well as amines are known to form hydrogen bonding with the solvent molecules. Such associations occur because of the presence of non bonding electrons on the heteroatom and thus, transition needs greater energy. Hydrogen bonding shifts the ultraviolet absorptions to shorter wavelengths.

UV-Visible Spectrophotometer

The instrument for measuring UV-visible radiation is called "spectrometers" or spectrophotometer. These are made up of the following components as shown in Fig. 3.7.

1. Radiation Sources (UV and visible)
2. Wavelength selector (filter or monochromator)
3. Sample containers cell
4. Detector
5. Signal processor and readout

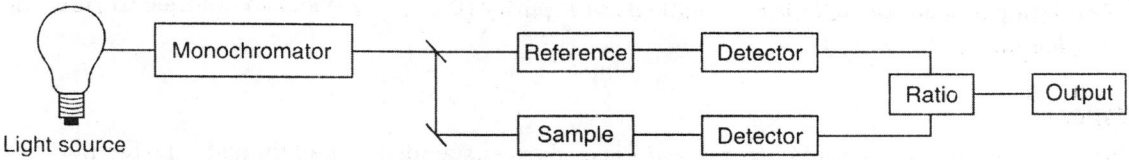

Fig. 3.7. UV-Visible spectrophotometer.

1. Radiation Sources (UV and Visible)

Radiation sources consist of materials that are electrically excited to high energy states which then emit the absorbed energy as photons while returning to their lower excited or ground energy states. A radiation source must meet certain requirements:

(i) It must possess sufficient intensity (photons/sec) to make detection.

(ii) It should be continuous that its spectrum should provide the desired wavelength required for analysis.

(iii) The source must be stable and must provide radiation of constant intensity.

UV Radiation Source

Hydrogen discharge lamp is used as UV source. It consists of pair of electrodes enclosed in a glass tube containing hydrogen gas or deuterium at a reduced pressure. When constant high voltage is applied across the electrode, the electrons of hydrogen gas molecules are excited to high energy state. This return to ground energy state, the electron emits continuous radiation in the region between 180 and 350 nm. Quartz windows must be employed in deuterium and hydrogen lamps, because glass absorbs strongly at wavelength less than 350 nm.

Visible Radiation Sources

For the simple analysis, the ordinary daylight is used as the source but it lacks in providing constant intensity. Hence, a glass enclosed tungstem filament lamp is used. It is heated to about 2300°C to get the radiation in the range of 350–2500 nm.

Tungston halogen lamp contains a small quantity of iodine within a quartz envelop that houses the tungsten filament. Quartz is required due to high operating temperature of lamp. The lifetime of tungsten filament is increased due to the use of iodine. This added life results from the reaction of iodine with gaseous tungsten that forms by sublimation and ordinary limits the life of the filament; the product is the volatile WI_2. When molecule of this volatile compound strikes the filament, decomposition occurs which redeposit tungsten at the filament to enhance the life of lamp.

2. Wavelength Selector (filter or monochromator)

It is a device for resolving the radiation from the source into component wavelength or band of wavelengths. Two devices are used - filters and monochromators. Filters are used in simple analysis and function by absorbing large portion of spectrum and transmit relatively limited wavelength (10–50 nm). Monochromator are used for ultraviolet, visible and infrared radiation. They are capable of isolating a beam of radiation of high spectral purity (0.1–10 nm) and in contrast to filter, their wavelength can be varied.

Filters

Filters used most commonly are colored glass, dyes suspended in gelatin and interference filters (Fig. 3.8). The colored glass and gelatin filters are used in the visible region and usually provide effective bandwidth from 20–50 nm. Interference filter consist of two extremely thin semi-transparent metallic film separated by very thin transparent material.

When a perpendicular ray of light strikes this arrangement a portion of beam passed through the first layer and a portion is reflected. The portion passing through the first layer under-goes a similar partition when it strikes the second layer. Through this process effective bandwidth of order of 10 nm are obtainable with interference filter.

Monochromators

These are most efficient and able to isolate the narrow band in comparison to filters.

Polychromatic radiation from the source enters the monochromator system through the entrance slit and collimated by either a lens or a mirror. This collimated beam of radiation is then dispersed by using either a prism or a grating. The desired portion of dispersed spectrum is then focussed by a lens or mirror on the exit slit on the test sample (Fig. 3.9).

The entire assembly is contained in a light base. A number of factors influence the effective bandwidth of radiation emerging from the monochromator's assembly. These include the structural

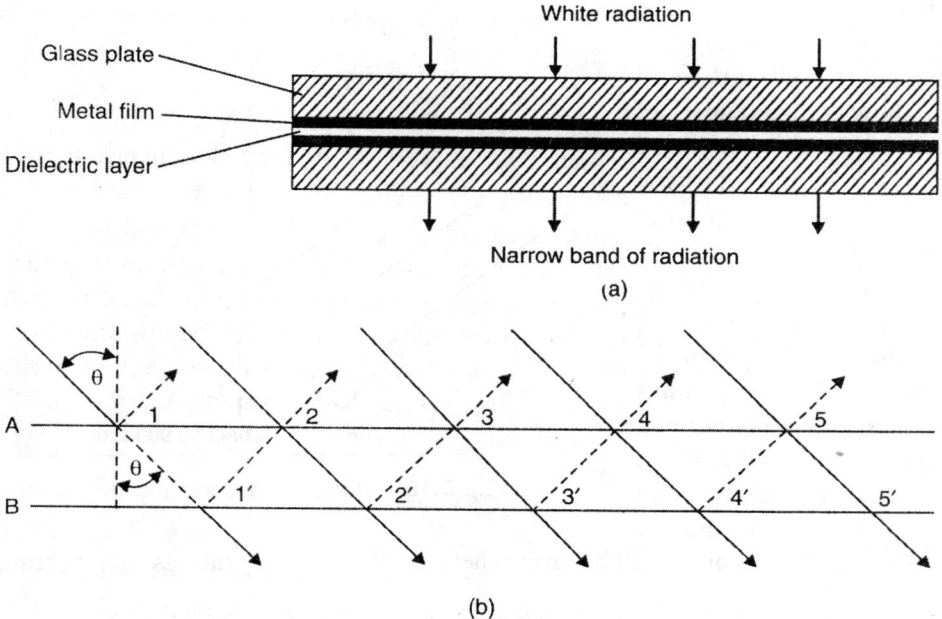

Fig. 3.8. (a) Cross-section of interference filter; (b) Schematic diagram of constructive interference.

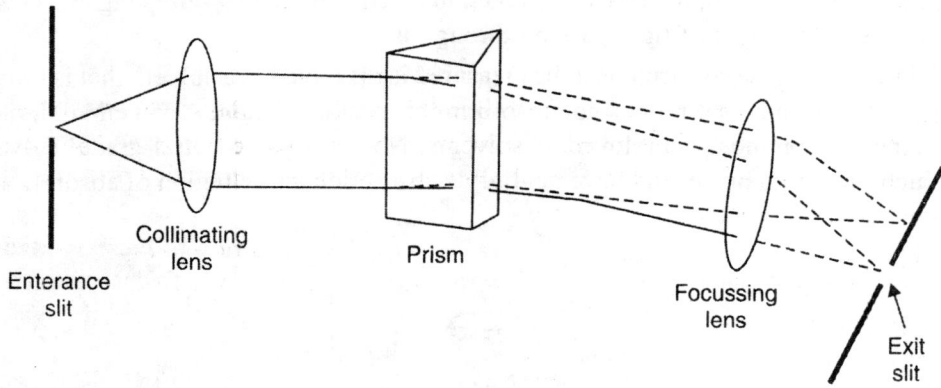

Fig. 3.9. Schematic diagram of prism monochromator.

nature of dispersing element (prism or grating) and width of exit slit. In general, narrow slit width isolate narrow bandwidth. However, a reduction in slit width results in the decrease in the radiant power. The dispersion of radiation by a prism is based on the phenomenon of refraction. A prism resolves polychromatic radiation into narrow band of wavelength by its rotation in the monochromator assembly. The dispersion is because of the variation of refractive index of prism material that is a function of the wavelength.

Diffraction gratings that are used dispersing polychromatic radiation in the UV, visible and IR region are based on reflection. These gratings consist of a highly polished reflective aluminized surface upon which are elected a large number of equally spaced parallel grooves (Fig. 3.10). The spacing between the rulings of a grating must be approximately the same order of magnitude as the wavelength in the region of spectrum. Typical gratings have between 800–2000 lines per mm (Fig. 3.10 depending upon the region of spectrum used. The diffraction gratings partitions polychromatic radiations striking it into as many small beams as there are lines on the gratings sample containers.

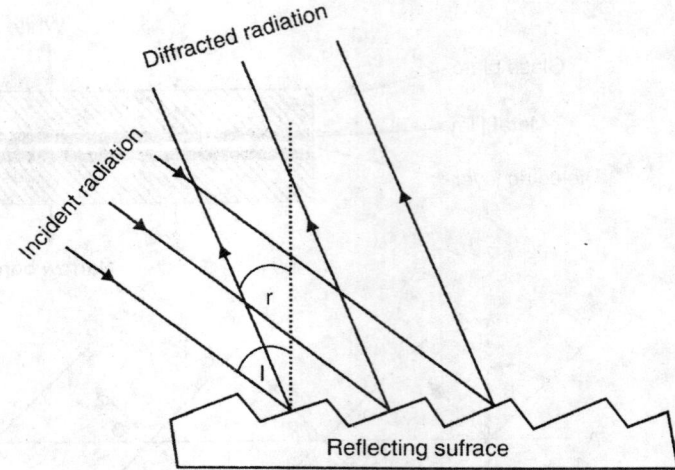

Fig. 3.10. Diffraction of radiation by grating.

3. Sample containers cell

The UV-visible absorption spectra are usually determined either in vapour phase or in solution. In order to take the UV spectrum, the analyte is taken in a cell, called a **cuvette** (Fig. 3.11) which is transparent to the wavelength of light passing through it.

The solid sample whose spectrum is to be measured is dissolved in a solvent that is transparent in the UV region. It means that it does not absorb in this region. Hexane, 95% ethanol, methanol and 1,4 dioxane are commonly employed as solvents. Now a days 'spectral grade' solvents are available which have high purity and have negligible absorption in the region of absorption by the chromophore.

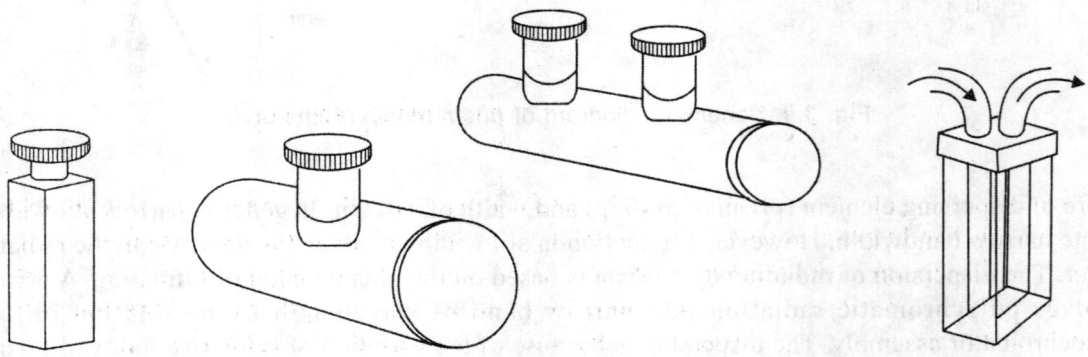

Fig. 3.11. Quartz cuvettes for measurements in solution and in vapour phase.

4. Detectors used in UV-Visible Spectrophotometer

The detectors are used to convert a light signal to an electrical signal which can be suitably measured and transformed into an output. The detectors used in most of the instruments generate a signal, which is linear in transmittance i.e. they respond linearly to radiant power falling on them. The transmittance values can be changed logarithmically into absorbance units by an electrical or mechanical arrangement in the signal read out device. There are three types of detectors, used in modern spectrophotometers. These are as follows.

(i) Phototube

It consists of semi-cylindrical cathode and central metal wire anode sealed inside and an evacuated glass envelope (Fig. 3.12). Concave face of cathode is coated with a layer of photo emissive material (containing loosely bound electrons) such as alkali metal. A potential difference is applied between the anode and the cathode, the anode being positive with respect to cathode. When photons strike to the photoemissive cathode, they transfer their energy to the photo emissive material on the cathode surface to release electrons. The loosely bound electrons leave the cathode surface and are collected at the anode, causing current to flow in the phototube circuit. The current from the phototube are quite small (10^{-10} amp) and require amplification so it is amplified before taken up by the recording device.

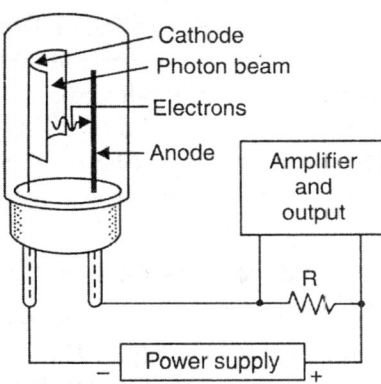

Fig. 3.12. Phototube.

(ii) Photomultiplier tube

The photomultiplier tube is a commonly used detector in UV-visible spectroscopy. It consists of a *photoemissive cathode* (a cathode which emits electrons when struck by photons of radiation), several *dynodes* (which emit several electrons for each electron striking them) and an *anode* (Fig. 3.13).

A photon of radiation entering the tube strikes the cathode, causing the emission of several electrons. These electrons are accelerated towards the first dynode (which is 90 V more positive than the cathode). The electrons strike the first dynode, causing the emission of several electrons for each incident electron. These electrons are then accelerated towards the second dynode, to produce more electrons which are accelerated towards dynode three and so on. Eventually, the electrons are

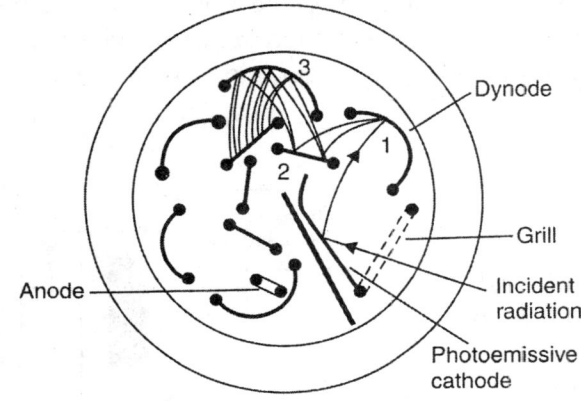

Fig. 3.13. Cross sectional diagram of a photo-multiplier tube.

collected at the anode. By this time, each original photon has produced 10^6–10^7 electrons. The resulting current is amplified and measured.

Photomultipliers are very sensitive to UV and visible radiation. They have fast response times. Intense light damages photomultipliers; they are limited to measuring low powder radiation.

(iii) Diode array detector

These detectors employ a large number of silicon diodes arranged side by side on a single chip. When a UV-visible radiation falls on the diode, its conductivity increases significantly. This increase in conductivity is proportional to the intensity of the radiation and can be readily measured. Since a large number of diodes can be arranged together, the intensity at a number of wavelengths can be measured simultaneously. Though the photodiode array is not as sensitive as the photomultiplier tube, the possibility of being able to measure a large number of wavelengths makes it a detector of choice in the modern fast instruments.

5. Signal Processing and Output Devices

The electrical signal from the transducer is suitably amplified or processed before it is sent to the recorder to give an output. The subtraction of the solvent spectrum from that of the solution is done electronically. The output plot between th wavelength and the intensity of absorption is the resultant of the subtraction process and is characteristic of the absorbing species.

TYPES OF UV-VISIBLE SPECTROPHOTOMETERS

There are main mainly three types of spectrometers:

1. Single Beam UV-Visible Spectrometers

As the name suggests, these instruments contain a single beam of light. The same beam is used for reading the absorption of the sample as well as the reference. The schematic diagram of a typical single beam UV-visible spectrometer is given in Fig. 3.14. The radiation from the source is passed through a filter or a suitable monochromator to get a narrow band of radiation or a monochromatic

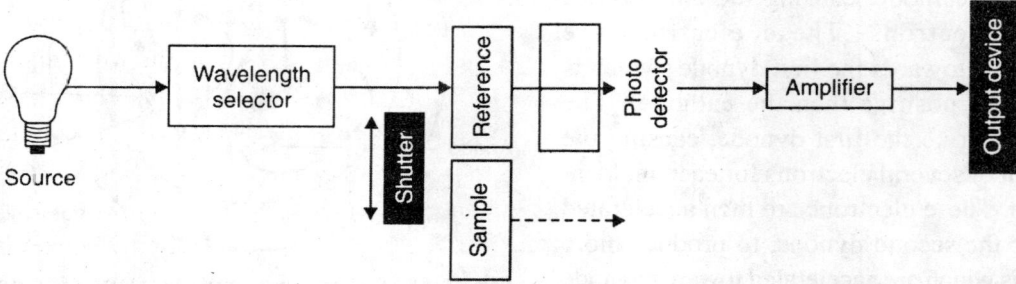

Fig. 3.14. Schematic diagram for a single beam UV-visible spectrometer.

radiation. It is then passed through the sample (or the reference) and the transmitted radiation is detected by the photodetector. The signal so obtained is sent as a read out or is recorded.

Typically, two operations have to be performed – first, the cuvette is filled with the reference solution and the absorbance reading at a given wavelength or the spectrum over the desired range is recorded. Second, the cuvette is taken out and rinsed and filled with sample solution and the process is repeated. The spectrum of the sample is obtained by subtracting the spectrum of the reference from that of the sample solution.

2. Double Beam UV-Visible Spectrometers

In a double beam spectrometer, the radiation coming from the monochromator is split into two beams with the help of a beam splitter. These are passed simultaneously through the reference and the sample cell. The transmitted radiations are detected by the detectors and the difference in the signal at all the wavelengths is suitably amplified and sent for the output. The general arrangement of a double beam spectrometer is shown in Fig. 3.15. There could be variations depending on the manufacturer, the wavelength regions for which the instrument is designed, the resolutions required etc.

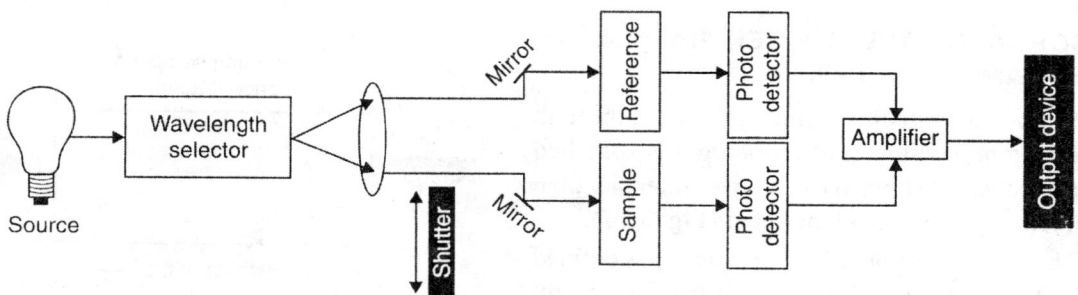

Fig. 3.15. Schematic diagram for a double beam UV-visible spectrometer.

3. Photodiode Array Spectrometer

In a photodiode array instrument, also called a multi-channel instrument, the radiation output from the source is focussed directly on the sample. This allows the radiations of all the wavelengths to simultaneously fall on the sample. The radiation coming out of the sample after absorption (if any) is then made to fall on a reflection grating. The schematic arrangement of a diode array spectrometer is given in Fig. 3.16.

The grating disperses all the wavelengths simultaneously. These then fall on the array of the photodiodes arranged side by side. In this way the intensities of all the radiations in the range of the spectrum are measured in one go. The advantage of such instruments is that a scan of the whole range can be accomplished in a short time.

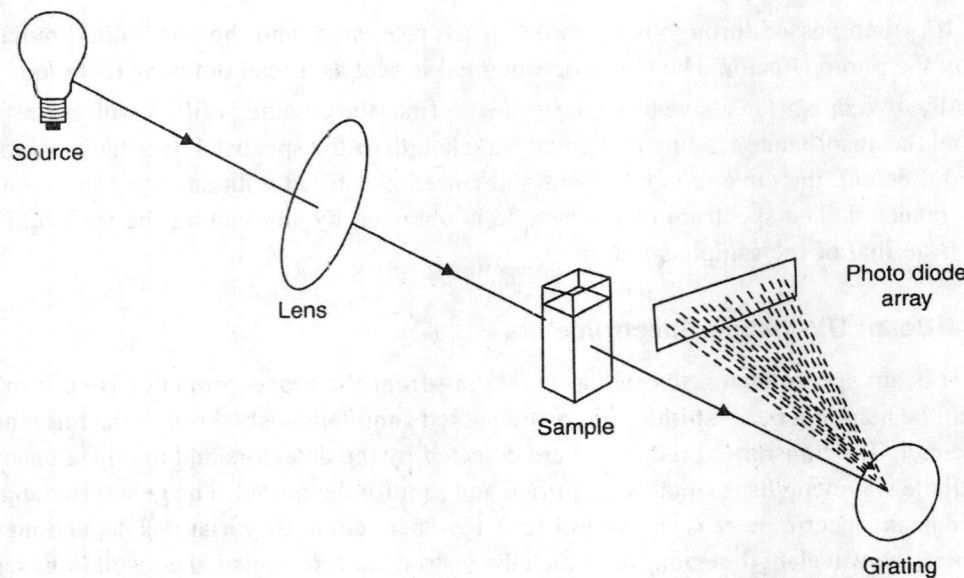

Fig. 3.16. Schematic diagram for a photodiode array spectrometer.

ABSORBANCE AND CONCENTRATION: BEER-LAMBERT'S LAW

When a beam monochromatic light passes through a transparent medium, part of the light is absorbed and the transmitted beam has a lower intensity than the intensity of the incident beam (Fig. 3.17).

The **Transmittance, T** of the solution is defined as the ratio of the intensities of the transmitted beam, I to the intensity, I_0 of the incident beam:

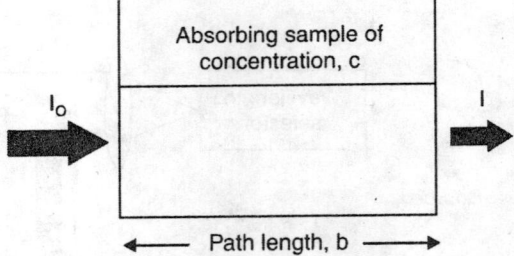

Fig. 3.17. Absorption of UV-visible light.

$$T = \frac{I}{I_0}$$

The **Absorbance, A** of a solution is defined as $A = -\log_{10} T$. Since A is a logarithmic, it is dimensionless.

The Beer-Lambert law

The Beer-Lambert law (also called Beer's law) is the linear relationship between absorbance and concentration of an absorber of electromagnetic radiation. The general Beer-Lambert law is usually written as:

$$A = a_\lambda \times b \times c$$

where A is the measured absornance, a_λ is a wavelength-dependent absorptivity coefficient, b is the path length, and c is the analyte concentration. When working in concentration units of molarity, the Beer-Lambert law is written as:

$$A = \varepsilon_\lambda \times b \times c$$

where ε_λ is the wavelength-dependent molar coefficient with units of $M^{-1}\,cm^{-1}$. The molar extinction coefficient is constant for a particular solute, and varies with the wavelength of the light. The λ subscript is often dropped with the understanding that a value for ε is for a specific wavelength. If multiple species that absorb light at a given wavelength are present in a sample, the total absorbance at that wavelength is the sum due to all absorbers:

$$A = (\varepsilon_1 \times b \times c_1) + (\varepsilon_2 \times b \times c_2) + \ldots$$

The Beer-Lambert law is readily applicable to the determination of the concentration of numerous substances, provided that (i) the molecular extinction coefficient ε for the substance is known at the wavelength at which the measurements are carried out, and (ii), that the path length of the solution is known accurately. Commonly, cuvettes with a path length of 1 cm are used, then, the molar concentration c is simply:

Example 1

Find out the concentration for a solution with absorbance of 0.16, a molar absorbivity of 960/mol/cm, in a cuvette with path length of 1 cm.

A = εbc
C = A/bc
C = 0.16/960 × 1
  = 1.67 × 10^4 mol/L

Example 2

Tryptophan has a molar extinction coefficient at 180 nm (ε_{280}) of 500 $M^{-1}\,cm^{-1}$. A solution of tryptophan has an absorbance at 280 nm of 0.225. What is the concentration of tryptophan in that solution?

Solution

From the Beer-Lambert law, $c = \dfrac{A}{\varepsilon} = \dfrac{0.225}{500} = 4.5 \times 10^{-4}$ M.

Example 3

The molar absorptivity of a substance is $2.0 \times 10^4\,cm^{-1}\,mol^{-1}\,dm^3$. Calculate the transmittance through a cuvette of path length 5.0 cm containing 2.0×10^{-6} mol dm^{-3} solution of the substance.

Solution

As per the Lambert Beer's law,

Absorbance, $A = \varepsilon c b$

Given: $\varepsilon = 2.0 \times 10^4$ cm^{-1} mol^{-1} dm^3, $c = 2.0 \times 10^{-6}$ mol dm^{-3} and $b = 5.0$ cm

Substituting the values we get, $A = 2.0 \times 10^4 \times 2.0 \times 10^{-6} \times 5.0 = 0.2$

$$\Rightarrow \log 1/T = 0.2 \quad \therefore \quad A = \log 1/T$$

Taking antilog on both sides, we get

$1/T = 1.585$

$\therefore T = 0.63$

Example 4

A solution containing 36.5 mg of potassium dichromate per 500 cm^3 was taken in a cuvette having a path length of 2 cm and its transmittance was measured at 455 nm. If the percentage transmittance is found to be 12, calculate the molar absorptivity of potassium dichromate.

Solution

The molarity of given potassium dichromate solution can be calculated as:

$$= \frac{1000 \times 0.0365}{500 \times 294} = 2.48 \times 10^{-4} \text{ mol dm}^3$$

(mm of potassium dichromate = 294 g mol^{-1})

12% transmittance means $T = 0.12$

$$\therefore A = \frac{1}{0.12} = 0.921$$

$$\therefore \varepsilon = \frac{A}{cb} = \frac{0.921}{(2.48 \times 10^{-4} \times 2)} = \frac{0.921}{4.96 \times 10^{-4}}$$

$\therefore 1.86 \times 10^3$ cm^{-1} mol^{-1} dm^3

Deviation from Beer-Lambert's Law

As per the Beer's law discussed above, there is a direct proportionality between the absorbance and concentration. A plot of absorbance versus concentration is expected to be a straight line passing through origin. However, this is not always true; there are certain limitations. The law does not hold for all species under every condition. Many a times instead of a straight line, a curvature in the plot may be observed as shown in Fig. 3.18. The upward curvature, curve (a), is known as **positive deviation** and the downward curvature, curve (c), as **negative deviation**.

Some of the factors responsible for the deviation from Beer's law are as follows:

Presence of Electrolytes

The presence of small amounts of colorless electrolytes which do not react chemically with the colored components, does not affect the light absorption as a rule. However, large amounts of electrolytes may affect the absorption spectrum qualitatively as well as quantitatively. This is due to the physical interaction between the ions of the electrolyte and the colored ions or molecules. This interaction results in a deformation of the later, thereby causing a change in its light absorption property.

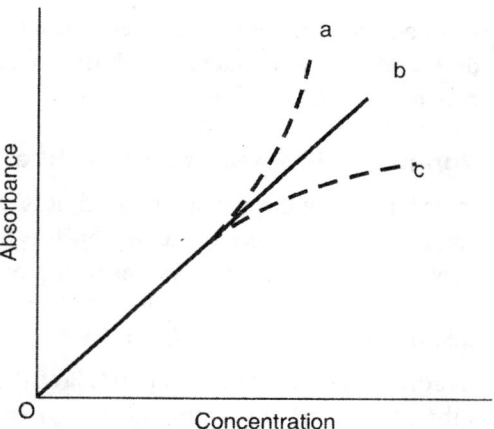

Fig. 3.18. Beer-Lambert law plots; the curvatures show deviations from the law.

Hydrogen Ion Concentration

There are a number of substances whose ionic state in solution is greatly influenced by the presence of hydrogen ions. For example, the aqueous solution of potassium dichromate involves the chromate ion-dichromate ion equilibrium as shown below:

$$2CrO_4^{2-} + 2H \rightleftharpoons Cr_2O_7^{2-} + H_2O$$

Chromate ion (λ_{max} 375 mm)   Dichromate ion (λ_{max} 350, 450 mm)

The chromate ion has a single λ_{max} at 375 nm whereas dichromate ion has two peaks in the spectra; λ_{max} at 350 and 450 nm. The position of equilibrium depends on the pH of the solution and yellow color of solution changes to orange on increasing the concentration of hydrogen ions. Therefore, the results of the determination of chromate ion concentration will depend on the pH. Thus, it is imperative that substances, whose color is influenced by change in hydrogen ion concentration, must be studied under the same pH.

Complexation, Association or Dissociation

Some salts have a tendency to form complexes whose colors are different from those of the simple compounds. For example, the color of cobalt chloride changes from pink to blue due to the following complex formation.

$$2CoCl_2 \rightleftharpoons Co[CoCl]_4$$

Pink   Blue

The degree of complex formation increases with increase in concentration, therefore, Beer's law does not hold at high concentrations. Similar discrepancies are found when the absorbing solute dissociates or associates in solution because the nature of the species in solution depends on the concentration.

Non-monochromatic Nature of the Radiation

In order for the Beer's law to hold, it is necessary that monochromatic light is used. The wider the bandwidth of radiation passed by the filter or other dispersing devices, the greater will be the apparent deviation of a system from adherence to Beer's law.

Concentration of the Analyte

According to Beer and Lambert's law, the plot of absorbance versus the concentration of absorbing substance should be a straight line when ε and b are constant. The path length can always be held constant but there are some factors which affect ε and it is found that at high concentration, ε is not constant. Therefore, at higher concentrations ($>10^{-3}$ mol dm^{-3}) there may be deviation from the law.

APPLICATIONS OF ULTRAVIOLET SPECTROSCOPY

The main applications of ultraviolet spectroscopy are as follows:

1. Detection of Conjugation

It helps to show the relationships between different groups, particularly with respect to conjugation that usually can occur between:

- Two or more carbon-carbon double or triple bonds
- Between carbon-carbon and carbon-oxygen double bonds
- Between double bonds and an aromatic ring

It can reveal the presence of an aromatic ring itself and the number and locations of substituents attached to the carbons of the conjugated system.

For example, nitrobenzene shows its λ_{max} at 252 nm with extinction coefficient ε 8620. It absorbs at longer wavelength due to extended conjugation, o-nitotouene shows max at 250 nm with extinction coefficient ε 5950. Here, placement of the substituent at ortho position causes steric hindrance to coplanarity and so effect of conjugation thus decreased.

For diens and trienes, the position of the most intense band can be predicted in most of the cases with the substituents present. Table 3.3 summarises these empirical relationships (usually called the Woodward rules since they were first used by Nobel R.B. Woodward in 1941.

UV-Visible Spectroscopy

Table 3.3. Conjugated dienes and trienes (in ethanol) λ_{max} for $\pi-\pi^*$ transition

Acyclic and heteroannular dienes	215 nm
Homoannular dienes	253 nm
Acyclic trienes	245
Addition for each substituent	
– R alkyl (including part of a carbocyclic ring)	5 nm
– OR alkoxy	6 nm
– SR thioether	30 nm
– Cl, –Br	5 nm
– OCO acyloxy	0 nm
– CH = CH– and additional conjugation	30 nm
If one double bond is exocyclic to one ring	5 nm
If exocyclic to two rings simultaneously	10 nm

The following examples will illustrate the method:

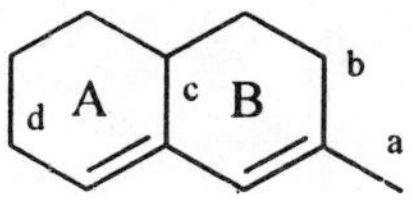

I 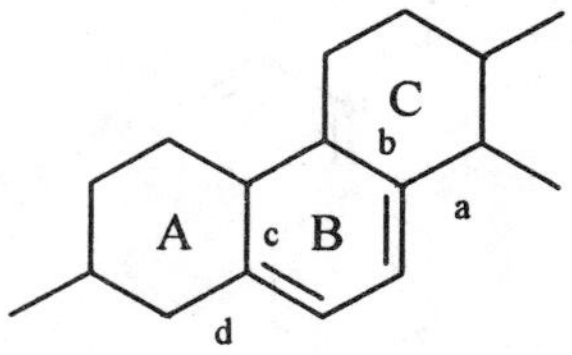   II 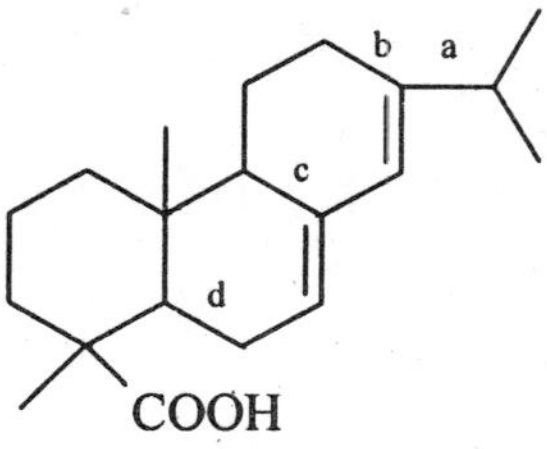   III

For compound I (*heteroannular diene*), the base value is 214 nm. There are 4 alkyl substituents (the ring residues a, b, c and the methyl group d), adding 4 × 5 nm, the double bond in ring A is exocyclic to ring B, adding 5 nm the total is 214 + 20 + 5 = 239 nm.

For compound II

The base value: (*homoannular diene*)	= 253 nm
four ring residues a, b, c and d: 4 × 5	= 20
Two exocyclic bond to A and C ring, 2 × 5	= 10
Total	= 283 nm

For compound III

Heteroannular diene	= 214 nm
4 alkyl residues (4 × 5)	= 20 nm
1 exocyclic bond	= +5 mm
	239 mm

2. Detection of Functional Groups

It is possible to detect the presence of certain functional groups with the help of UV spectrum specially α, β-unsaturated carbonyl system.

Table 3.4 shows the correlation of α, β-unsaturated carbonyl compounds with various substituents. These data were compiled by Woodward.

Following examples will illustrate the method for calculating λ_{max}:

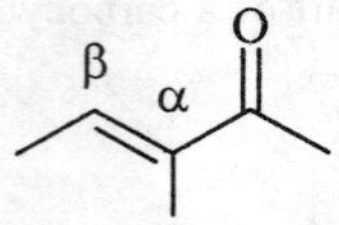

I

Base value	215 nm
One-β-alkyl group	12 nm
α-alkyl group	10 nm
Total	237 nm

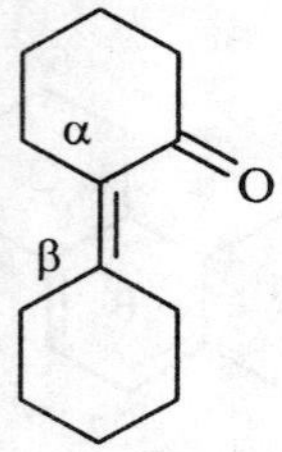

II

Base value	=	215 nm
α-alkyl group	=	10 nm
Two β-alkyl group 2 × 12 nm	=	24 nm
Double bond exocyclic to two rings, 2 × 5	=	10 nm
Total	=	259 nm

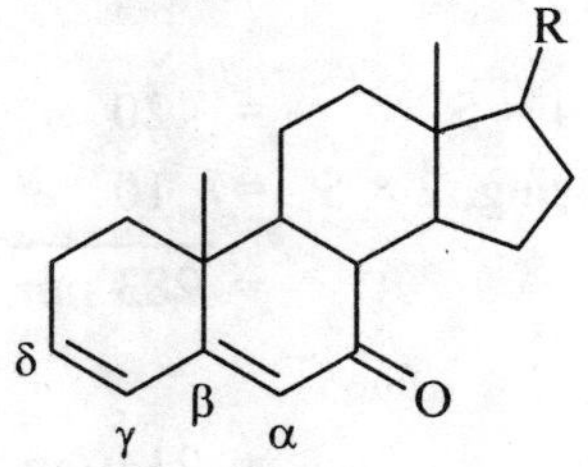

III

Cyclic enone	=	215 nm
Extended conjugation	=	30 nm
β ring residue	=	12 nm

δ ring residue   = 18 nm
Exocyclic double bond = 5 nm
Total   = 280 nm

3. Qualitative UV-Visible Spectroscopy

UV absorption spectroscopy can characterize those types of compounds which absorbs UV radiation. Identification is done by comparing the absorption spectrum with the spectra of known/standard compounds. A record of UV absorption curves is found in certain reference books.

Table 3.4. α, β-unsaturated carbonyl compounds (in ethanol) λ_{max} for π-π^* transition

Ketones–$\overset{\beta}{C}=\overset{\alpha}{C}$–CO–acyclic or 6-membered cyclic	215 nm
Aldehydes–$\overset{\beta}{\underset{\|}{C}}=\overset{\alpha}{\underset{\|}{C}}$–CHO	207 nm
Acid and esters–$\overset{\beta\|}{C}=\overset{\alpha\|}{C}$–CO$_2$H (R)	193 nm
$\overset{\delta}{\underset{\|}{}}-\overset{\lambda}{C}=\overset{}{C}-\overset{\beta}{C}=\overset{\alpha}{C}$–CO– etc., extender conjugation	30 nm

Addition for each substituent   Add

	α	β	γ	δ
– R alkyl	10 nm	12 nm	17 nm	17 nm
– OR alkoxy	35 nm	30 nm	17 nm	31 nm
– OH hydroxy	35 nm	30 nm	30 nm	50 nm
– SR trioether	–	80 nm	–	–
– Cl chloro	15 nm	12 nm	2 nm	12 nm
– Br bromo	25 nm	30 nm	25 nm	25 nm
– NH$_2$, – NHR, – NR$_2$ amino	–	95	–	–
If one double bond is exocyclic to one ring		5 nm		
If one double bond is exocyclic to two rings		10 nm		

Solvent effect

Above values shifted to longer (+) wavelength in water and to shorter (–) wavelength in less polar solvents. For example:

Water	+8 nm
CH$_3$OH	0
Chloroform	–1 mm
Dioxan	–5 nm
Diethyl ether	–7 nm
Hexane	–11 nm
Cyclohexane	–11 nm

4. Detection of Impurities by UV-Visible Spectroscopy

UV absorption spectroscopy is one of the best methods for determination of impurities in organic molecules. Additional peaks can be observed due to impurities in the sample and it can be compared with that of standard raw material. By also measuring the absorbance at specific wavelength, the impurities can be detected. Benzene appears as a common impurity in cyclohexane. Its presence can be easily detected by its absorption at 255 nm. In nylon manufacture, the starting materials like adiponitrile and hexamethylenediamine should be very pure. If these starting materials are not pure, the nylon obtained will be of very poor quality. The purity of these materials can be tested of UV absorption spectroscopy. Traces of unsaturated and aromatic impurities can be detected because the starting materials are transparent in the near ultraviolet region.

5. Quantitative UV-Visible Spectroscopy

UV absorption spectroscopy can be used for the quantitative determination of compounds that absorb UV radiation. This determination is based on Beer-Lambert's law which is as follows:

$$A = \log \frac{I_0}{I} = \log \frac{1}{T} = -\log T = abc = \varepsilon bc$$

where ε is extinction co-efficient, c is concentration, and b is the length of the cell that is used in UV spectrophotometer.

Many drugs either in the form of raw material or in the form of formulation, can be assayed by making a suitable solution of the drug in a solvent measuring the absorbance at specific wavelength. Diazepam tablet can be analyzed by measuring the absorbance of diazepam in 0.5% H_2SO_4 solution in methanol at the wavelength of 284 nm (λ_{max}). Paracetamol tablet can be analyzed in neutral, acidic and alkaline media at λ_{max} 242, 243 and 257 nm respecctively.

Quantitative Determination Methodology

The methodology followed for the quantitative determinations have certain essential steps which are as follows:
- Formation of an absorbing species
- Selection of the specific measurement wavelength
- Controlling factors influencing absorbance
- Validation of Beer-Lambert's law

Formation of an absorbing species

There are only a few analytes that have a strong absorption in the UV or visible region and can be subjected to quantitative determinations directly. However, for most of the analytes we have to form a absorbing species by reacting them with a suitable reagent. In any case, the absorbance of the solution should be stable and should not change with minor variations in the pH, temperature and the ionic strength of the solution. Further, the reagent should be selective towards the analyte and its reaction with the analyte should be quantitative i.e. 100%.

Selection of the specific measurement wavelength

In the absence of interfering substances, the measurements are made at the wavelength of the maxima λ_{max} of the largest peak in the spectrum. At this wavelength, the absorbance is most sensitive to be concentration. Further, as in many cases there is broadening of peak so within certain interval of wavelength near the λ_{max}, there is no appreciate change in the value of absorbance i.e. the measurement is not very sensitive to the wavelength. This is quite advantageous because even if the spectrophotometer fails to resolve λ_{max}, the determination does not suffer. However, in systems where the reagent, metal and products all absorb light, it may so happen that at λ_{max} there is not much of difference in the absorbance value for pure reagent and the metal complex. In such cases we need to identify such a wavelength at which there is large difference in the absorbance values of pure reagent and the complex.

Controlling factors influencing absorbance

As discussed earlier, a number of factors can effect the absorption spectrum of the analyte. These include solvent polarity, pH, temperature, ionic strength and interferences from other absorbing species. It is therefore, essential for a reliable quantitative determination that the conditions of the determination are so chosen that there is minimal effect of these factors.

Validation of Beer-Lambert's Law

The expression for the Beer and Lambert's law is written as:

$$A = \log \frac{I_0}{I} = A = abc \text{ or } \varepsilon bc$$

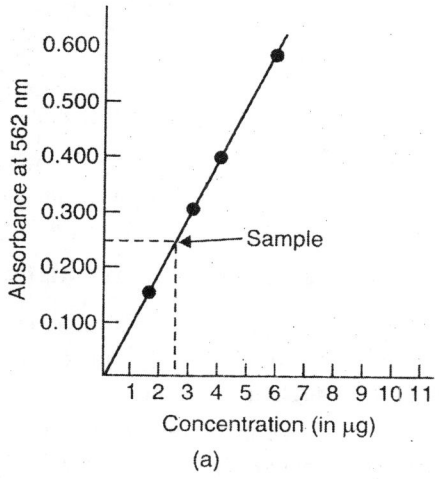

Fig. 3.19. Calibration curve: (a) Standard solution method.

According to this expression, if we know the values of a (or ε) and b then we can determine the concentration directly from the absorbance value. However, generally the value of ε is not known accurately for the species being determined under conditions of the determination. Quite often even the validity of the Beer-Lambert's law expression is questionable. Therefore in most of the methods, a calibration curve is obtained by measuring the absorbance values for a series of standard solutions of the analyte being determined at a fixed wavelength. These solutions should be under similar solution conditions and in the range of the concentration of the analyte. For the law to be valid, the plot of absorbance, A versus the concentration, c for the standard solutions should be a straight line passing through origin. Such a curve is known as **calibration curve** and is handy in determination of concentration of unknown solution from a measurement of absorbance value. For example, the unknown concentration of a solution of iron can be determined by using a calibration curve obtained by plotting the absorbance values of a series of standard solutions of iron measured at 562 nm depicted in Fig. 3.19(a).

76 Pharmaceutical Analysis

Sometimes, it may so happen that all the constituents in the sample may not be known and so a standard solution with the same chemical composition cannot be prepared. In such a case, a method called **standard addition method** is used which eliminates any error arising from the molar absorptivities (ε) being different in the standard solution from that in the sample solution. In this method known amounts of the standard is added to identical aliquots of the sample and the absorbance is measured. The first reading is the absorbance of sample alone and the second reading is absorbance of sample containing analyte plus, a known amount of analyte and so on. The readings so obtained are then plotted to obtain the calibration curve. If the Beer's law is obeyed, i.e. a straight line is obtained; the unknown concentration of the solution can then be obtained by the extrapolation of the calibration curve as shown in Fig. 3.19(b).

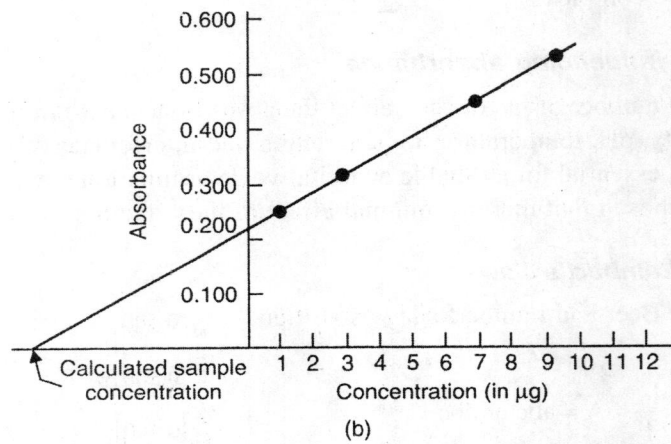

Fig. 3.19. Calibration curve: (b) Standard addition method.

6. Molecular Weight Determination

Molecular weight of compounds can be measured spectrophotometrically provided that suitable derivatives of these compounds could be prepared. This method is based upon the formation of a derivative such as a picrate.

Suppose we are interested in determining the molecular weight of any amine. First of all it is converted into amine picrate. Then, a known concentration of the amine picrate is dissolved in a litre of solution and its optical density is measured at its λ_{max} 380 nm.

$$c = \frac{\log \frac{I_0}{I}}{\varepsilon \times b}$$

where I_0 and I are the radiant power of incident and transmitted radiation. The 'b' is the path length of cell.

From the above equation, concentration 'c' can be calculated. The weight w of the amine picrate is also known. From c and w, the molecular weight of the amine picrate can be calculated. From the molecular weight of the amine picrate, one can calculate the molecular weight of the parent compound.

7. As HPLC detector

A UV-Visible spectrophotometer may be used as a detector for HPLC. The presence of an analyte gives a response which can be assumed to be proportional to the concentration. For more accurate results, the instrument's response to the analyte in the unknown should be compared with the response to a standard; as in the case of calibration curve.

8. Chemical kinetics

Kinetics of reaction can also be studied using UV spectroscopy. The UV radiation is passed through the reaction cell and the absorbance changes can be observed.

9. Dissociation constants of acids and bases

$$pH = P_{Ka} + \log \frac{[A^-]}{[HA]}$$

From the above equation, the pK_a value can be calculated if the ratio of $[A^-]/[HA]$ is known at a particular pH and the ratio of $[A^-]/[HA]$ can be determined spectrophotometrically from the graph plotted between absorbance and wavelength at different pH values.

CHAPTER 4

Infrared Spectroscopy

Infrared (IR) spectroscopy is one of the most common spectroscopic techniques used by organic and inorganic chemists. Simply, it is the measurement of different IR frequencies absorbed by a sample positioned in the path of an IR beam. Infrared radiation absorbed by organic molecules, is converted into energy of molecular vibration, either stretching or bending (Fig. 4.1).

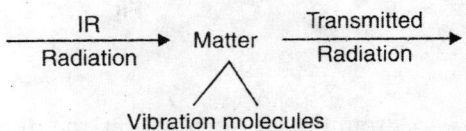

Fig. 4.1. Interaction of IR radiation with matter.

Different types of bonds, and thus different functional groups, absorb infrared radiation at different wavelength to give the *IR spectrum*. The IR spectrum is a plot of wavenumber/wavelength (X-axis) vs percent transmittance, Y-axis (Fig. 4.2). The main goal of IR spectroscopic analysis is to determine the chemical functional groups in the sample. Different functional groups absorb at characteristic frequencies/wavelength of IR radiation. Using various sampling accessories, IR spectrometers can accept a wide range of sample types such as gases, liquids and solids. Thus, IR spectroscopy is an important and popular tool for structural elucidation and compound identification.

IR REGION

Infrared radiation is that part of the electromagnetic spectrum between the visible and microwave regions (Fig. 4.3). The IR region is commonly divided into three smaller areas: near IR, mid IR and far IR.

Type of region	Wavelength (μm)	Wave number (cm^{-1})
Near IR	0.78–3	12820 to 4000
Mid IR	3–30	4000–200
Far IR	30–300	200–10

Note: cm = 10^{-2} m, mm = 10^{-3} m, μm = 10^{-6} m

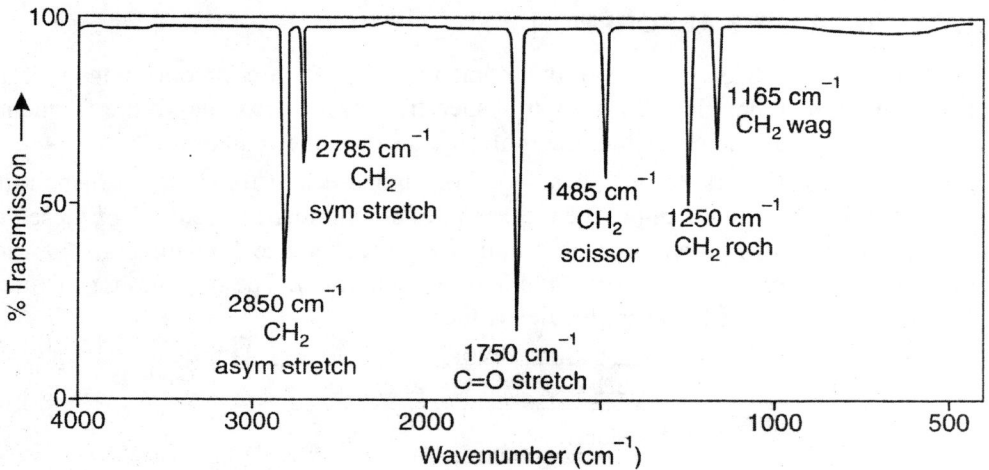

Fig. 4.2. Infrared spectrum of Formaldehyde.

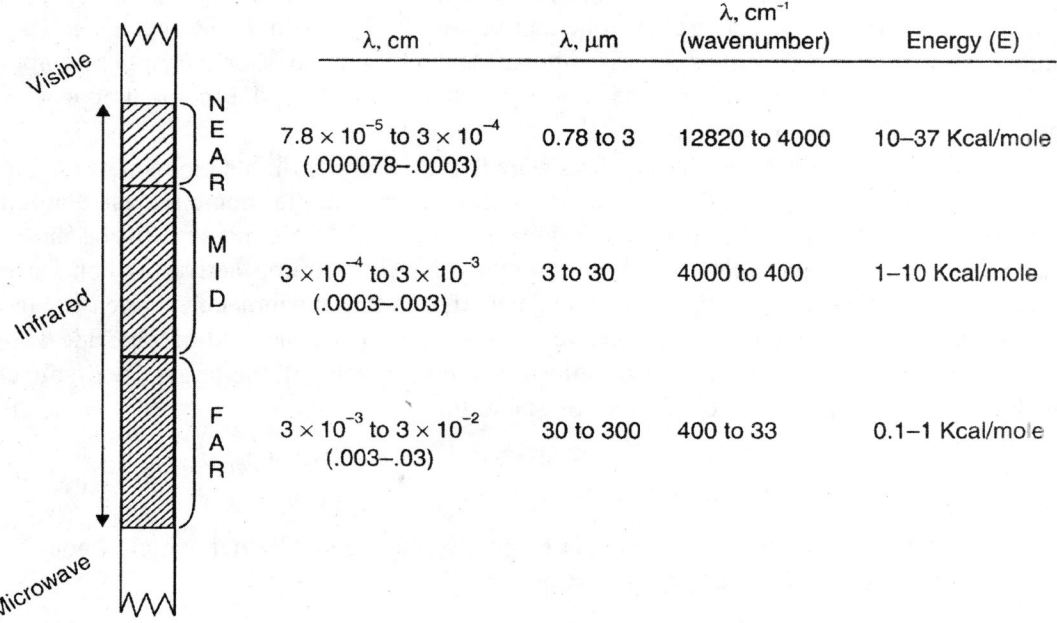

Fig. 4.3. IR regions of the electromagnetic spectrum.

The infrared region, 3–30 μm (4000–400 cm^{-1}) is commonly used for analysis. The region from 4000–1300 cm^{-1} is known as Functional group region, particularly useful for identifying the presence of specific functional groups. IR spectra are also analyzed by comparing observed spectra with spectra of known compounds. The *fingerprint region* to the right of 1300 cm^{-1} (1300–400 cm^{-1}) is particularly useful in the compound identification. It is specific to the structure of the compound.

THEORY OF INFRARED ABSORPTION

At temperatures above absolute zero, all the atoms in molecules are in continuous vibration with respect to each other. When the frequency of a specific vibration is equal to the frequency of the IR radiation, directed on the molecule, the molecule absorbs the radiation.

A molecule consisting of n atoms, has a total of $3n$ degrees of freedom, corresponding to the Cartesian coordinates of each atom in the molecule. In a nonlinear molecule, 3 of these degres are rotational and 3 are translational and the remaining correspond to fundamental vibrations; in a linear molecule, 2 degrees are rotational and 3 are translational. The net number of fundamental vibrations for nonlinear and linear molecules is therefore:

Molecule	Degrees of freedom
Nonlinear	$3n - 6$
Linear	$3n - 5$

Calculation reveals that a sample molecule such as propane, C_3H_8, has 27 ($11 \times 3 - 6$) fundamental vibrations, and therefore, one can predict 27 bands in an IR spectrum. The actual number is sometimes different as discussed in part later. All the vibrational changes do not appear as band. Only those vibrational changes that result in change in dipole moment appear as band. This is referred as **Selection rule**.

Selection rule for vibrational transitions state that the electric dipole moment of the molecule must change in the course of the vibrational motion. For example, homonuclear diatomics are infrared inactive if stretching of the bond does not alter the dipole moment of the molecule, it remains at zero. However, heteronuclear diatomics may be infrared active, as bond stretching increases the distance between the positive and negative ends of the molecule, increasing its dipole moment. On the following linear molecules, carbon monoxide and iodine chloride absorb IR radiation, while hydrogen, nitrogen and chlorine do not. In general, the larger the dipole change, the strong the intensity of the band in an IR spectrum.

$C\equiv O$ $I-Cl$ H_2 N_2 Cl_2
Absorb in IR   Do not absorb in IR

The fundamental vibrations for water, H_2O are given in Fig. 4.4. Water, which is nonlinear, has three fundamental vibrations as per prediction ($3 \times 3 - 6 = 3$).

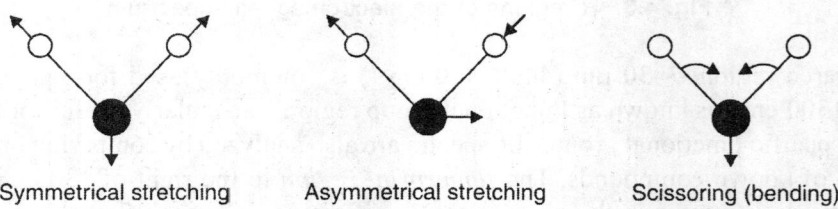

Symmetrical stretching   Asymmetrical stretching   Scissoring (bending)

Fig. 4.4. Stretching and bending vibrational modes for H_2O.

Carbon dioxide, CO_2 is linear and hence should have four fundamental vibrations (Fig. 4.5) as per prediction but IR spectrum reveals only two instead of four. The asymmetrical stretch of CO_2 gives a strong band in the IR at 2350 cm^{-1}. This band can be noticed in samples on running the instruments in the teaching labs, since CO_2 is present in the atmosphere. The two scissoring or bending vibrations are equivalent and therefore, have the same frequency and are said to be *degenerate*, appearing in an IR spectrum at 666 cm^{-1}. The symmetrical stretch of CO_2 is inactive in the IR (Fig. 4.4) because this vibration produces no change in the dipole moment of the molecule. In order to be IR active, a vibration must cause a change in the dipole moment of the molecule.

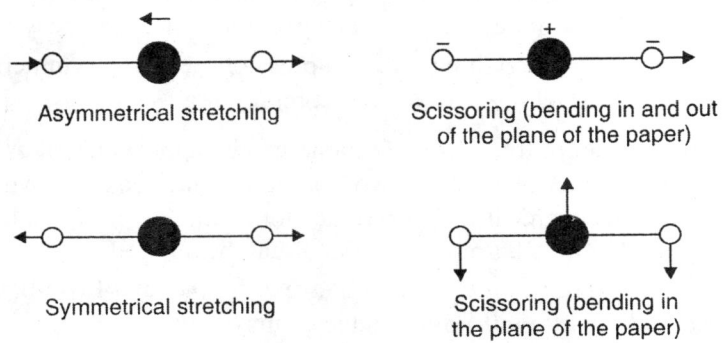

Fig. 4.5. Stretching and bending vibrational modes for CO_2.

Hence, two IR bands (2350 and 666 cm^{-1}) are seen for carbon dioxide, instead of predicted four fundamental vibrations. Carbon dioxide is an example of why one does not always seen as many bands as predicted by our simple calculation. Other reasons why fewer than the theoretical number of IR bands are seen include an absorption is not in the 4000–400 cm^{-1} range; an absorption is too weak to be observed; absorptions are too close to each other to be resolved on the instrument.

Conversely, additional bands are generated by the appearance of overtones (integral multiples of the fundamental absorption frequencies), combinations of fundamental frequencies, differences of fundamental frequencies, coupling interactions of two fundamental absorption frequencies and coupling interactions between fundamental vibrations and overtones or combination bands (Fermi resonance). The intensities of overtone, combination, and difference bands are less than those of the fundamental bands. The combination and blending of all the factors thus create a unique IR spectrum for each compound.

TYPES OF MOLECULAR VIBRATIONS

The bond of a molecule experiences various types of vibrations and rotations. This causes the fluctuation of atom continuously. There are two types of molecular vibrations – fundamental and non-fundamental vibrations which are likely to be changed when molecule interact the electromagnetic radiation in the IR region.

1. Fundamental Vibrations

These are classified as follows:

(i) Stretching vibrations
(ii) Bending vibrations

A CH_2 group is used as an example to illustrate stretching and bending vibrations in Fig. 4.7.

(i) Stretching vibrations

These occur along the bond axis where inter atomic distance increases or decreases but atomic position remain as such. Two types of stretching vibrations occur along the bond axis, when the inter atomic distance increases or decreases. These are: symmetrical and asymmetrical stretching.

In *symmetrical stretching*, stretching and compression occur in symmetrical fashion but in *asymmetrical* one bond is stretching and other is compressing.

Hook's law: The stretching frequency of a bond can be approximated by Hook's law. Let us consider a simple diatomic molecule in which two atoms are connected by a covalent bond. Assuming the covalent bond to be a mechanical spring and the atomic masses as two spheres at either end of the spring, the concept of simple harmonic oscillator can be applied.

Hook's law applied here gives the relation between frequency of oscillation, atomic masses and the force constant (bond strength) of the bond. Thus:

$$\text{Vibrational frequency (cm}^{-1}) = \frac{1}{2\pi C}\sqrt{\frac{f}{\mu}}$$

$$\mu = \frac{M_x M_y}{M_x + M_y}, \text{ masses of atoms in grams}$$

or

$$\frac{M_x M_y}{(M_x + M_y)(6.02 \times 10^{23})}, \text{ masses of atoms in amu}$$

where C is velocity of light (3×10^{10} cm/s), f is the constant (dyne/cm) and M_x and M_y are the mass (g) of atoms x and y. Since the force constant 'f' measures the stiffness (i.e. strength) of bond, the value of 'f' becomes double and triple for the double and triple bonds respectively.

The force constants (f) for bonds are:

Single bond	5×10^5 dyne/cm
Double bond	10×10^5 dyne/cm
Triple bond	15×10^5 dyne/cm

As the mass of the atoms increases, the vibration frequency decreases. Using the following mass value:

C, carbon	$12/6.02 \times 10^{23}$
H, hydrogen	$1/6.02 \times 10^{23}$

The frequency for a C–H bond is calculated to be 3032 cm^{-1} as per calculation shown below. The actual range for C–H absorptions is 2850–3000 cm^{-1}.

$$\mu = \frac{M_x M_y}{M_x + M_y} = \frac{12 \times 1}{12 + 1} = 0.9238 \text{ g/atom}$$

$$f = 5 \times 10^5 \text{ dyne/cm}$$

$$\text{Vibrational frequency (cm}^{-1}) = 4.12 \sqrt{\frac{5 \times 10^5}{0.923}} = 3023 \text{ cm}^{-1}$$

The appearance of band due to changes in bond stretching vibrations depend primarily on whether the bonds are single, double, or triple or bonds to hydrogen. The reasons explaining why C–H bending vibrations are at *lower frequency* than C–H stretching vibrations are also related to Hooke's Law. An H–C–H bending vibration involves three atoms, not just two, so the mass involved is greater than a C–H stretch.

Example 1: Calculate the fundamental frequency expected in IR spectrum for –CO stretching vibration.

$$\text{Vibrational frequency (cm}^{-1}) = \frac{\sqrt{\frac{(5 \times 10^5)(12+16)(6.023 \times 10^{23})}{12 \times 16}}}{2 \times 3.1416 \times 3 \times 10^{10}} = 1110 \text{ cm}^{-1}$$

The Fig. 4.6 gives an approximate outline of where specific types of bond stretches may be found as per Hook's law.

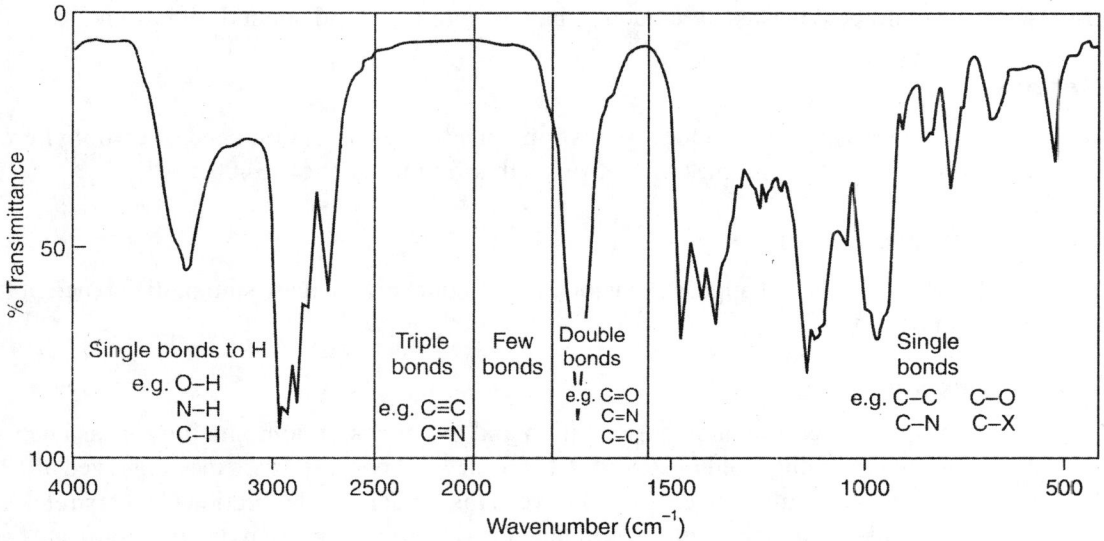

Fig. 4.6. Position of various bonds as per Hook's law.

In conclusion, according to Hook's law, it means:
- Stronger bonds absorb at higher frequencies.
- Weaker bonds absorb at lower frequencies.
- Bonds between lighter atoms absorb at higher frequencies.
- Bonds between heavier atoms absorb at lower frequencies.

(ii) Bending vibrations

Bending vibrations occur due to the changes in the bond angle. Two types of bending vibrations are possible:
- in plane bending: scissoring and rocking
- out of the plane bending: twisting and wagging

Scissors: When the two atoms joined to a central atom move toward and away from each other like scissor, then deformation is known as scissoring.

Rocking: In this two atoms joining a central atom move back and forth in the plane of the molecule.

Wagging: In this deformation, the structural unit moves back and forth out of the plane of the molecule.

Twisting: When the structural unit rotates about the bond which joins to the rest of the molecule, the deformation produced is known as twisting.

2. Non-Fundamental vibrations

Absorption bands can also resulted in addition to those predicted by the number of degree of freedom possessed by the molecule. These are due to changes into non-fundamental vibrations.

Overtones

These are observed at twice the frequency of strong band. The absorption band of carbonyl group appears at $1700\ cm^{-1}$ but sometimes also at twice this frequency (near $3400\ cm^{-1}$).

Combination tones

These are also weak bands that appear occasionally at frequencies that are sum or difference of two or more fundamental bands.

Fermi resonance

It is an interaction between fundamental vibration and overtones or combination tones. The CO_2 shows symmetrical stretching band observed at $1340\ cm^{-1}$ but two bands are also observed at 1286 and $1388\ cm^{-1}$. The split result from coupling between the fundamental vibration $C = O$ (stretching) and first overtone of bending vibration. The fundamental bending vibration occurs at $666\ cm^{-1}$ and Ist overtone near $1344\ cm^{-1}$.

FACTORS AFFECTING ABSORPTION FREQUENCIES

Here, structural factors affecting the position of absorption bands are discusses by taking and example of carbonyl functional group:

1. **Electron effect:** The carbonyl has double bond to produce an absorption band with high intensity at a large wavenumber, whose shift produced by a structural change is evident. Therefore, IR bands of carbonyl functional group can be used as an example. If a structural change induces it from (d+)C = O(d−) towards (+)C − O(−), this can displace the absorption band towards a smaller number.

   (i) *Induction effect*: The normal absorption band of aliphatic ketone is situated at 1715 cm^{-1}. The substitution of a carbonyl by a halogen atom increases the double bond tendency of the carbonyl (it has more difficulty toward C − O) so that the IR absorption of the carbonyl group will shift to a large wavenumber.

   The following structural change illustrates the effect of substitution of the carbonyl by a halogen atom, which is mainly the inductive effect.

R–C(=O)–R	R–C(=O)–Cl	R–C(=O)–Br	R–C(=O)–F
1715 cm^{-1}	1785 cm^{-1}–1815 cm^{-1}	1815 cm^{-1}	1869 cm^{-1}

   (ii) *Mesomeric effect*: The mesomeric effect is also called resonance effect. The most typical example is the IR absorption of amides. According to the mesomeric effect, the connection of an amine group with a carbonyl group will produce the following reaction:

   $$R-\overset{O}{\underset{\|}{C}}-NH_2 \longleftrightarrow R-\overset{O^-}{\underset{|}{C}}=NH_2$$

   The resonance reduces the double bond tenency of the amide so its absorption band is displaced towards a rather smaller wavenumber. All amides have an IR absorption frequency lower than 1690 cm^{-1}.

   (iii) *Conjugation effect*: If carbonyl is conjugated with another double bond, the delocalization of electrons of the carbonyl group decreases the bond order of the carbonyl double bond. Therefore, its absorption is displaced towards a smaller wavenumber. The absorption bands of unsaturated ketones and those of aromatic ketones are visible at 1675 cm^{-1} and 1690 cm^{-1} respectively.

2. **Steric effect:** Generally speaking, the stronger tension a cyclic ring has, the large wavenumber its an absorption band shift. A typical example is the IR absorption of a CH$_2$ in a ring.

   Cyclohexane (2925 cm^{-1}, due to steric hinderance)

   Cyclopropane (3050 cm^{-1})

   Influence of hydrogen bond: Both inter- and intra-hydrogen bonds weaken the bond which participates in the formation of hydrogen bond. As a result, the absorption band of the bond shifts into smaller wavenumber. However, the dipolar moment change of the bond affected

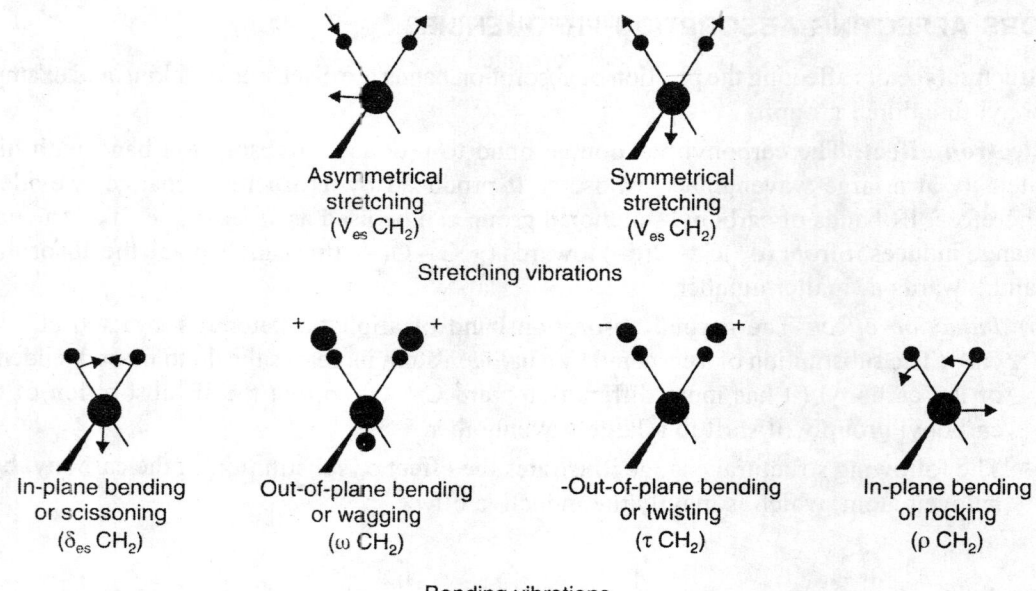

Fig. 4.7. Types of molecular vibrations of CH_2 group.

by the hydrogen bond increases so that its absorption intensity increases. The absorption bands of alcohol can be listed as an example.

Isolated (3610–3640 cm^{-1})   **Dimer** (3500–3600 cm^{-1})   **Polymer** (3200–3400 cm^{-1})

The strong hydrogen bond between carboxylic acid molecules can shift the absorption band to about 3000 cm^{-1} with its tail about 2500 cm^{-1}.

3. **Mass effect (Deuteration effect):** If a group containing hydrogen atom is deuterated, its absorption frequency will decrease as per Stokes equation.

COUPLED INTERACTIONS

Vibrational frequencies are affected with new type of interaction called **coupled interactions**. When two bond oscillators share a common atom, they seldom behave as individual oscillators unless the individual oscillation frequencies are widely different. This is because there is mechanical coupling interaction between the oscillators. For example, the carbon dioxide molecule, which consist of two C = O bonds with a common carbon atom, has two fundamental stretching vibrations, as asymmetrical and a symmetrical stretching vibration.

The requirements for effective coupling interaction are:
- The vibrations must be of the same symmetry species for interaction to occur.
- Strong coupling between stretching vibrations requires a common atom between the groups.
- Interaction is greatest when the coupled absorb almost near the same frequency.
- Coupling between bending and stretching vibrations can occur if the stretching bond forms one side of the changing angle.

- A common bond is required for coupling of bending vibrations.
- Coupling is negligible when groups are separated by one or more carbon atoms and vibrations are mutually perpendicular.

FACTORS AFFECTING ABSORPTION FREQUENCIES

EFFECT OF HYDROGEN BONDING ON IR ABSORPTION

Hydrogen bonding occurs in a system containing a proton donor group and a proton acceptor group if the s orbital of the proton donor group can overlap with the p orbital of the proton acceptor group. The common proton donor groups are carboxyl, hydroxyl, amine or amide group. The common proton acceptor groups are oxygen, nitrogen, halogens and unsaturated group like C = C bonds. It may be intermolecular (involves association of two or more molecules of same or different compounds) or intra-molecular (proton donor and acceptor are present in a single molecule).

Intermolecular

p-Hydroxy acetophenone
3600 cm^{-1} (OH)

o-Hydroxy acetophenone
3077 cm^{-1} (OH)
Broad peak due to intra-molecular hydrogen bonding

The strength of the hydrogen bonding is maximum, when the proton donor group and the lone pair of the proton acceptor group are collinear. As the distance between these decreases, the strength of the bond decreases. Since hydrogen bonding alters the force constant, the frequencies of both bending and stretching vibrations are altered. The X–H stretching bands move to the longer wavelength or lower frequencies, whereas the bending vibrations of H–X vibrations shift to shorter wavelength or higher frequencies. In the absence of hydrogen bonding, the absorption band is weak, but strong hydrogen bonding, resulted in broader and sharp absorption band.

Both intermolecular and intra-molecular hydrogen bonding are temperature dependent. Intermolecular H-bonding is concentration dependent and gives rise to broad bands. On dilution intermolecular H-bonding decreases and consequently the intensities of the bands decreases. Intramolecular hydrogen bonding shows no comparable effect. Ring strain, molecular geometry and the relative acidity and basicity of the proton donor and acceptor groups also affect the strength of hydrogen bonding.

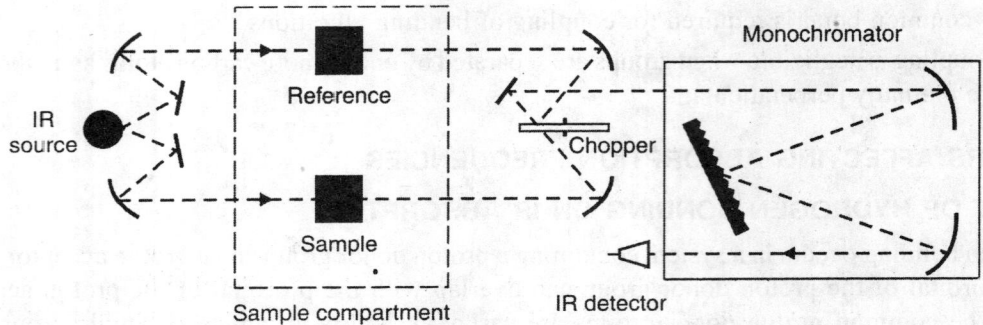

Fig. 4.8. Schematic of typical dispersive IR absorption spectrometer.

IR INSTRUMENTATION

IR spectra are obtained by detecting changes in transmittance (or absorption) intensity as a function of frequency. Most commercial instruments record the IR spectrum using dispersive spectrometers or Fourier transform spectrometers.

(i) Dispersive infrared spectophotometers

The IR spectrometer consists of three basic components. IR radiation source, monochromator, and detector. A schematic diagram of a typical dispersive spectrometer is shown in Fig. 4.8.

The instrument produces a beam of infrared radiation from a hot filament wire and uses mirrors to divide it into two parallel beams of equal intensity radiation. The sample is placed in one beam, and a reference in the other. The beam then passes into the monochromator which disperses it into a continuous spectrum of frequencies of IR light.

The monochromator consists of a beam chopper (a rapidly rotating sector) that passes the two beams alternatively to a diffraction grating. The slowly rotating diffraction grating varies the frequency of radiation reaching the thermocouple detector, which senses the ratio between the intensities of the reference and sample beams. In this way, the detector determines which frequencies have been absorbed by the sample. Once the signal from the detector is amplified, the recorder draws the resulting spectrum.

(a) IR sources

An inert solid is electrically heated to a temperature in the range 1500–2000°C to emit out infrared radiation. Some of the common IR sources are as follows:

(i) *Nernst glower*: It is a cylinder (1–3 mm diameter, approximately 20 mm long), made of rare earth oxides (ZrO_2, Y_2O_3 and thorium oxide) (Fig. 4.9).

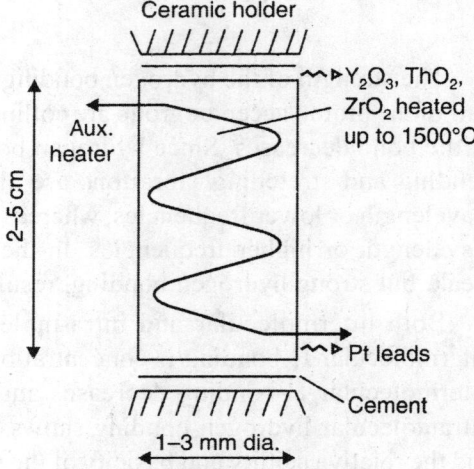

Fig. 4.9. Nernst glower.

Platinum wires are sealed to the ends, and a current passed through the cylinder for heating. The Nernst glower can reach temperatures of 2200°C.

(ii) *Globar source*: It is a silicon carbide rod (6 mm diameter, 50 mm long) (Fig. 4.10) which is electrically heated to about 1500°C. Water cooling of the electrical contacts is needed to prevent arcing. The spectral output is comparable with the Nernst glower, except at short wavelengths (less than 5 mm) where its output becomes larger.

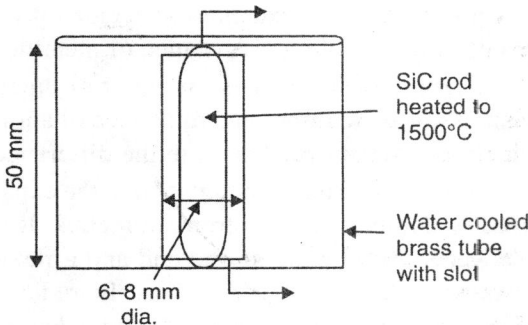

Fig. 4.10. Globar source.

(iii) *Incandescent wire source*: It is a tightly wound coil of nichrome wire, electrically heated to 1100°C. It produces a lower intensity of radiation than the Nernst or Globar sources, but has a longer working life.

(b) Monochromator

It is same as discussed in Chapter 3. The monochromator is a device used to disperse a broad spectrum of radiation and provide a continuous calibrated series of electromagnetic energy bands of determinable wavelength or frequency range. Prisms or gratings are the dispersive components used in conjunction with variable-slit mechanisms, mirrors, and filters. For example, a grating rotates to focus a narrow band of frequencies on a mechanical slit. Narrower slits enable the instrument to better distinguish more closely spaced frequencies of radiation, resulting in better resolution. Wider slits allow more light to reach the detector and provide better system sensitivity. Thus, certain compromise is exercised in setting the desired slit width.

Often double-beam recording instruments, employing diffraction gratings for dispersion of radiation are used. Radiation from the source is flicked between the reference and sample paths. Often, an *optical null* system is used. This is when the detector only responds if the intensity of the two beams is unequal. If the intensities are unequal, a light attenuator restores equally by moving in or out of the reference beam. The recording pen is attached to this attenuator.

(c) Detectors used in IR instrumentation

There are three categories of detector:
- Thermal
- Pyroelectric
- Photoconducting

Thermal detectors include thermocouples, thermistors, and pneumatic devices (Golay detectors). They measure the heating effect produced by infrared radiation. A variety of physical property changes are quantitatively determined: expansion of a nonabsorbing gas (Golay detector), electrical resistance (bolometer), and voltage at junction of dissimilar metals (thermocouple).

Bolometer is an excellent detector for measuring IR radiation. It gives electrical signal as a result of the change in resistance of metallic conductor with temperature.

Thermocouples consist of a pair of junctions of different metals; for example, two pieces of bismuth fused to either end of a piece of antimony. The potential difference (voltage) between the junctions changes according to the difference in temperature between the junction.

Golay cell: This detector utilizes the expansion of the gas as the basis for detection. It is mostly used in commercial spectrophotometres. It consists of a small metal cylinder closed by a rigid blackened metal plate at one end and a flexible silvered diaphragm at the other end. The whole chamber is filled with xenon gas. IR radiation passes through a radiation transmitting window. Heat conducted causes the gas to expand and causes the flexible metal diaphragm to deform. Light from lamp is made to fall on the metalized diaphragm which reflects the light on the photo cell. Motion of diaphragm changes the output of cell. The signal seen by the phototube is modulated in accordance with the power of the radiant beam incident on the gas cell.

Thermal detectors provide a linear response over a wide range of frequencies but exhibit slower response times and lower sensitivities than photon detectors.

Pyroelectric detectors are made from a single crystalline wafer of a pyroelectric material, such as triglycerine sulphate. The properties of a pyroelectric material are such that when an electric field is applied across it, electric polarisation occurs (this happens in any dielectric material). In a pyroelectric material, when the field is removed, the polarisation persists. The degree of polarisation is temperature dependent. So, by sandwiching the pyroelectric material between two electrodes, a temperature dependent capacitor is made. The heating effect of incident IR radiation causes a change in the capacitance of the material. Pyroelectric detectors have a fast response time. They are used in most **Fourier transform IR spectrometers**.

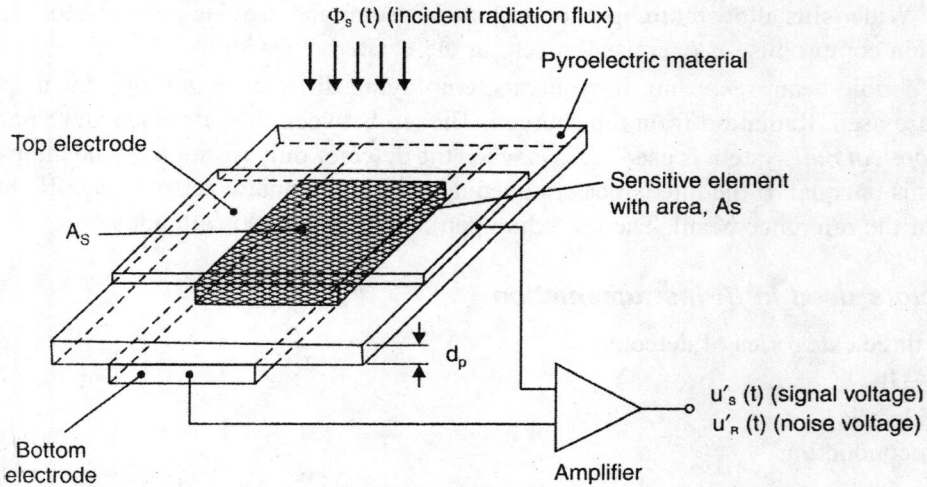

Fig. 4.11. Principle set-up of a pyroelectric infrared detector.

Photoelectric detectors such as the mercury cadmium telluride detector comprise a film of semiconducting material deposited on a glass surface, sealed in an evacuated envelope. Absorption of IR promotes nonconducting valence electrons to a higher, conducting, state. The electrical resistance of the semiconductor decreases. Thus, a small current or voltage can be generated. It serves as measure of power of radiation. These detectors have better response characteristics than pyroelectric detectors and are used in FT-IR instruments - particularly in GC-FT-IR.

(ii) Fourier-transform spectrometers

Fourier transform spectrometers have recently replaced dispersive instruments for most applications due to their superior speed and sensitivity. They have greatly extended the capabilities of infrared spectroscopy and have been applied to many areas that are very difficult or nearly impossible to analyze by dispersive instruments. Instead of viewing each component frequency sequentially, as in a dispersive IR spectrometer, all frequencies are examined simultaneously in Fourier transform infrared (FT-IR) spectrometer. In FT-IR, the light beam is passed through the sample and the absorbances at all frequencies are received at the detector simultaneously. A computerized mathematical manipulation (known as 'Fourier transform') is performed on this data to obtain absorption data for each and every wavelength. Dispersive IR instruments operate in the frequency domain while FT-IR operate FT-IR in the time domain (gives interferrogram) followed by computer transformation into the frequency domain.

There are three basic spectrometer components in an FT system: radiation source, interferometer and detector.

The same types of radiation sources are used for both dispersive and Fourier transform spectrometers. However, the source is more often water-cooled in FTIR instruments to provide better power and stability. In contrast, a completely different approach is taken in an FTIR spectrometer to differentiate and measure the absorption at component frequencies. The monochromator is replaced by an interferometer, which divides radiant beams, generates an optical path difference between the beams, then recombines them in order to produce repetitive interference signals measured as a function of optical path difference by a detector. As its name implies, the interferometer produces interference signals, which contain infrared spectral information generated after passing through a sample.

The most commonly used interferometer is a *Michelson interferometer*. It consists of three active components: a moving mirror, a stationary mirror, and a beam splitter (Fig. 4.12). The two mirrors are perpendicular to each other. The beam splitter is a semi-reflecting device and is often made by depositing a thin film of germanium onto a flat KBr substance.

Radiation leaves the source and is split. Half is reflected to a stationary mirror and then back to the splitter. This radiation has travelled a fixed distance. The other half of the radiation from the source passes through the splitter and is reflected

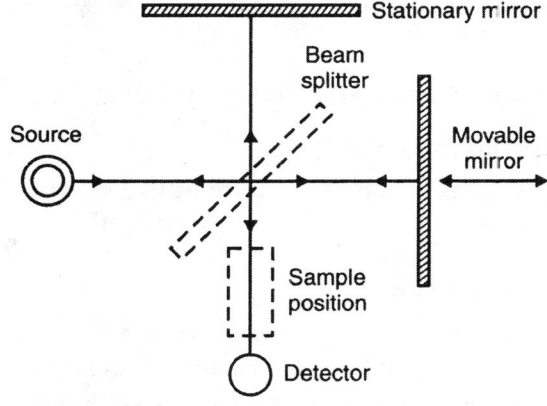

Fig. 4.12. Michelson interferometer.

back by a **movable mirror**. Therefore, the path length of this beam is variable. The two reflected beams recombine at the splitter, and they interfere (e.g. for any one wavelength, interference will be constructive if the difference in path lengths is an exact multiple of the wavelength. If the difference in path lengths is half the wavelength then destructive interference will result). If the movable mirror moves away from the beam splitter at a constant speed, radiation reaching the detector goes through a steady sequence of maxima and minima as the interference alternates between constructive and destructive phases. If monochromatic IR radiation of frequency, $f(ir)$ enters the interferometer, then the output frequency, f_m can be found by:

$$f_m = \frac{v}{1.5 \times 10^{11}} \times f(ir)$$

where v is the speed of mirror travel in mm/s

In the FT-IR instrument, the sample is placed between the output of the interferometer and the detector. The sample absorbs radiation of particular wavelengths. Therefore, the interferogram contains the spectrum of the source minus the spectrum of the sample. An interferogram of a reference (sample cell and solvent) is needed to obtain the spectrum of the sample. After the interferogram has been collected, a computer performs a *Fast Fourier Transform*, which results in a frequency domain trace (i.e. intensity vs. wave number). The detector used in an FT-IR instrument must respond quickly because intensity changes are rapid (the moving mirror moves quickly). Pyroelectric detectors or liquid nitrogen cooled photon detectors must be used.

Advantage of Fourier transform IR over dispersive IR spectrometer

- Improved frequency resolution.
- Improved frequency reproducibility (older dispersive instruments must be recalibrated for each session of use).
- Higher energy throughput.
- Faster operation.
- Computer based (allowing storage of spectra and facilities for processing spectra).
- Easily adapted for remote use (such as diverting the beam to pass through an external cell and detector, as in GC-FT-IR).

SAMPLE PREPARATIONS IN IR SPECTROSCOPY

Gaseous samples

The gaseous samples require little preparation beyond purification, but a sample cell with a long path length (typically 5–10 cm) is normally needed, as gases show relatively weak absorbances.

Liquid samples

These can be sandwiched between two plates of a high purity salt (commonly sodium chloride, or common salt, although a number of other salts such as potassium bromide or calcium fluoride are also used). The plates are transparent to the infrared light and don't not introduce any lines onto the spectra. Some salt plates are highly soluble in water, so the sample and washing reagents must be anhydrous (without water).

Solid samples

The KBr press method and the nujol mull methods are usually used to analyze solid samples of organic compounds.

In the KBr press method about 1–2 mg quantity of the sample is with a 100 times quantity of specially purified salt (usually potassium bromide) finely (to remove scattering effects from large crystals). This powder mixture is then pressed in a mechanical die press to form a translucent pellet through which the beam of the spectrometer can pass.

Mulls are used as alternatives for pellets. The sample (1 to 5 mg) is ground with a mulling agent (1 to 2 drops) to give a two-phase mixture that has a consistency similar to toothpaste. This mull is pressed between two IR-transmitting plates to form a thin film. The common mulling agents include mineral oil or Nujol (a high-boiling hydrocarbon oil), Fluorolube (a chlorofluorocarbon polymer), and hexachlorobutadiene. To obtain a full IR spectrum that is free of mulling agent bands, the use of multiple mulls (such as Nujol and Fluorolube) is generally required. Thorough mixing and reduction of sample particles of 2 μm or less in size is very important for obtaining a satisfactory spectrum.

The third technique is the **Cast Film technique**, which is used mainly for polymeric materials. The sample is first dissolved in a suitable, non-hygroscopic solvent. A drop of this solution is deposited on surface of KBr or NaCl cell. The solution is then evaporated to dryness and the film formed on the cell is analysed directly. Care is important to ensure that the film is not too thick otherwise light cannot pass through. This technique is suitable for qualitative analysis.

The fourth method is to use microtomy to cut a thin (20–100 micron) film from a solid sample. This is one of the most important ways of analysing failed plastic products for example because the integrity of the solid is preserved.

A more recent development in a sample preparation is the use of **diffuse reflectance technique**, often called diffuse reflectance infrared Fourier transform spectroscopy (DRIFTS). It is observed when light is reflected off a material surface the light observed is of same intensity no matter what the angle of observation. Samples for diffuse reflectance are treated in a same way as those prepared for KBr disc formation except that instead of being compressed is loaded into a small cup, which is placed in the path of sample beam. The incident radiation is reflected from the base of the cup and during its passage through the powdered sample, back absorption of radiation takes place- yielding an infrared spectrum which is similar to that obtained from the KBr technique. In fact the spectrum produced is an absorbance spectrum rather than a transmitt-ance spectrum but it can be easily converted into a transmittance spectrum if the instrument is attached to a computer. This technique is widely used in near IR spectrophotometry. It is useful technique for examining polymorphs since sample can be prepared with minimal grinding and compression which can cause interconversion of polymorphs. The principle of Diffuse Reflectance IR Fourier transform spectrometry is depicted in Fig. 4.13.

When incident light strikes a surface, there is occurrence of two types of reflections: specular reflectance, which directly reflects off the surface and has equal angles of incidence and reflectance, and diffuse reflectance, which penetrates into the sample lying on surface, then scatters in all directions. Special reflection accessories are designed to collect and refocus the resulting diffusely scattered light by large ellipsoidal mirrors, while minimizing or eliminating the specular reflectance, which complicates and distorts the IR spectra. As the light that leaves the surface has passed through a thin layer of the reflecting sample material, its wavelength content will have been modified by the optical properties of the sample material. Consequently, the wavelength and intensity distribution of the reflected light will contain structural information of the substance.

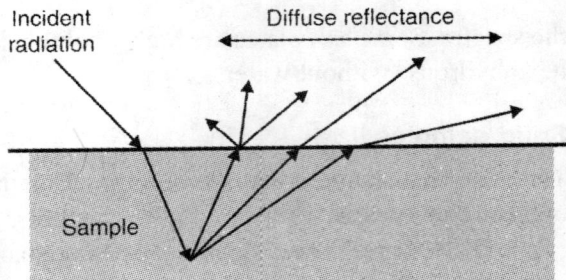

Fig. 4.13. Principle of diffuse reflectance IR spectroscopy.

QUANTITATIVE INFRARED SPECTROSCOPY

IR spectroscopy was generally considered to be able to provide only qualitative and semiquantitative analyses of common samples, especially when the data were acquired using the conventional dispersive instruments. However, the development of reliable FTIR instrumentation and strong computerized data-processing capabilities have greatly improved the performance of quantitative IR work. Thus, modern infrared spectroscopy has gained acceptance as a reliable tool for quantitative analysis.

The basis for quantitative analysis of absorption spectrometry is the Beer-Lambert law as discussed in Chapter 3. For a single compound in a homogeneous medium, the absorbance at any frequency is expressed as:

$$A = abc$$

where A is the measured sample absorbance at the given frequency, a is the molecular absorptivity at the frequency, b is the path length of source beam in the sample, and c is the concentration of the sample. This law basically states that the intensities of absorption bands are linearly proportional to the concentration of each component in a homogeneous mixture or solution.

Deviations from Beer's law occur more often in infrared spectroscopy than in UV-visible spectroscopy. These deviations stem from both instrumental and sample effects. Instrumental effects include insufficient resolution and stray radiation. Resolution is closely related to the slit width in dispersive IR instruments or the optical path difference between two beams in the interferometer of FTIR spectrometers. Stray light levels in FT instruments are usually negligible. Sample effects include chemical reactions and molecular interactions such as hydrogen bonding. The Beer's law deviations result in a nonlinear relationship for plots of absorbance (A) against concentration (c). It is therefore, a good practice to obtain calibration curves that are determined empirically from known standards.

Instead of the transmittance scale, absorbance is generally used in quantitative analysis. Absorbance (A) is defined as the negative logarithm of the transmittance (T). According to Beer's law, a linear relationship exists only between the sample concentration and absorbance, not between the sample concentration and transmittance. The linearity of Beer's law plots usually holds better when the absorbance is limited to less than 0.7 absorbance units, although in some cases good linearity has been achieved over more than 2 absorbance units. A number of quantification parameters, which include peak height, peak area, and derivatives, can be used in quantitative analysis. The integration limits for peak area determinations should be carefully chosen to ensure maximum accuracy.

In multicomponent quantitative analysis, the determination of the composition of mixtures involves the use of software packages. These analyses usually assume that Beer's law is additive for a mixture of compounds at a specified frequency. For a simple two-component mixture, the total absorbance, A_T, of the mixture at a given frequency is the sum of the absorbance of two component compounds, x and y, at the specified frequency:

APPLICATIONS OF IR SPECTROSCOPY

Infrared spectroscopy is widely used in industry as well as in research. It is a simple and reliable technique for measurement, quality control and structural elucidation. Some of the major applications of IR spectroscopy are as follows:

1. Identification of functional group and structural elucidation

Entire IR region is divided into group frequency region and fingerprint region. Range of group frequency is 4000–1300 cm^{-1} while that of finger print region is 1300–400 cm^{-1}. In group frequency region, the peaks corresponding to different functional groups can be observed. Each atom of the molecule is connected by bond and each bond requires different IR region so characteristic peaks are observed. These characteristic peaks are observed in finger print region of the molecule. The structural elucidation solely on the basis of IR spectrum is done by comparison with known spectra.

2. Identification of substances

IR spectroscopy is used to establish whether a given sample of an organic substance is identical with another or not. This is because large number of absorption bands is observed in the IR spectra of organic molecules and the probability that any two compounds will produce identical spectra is almost zero. So if two compounds have identical IR spectra then both of them must be samples of the same substances.

For example, an IR spectrum of benzaldehyde (Fig. 4.22) is observed as follows:

C–H stretching of aromatic ring	3073 cm^{-1}
C–H stretching of aldehyde	2827 cm^{-1} and 2745 cm^{-1}
C=O stretching of an aromatic aldehyde	1696 cm^{-1}
C=C stretching of an aromatic ring	1595 cm^{-1}
C–H bending	745 cm^{-1} and 685 cm^{-1}

None of the compound except benzaldehyde produces same IR spectra as shown above.

3. Studying the progress of the reaction

IR spectra of two enatiomeric compounds are identical. So IR spectroscopy fails to distinguish between enantiomers. Progress of chemical reaction can be determined by examining the small portion of the reaction mixture withdrawn from time to time. The rate of disappearance of a characteristic absorption band of the reactant group and/or the rate of appearance of the characteristic absorption band of the product group due to formation of product can be observed to monitor the progress of reaction.

4. Detection of impurities

IR spectrum of the test sample to be determined is compared with the standard compound. If any additional peaks are observed in the IR spectrum, then it may be due to impurities present in the compound.

5. Quantitative analysis

The quantity of the substance can be determined either in pure form or as a mixture of two or more compounds. In this, characteristic peak corresponding to the drug substance is chosen and log I_0. It of peaks for standard and test sample is compared. This is called base line technique to determine the quantity of the substance.

6. Identification of polymorphs

Drug polymorphism, where materials exhibit a different crystal structure while the chemical composition remains unchanged, is a very important phenomenon with a large number of Pharmaceutical substances. The selection of polymorph is important for getting appropriate solubility and dissolution for ideal pharmaceutical formulation. Familiar examples of polymorphic materials are diamond and graphite, which are both polymorphs of carbon. But while these polymorphs differ greatly, for instance in color and hardness, others are not always that easy to distinguish. It is often difficult to differentiate between pharmaceutical polymorphs, where sometimes the only reliable technique is x-ray crystallography. However, sometime it is a potentially hazardous due to the ionising nature of x-ray radiation. IR spectroscopy is a technique with enormous potential, which could provide a rapid and intrinsically safe alternative for polymorph identification. **DRIFT** technique is suitable for polymorph identification. The Fig. 4.14 shows the differences in IR spectra of some polymorphs e.g. (a) carbamazepine, (b) Enalapril maleate, (c) Sulphathiazole.

7. Study of Isotope effects

The different isotopes in a particular species may give fine detail in infrared spectroscopy. For example, the O–O stretching frequency of oxyhemocyanin is experimentally determined to be 832 and 788 cm^{-1} for $v(^{16}O-^{16}O)$ and $v(^{18}O-^{18}O)$ respectively.

By considering the O–O as a spring, the wavelength of absorbance, v can be calculated:

$$v = \frac{1}{2\pi}\sqrt{\frac{k}{\mu}}$$

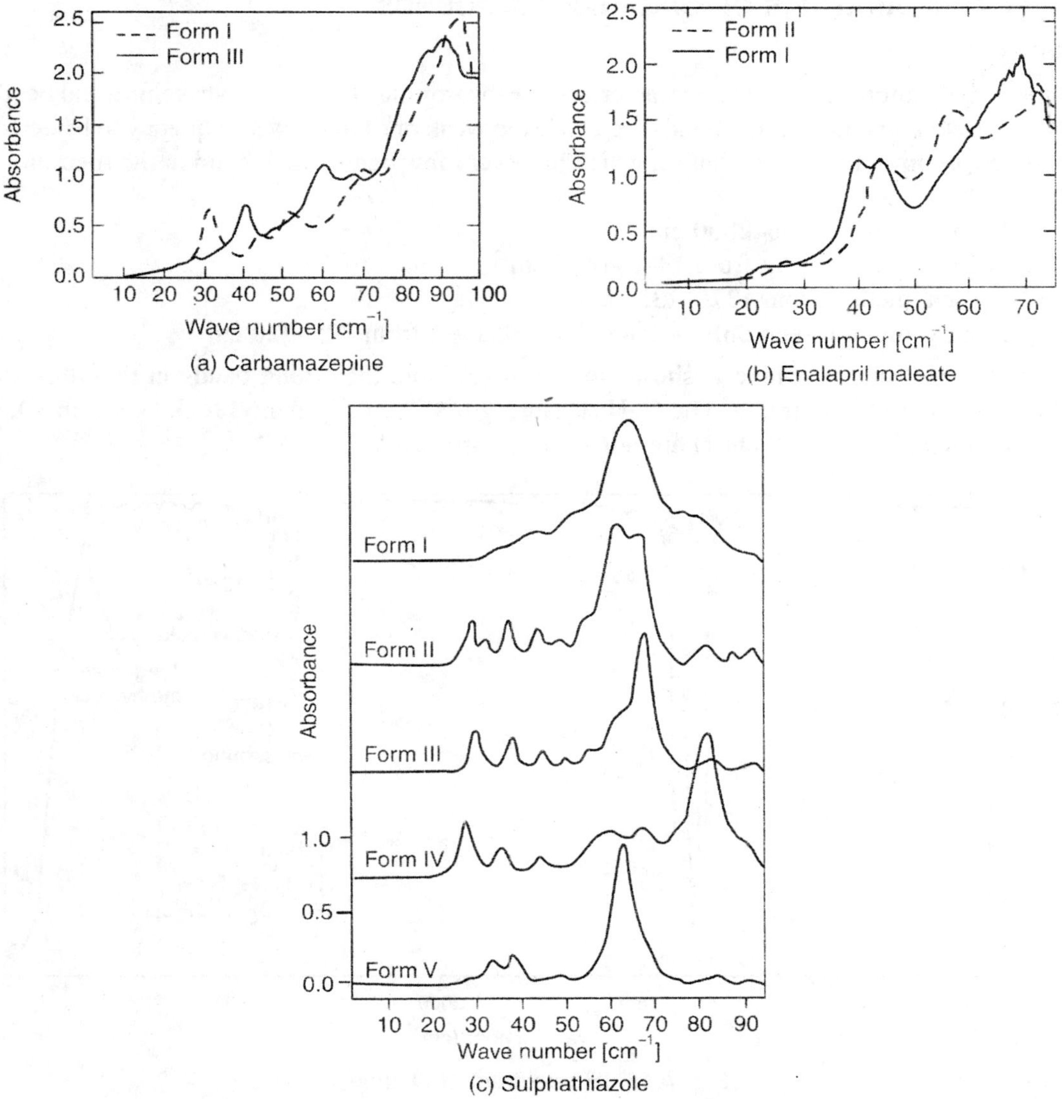

Fig. 4.14. IR spectra of some polymorphs (a) Carbamazepine, (b) Enalapril maleate, (c) Sulphathiazole.

where k is the spring constant for the bond, and m is the reduced mass of the A-B system:

$$\mu = \frac{m_A m_B}{m_A + m_B}$$

(m_i is the mass of atom i).

The reduced masses for $^{16}O-^{16}O$ and $^{18}O-^{18}O$ can be approximated as 8 and 9 respectively. Thus,

$$\frac{v^{16}O}{v^{16}O} = \sqrt{\frac{9}{8}} \approx \frac{832}{788}$$

IR SPECTRAL ANALYSIS OF ORGANIC COMPOUNDS

Alkanes

The spectra of simple alkanes are characterized by absorptions due to C–H stretching and bending (the C–C stretching and bending bonds are either too weak or of too low a frequency to be detected in IR spectroscopy). In simple alkanes, which have very few bands, each bond in the spectrum can be assigned.

- C–H stretch from 3000–2850 cm^{-1}
- C–H bend or scissoring from 1470–1450 cm^{-1}
- C–H rock, methyl from 1370–1350 cm^{-1}
- C–H rock, methyl, seen only in long chain alkanes, from 725–720 cm^{-1}

The IR spectrum of octane is shown in Fig. 4.15. Note the strong bands in the 3000–2850 cm^{-1} region due to C–H stretch. The C–H scissoring (1470 cm^{-1}), methyl rock (1383 cm^{-1}), and long-chain methyl rock (728 cm^{-1}) are noted in this spectrum.

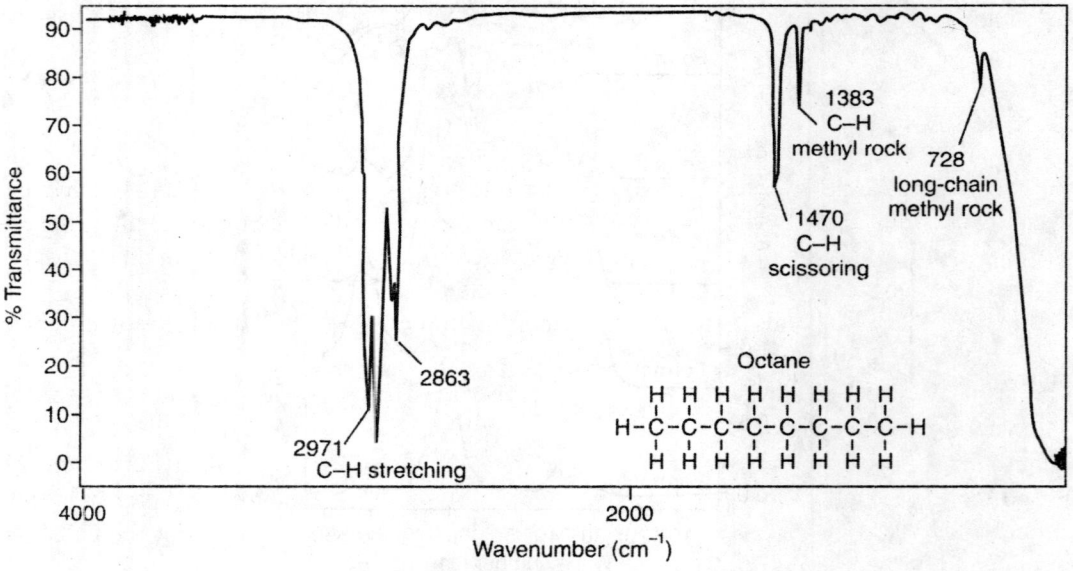

Fig. 4.15. IR spectrum of Octane.

Alkenes

Alkenes are compounds that have a carbon-carbon double bond, –C=C–. The stretching vibration of the C=C bond usually gives rise to a moderate band in the region 1680–1640 cm^{-1}. Stretching vibrations of the –C=C–H bond are of higher frequency (higher wavenumber) than those of the –C–C–H bond in alkanes.

The IR spectrum of 1-octene is shown in Fig. 4.16. Note the band greater than 3000 cm^{-1} for the =C–H stretch and the several bands lower than 3000 cm^{-1} for –C–H stretch (alkanes). The C=C stretch band is at 1644 cm^{-1}. Bands for C–H scissoring (1465 cm^{-1}) and methyl rock (1378 cm^{-1}) are marked in this spectrum.

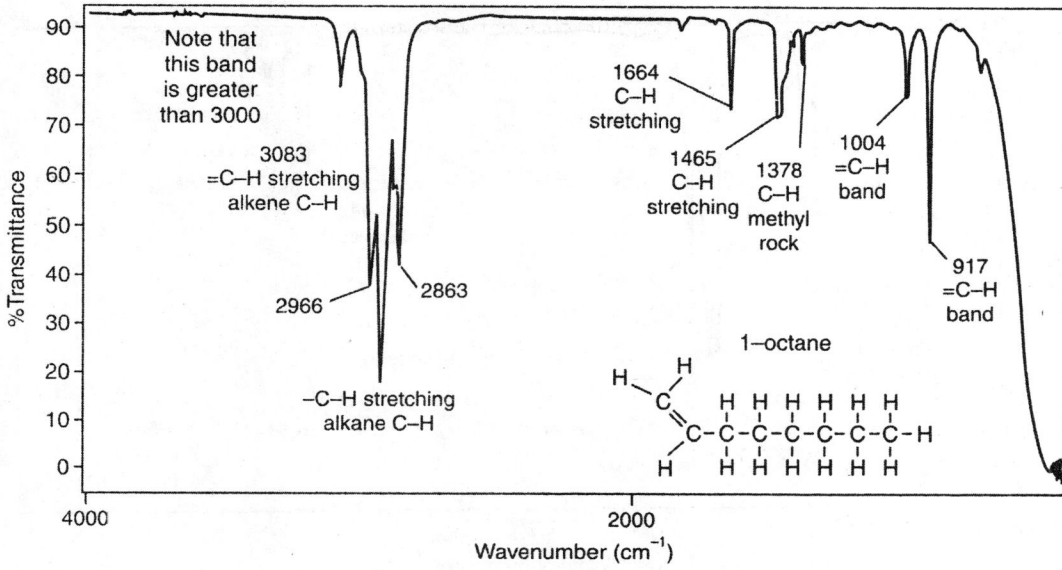

Fig. 4.16. IR spectrum of 1-Octene.

Alkynes

Alkynes are compounds that have a carbon-carbon triple bond (–C≡C–). The –C≡C– stretch appears as a weak band from 2260–2100 cm^{-1}. This can be an important diagnostic tool because very few organic compounds show an absorption in this region. A terminal alkyne (but not an internal alkyne) will show a C–H stretch as a strong, narrow band in the range 3330–3270 cm^{-1}. (Often this band is indistinguishable from bands resulting from other functional groups on the same molecule which absorb in this region, such as the O–H stretch.)

A terminal alkyne will show a C–H bending vibration in the region 700–610 cm^{-1}. The spectrum of 1-hexyne, a terminal alkyne, is shown in Fig. 4.17. Note the C–H stretch of the C–H bond adjacent to the carbon-carbon triple bond (3324 cm^{-1}), the carbon-carbon triple bond stretch (2126 cm^{-1}) and the C–H bend of the C–H bond adjacent to the carbon-carbon triple bond (636 cm^{-1}). The other bands noted are C–H stretch, scissoring, and methyl rock bands from the alkane portions of the molecule.

Aromatics

The =C–H stretch in aromatics is observed at 3100–3000 cm^{-1}. This appears slightly at higher frequency than is the –C–H stretch in alkanes. This is a very useful tool for interpreting IR spectra. Only alkenes and aromatics show a C–H stretch slightly higher than 3000 cm^{-1}. Compounds that do not have a C=C bond show C–H stretches only below 3000 cm^{-1}.

Aromatic hydrocarbons show absorptions in the region 1600–1585 cm^{-1} and 1500–1400 cm^{-1} due to carbon-carbon stretching vibrations in the aromatic ring. Bands in the region 1250–1000 cm^{-1} are due to C–H in-plane bending, although these bands are too weak to be observed in most aromatic compounds. Besides the C–H stretch above 3000 cm^{-1}, two other regions of the

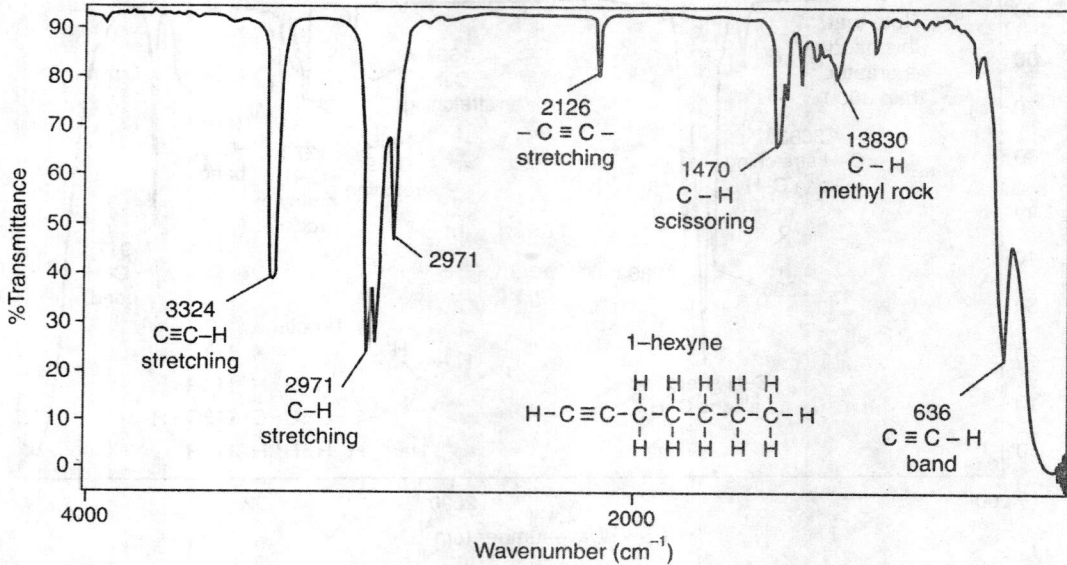

Fig. 4.17. IR spectrum of 1-Hexyne.

infrared spectra of aromatics distinguish aromatics from organic compounds that do not have an aromatic ring:

- 2000–1665 cm^{-1} (weak bands known as "overtones").
- 900–675 cm^{-1} (out-of-plane).

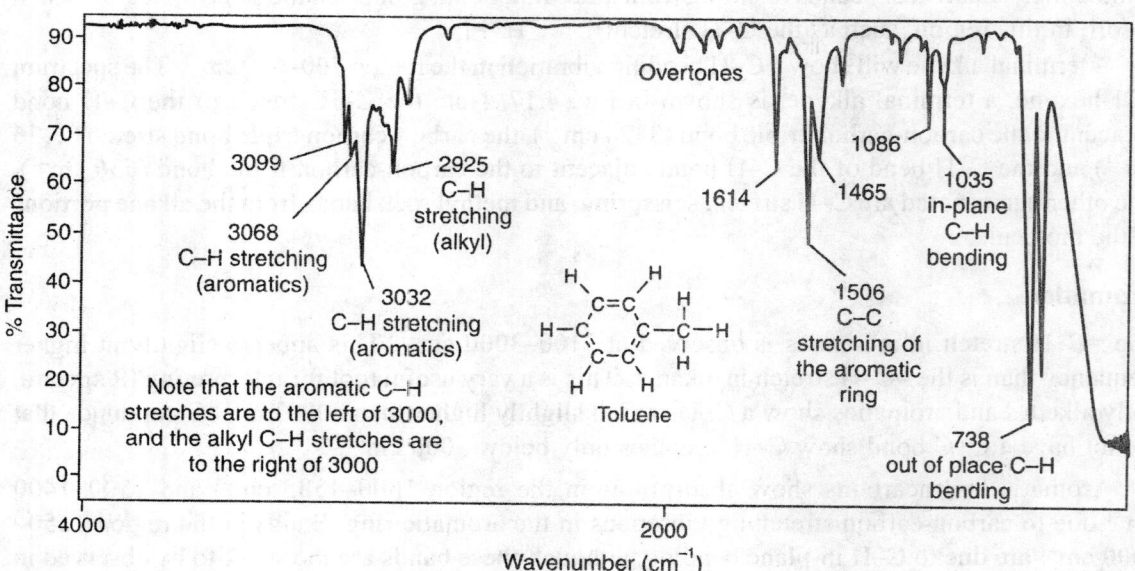

Fig. 4.18. IR spectrum of Toluene.

The spectrum of toluene is shown in Fig. 4.18. Note the =C–H stretches of aromatics (3099, 3068, 3032) and the –C–H stretches of the alkyl (methyl) group (2925 is the only one marked). The characteristic overtones are seen from about 2000–1665 cm^{-1}. Also note the carbon-carbon stretches in the aromatic ring (1614, 1506, 1465 cm^{-1}), the in-plane C–H bending (1086, 1035 cm^{-1}), and the C–H out of plane (738 cm^{-1}).

Alcohols

These have characteristic IR absorptions associated with both the O–H and the C–O stretching vibrations. When run as a thin liquid film, or "neat", the O–H stretch of alcohols appears in the region 3500–3200 cm^{-1} and is a very intense, broad band. The C–O stretch shows up in the region 1260–1050 cm^{-1}.
- O–H stretch, hydrogen bonded 3500–3200 cm^{-1}.
- C–O stretch 1260–1050 cm^{-1} (s).

The spectrum of ethanol is shown in Fig. 4.19. Note the very broad, strong band of the O–H stretch (3391 cm^{-1}) and the C–O stretches (1102, 1055 cm^{-1}).

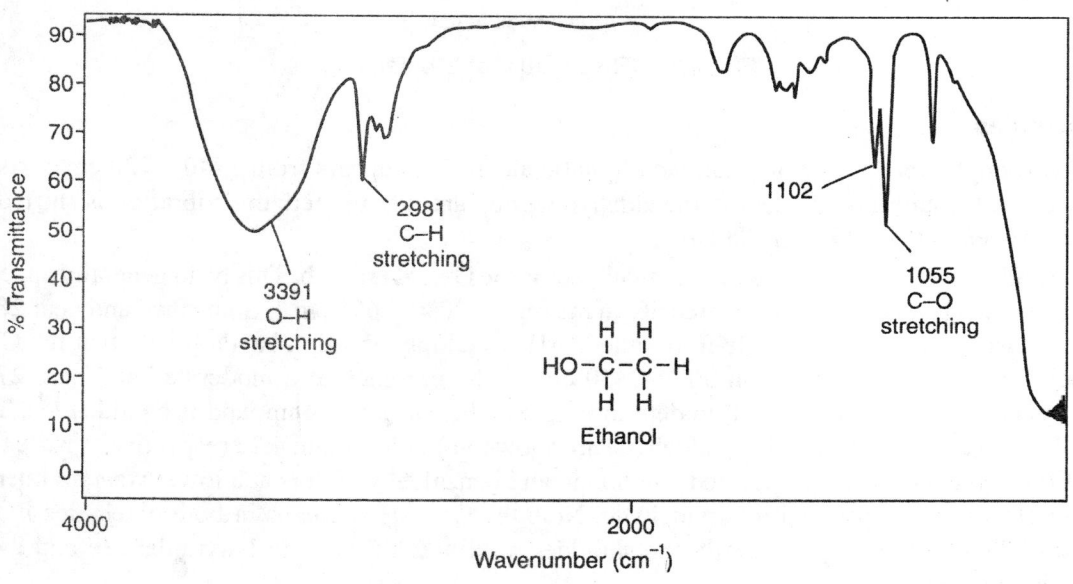

Fig. 4.19. IR spectrum of Ethanol.

Carbonyl compounds

The carbonyl stretching vibration band C=O of saturated aliphatic ketones appears at 1715 cm^{-1}. Conjugation of the carbonyl group with carbon-carbon double bonds or phenyl groups, as in α, β-unsaturated aldehydes and benzaldehyde, shifts this band to lower wavenumbers, 1685–1666 cm^{-1}. The spectrum of 2-butanone is shown in Fig. 4.20. This is a saturated ketone, and the C=O band appears at 1715 cm^{-1}. Note the C–H stretches (around 2991 cm^{-1}) of alkyl groups. It is usually not necessary to mark any of the bands in the fingerprint region (less than 1500 cm^{-1}).

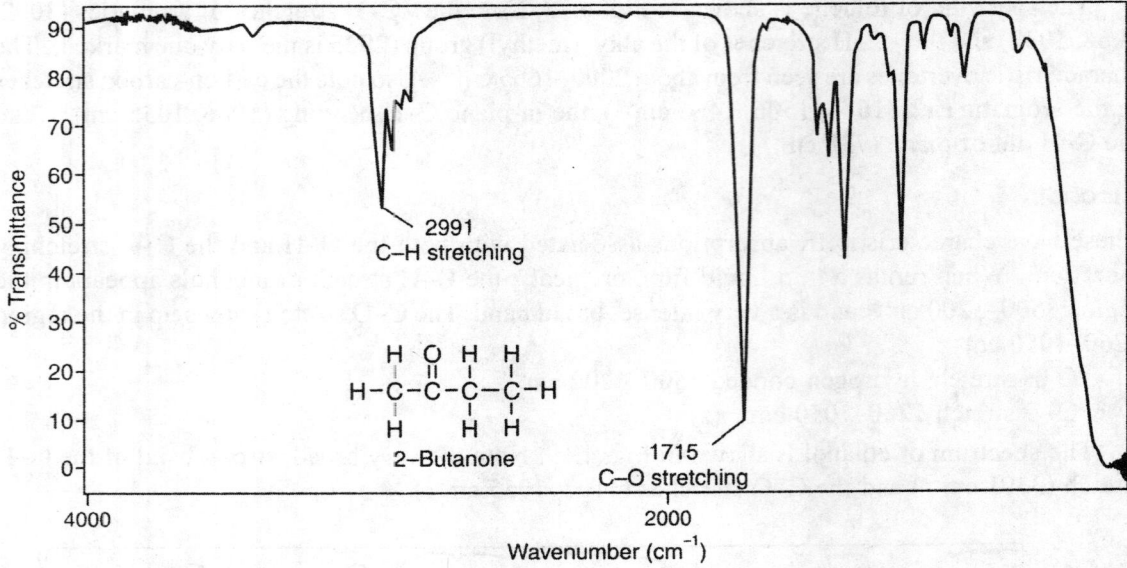

Fig. 4.20. IR spectrum of 2-Butanone.

Aldehydes

The carbonyl stretch C=O of saturated aliphatic aldehydes appears from 1740–1720 cm^{-1}. As in ketones, if the carbons adjacent to the aldehyde group are unsaturated, this vibration is shifted to lower wavenumbers, 1710–1685 cm^{-1}.

Another useful diagnostic band for aldehydes is the O=C–H stretch. This band generally appears as one or two bands of moderate intensity in the region 2830–2695 cm^{-1}. Since the band near 2830 cm^{-1} is usually indistinguishable from other C–H stretching vibration bands (recall that the C–H streches of alkanes appear from 3000–2850 cm^{-1}), the presence of a moderate band near 2720 cm^{-1} is more likely to be helpful in determining whether or not a compound is an aldehyde. The spectra of benzaldehyde and butyraldehyde are shown in Fig. 4.21 and 4.22 respectively. Note that the O=C stretch of α, β-unsaturated compound and benzaldehyde. It is at a lower wavenumber in comparison to the saturated butyraldehyde. Note the O=C–H stretches in both aldehydes in the region 2830–2695 cm^{-1}, especially the shoulder peak at 2725 cm^{-1} in butyraldehyde and 2745 cm^{-1} in benzaldehyde.

Carboxylic acids

These show a strong, wide band for the O–H stretch. Unlike the O–H stretch band observed in alcohols, the carboxylic acid O–H stretch appears as a very broad band in the region 3300–2500 cm^{-1}, centered at about 3000 cm^{-1}. This is in the same region as the C–H stretching bands of both alkyl and aromatic groups. Thus a carboxylic acid shows a somewhat "messy" absorption pattern in the region 3300–2500 cm^{-1}, with the broad O–H band superimposed on the sharp C–H stretching bands. The reason that the O–H stretch band of carboxylic acids is so broad is because carboxylic acids usually exist as hydrogen-bonded dimers.

Infrared Spectroscopy 103

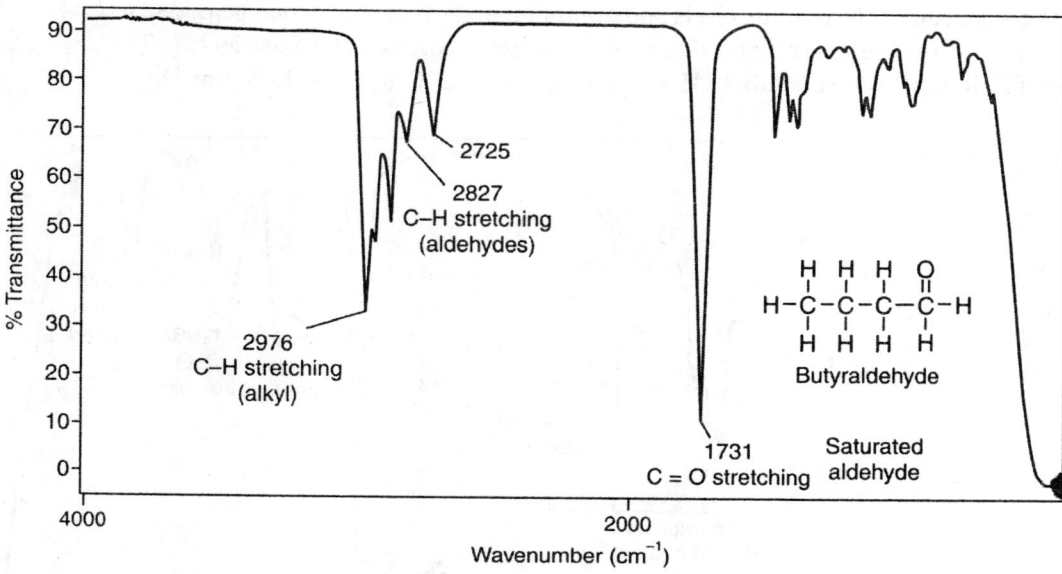

Fig. 4.21. IR spectrum of Butyraldehyde.

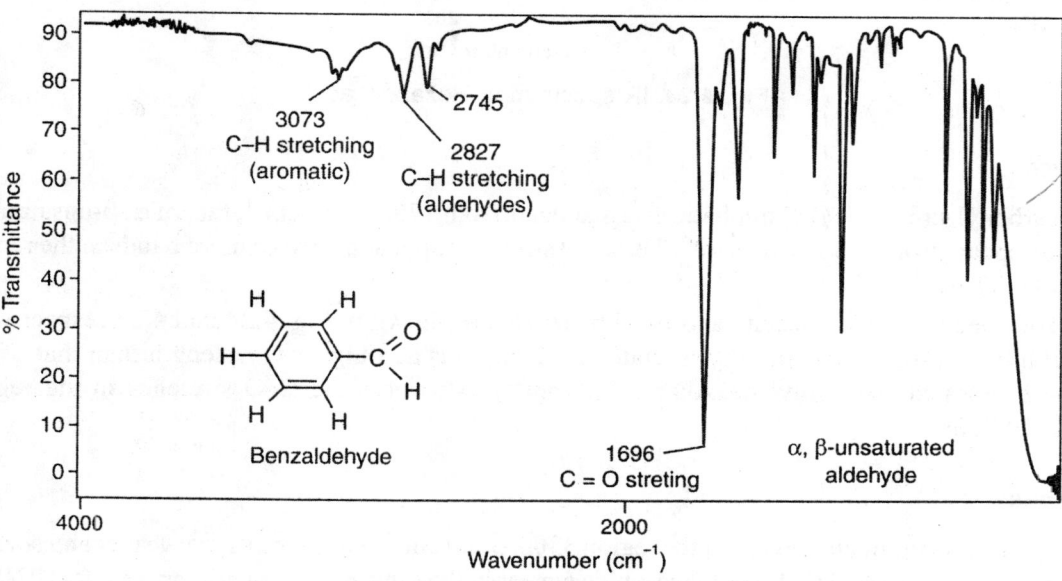

Fig. 4.22. IR spectrum of Benzaldehyde.

The carbonyl stretch C=O of a carboxylic acid appears as an intense band from 1760–1690 cm^{-1}. The exact position of this broad band depends on whether the carboxylic acid is saturated or unsaturated, dimerized, or has internal hydrogen bonding. The C–O stretch appears in the region 1320–1210 cm^{-1}, and the O–H bend is in the region 1440–1395 cm^{-1} and 950–910 cm^{-1}, although the 1440–1395 cm^{-1} band may not be distinguishable from C–H bending bands in the same region.

104 Pharmaceutical Analysis

The spectrum of hexanoic acid is shown in Fig. 4.23. Note the broad peak due to O–H stretch superimposed on the sharp band due to C–H stretch. Note the C=O stretch (1721 cm^{-1}), C–O stretch (1296 cm^{-1}, O–H bends (1419, 948 cm^{-1}), and C–O stretch (1296 cm^{-1}).

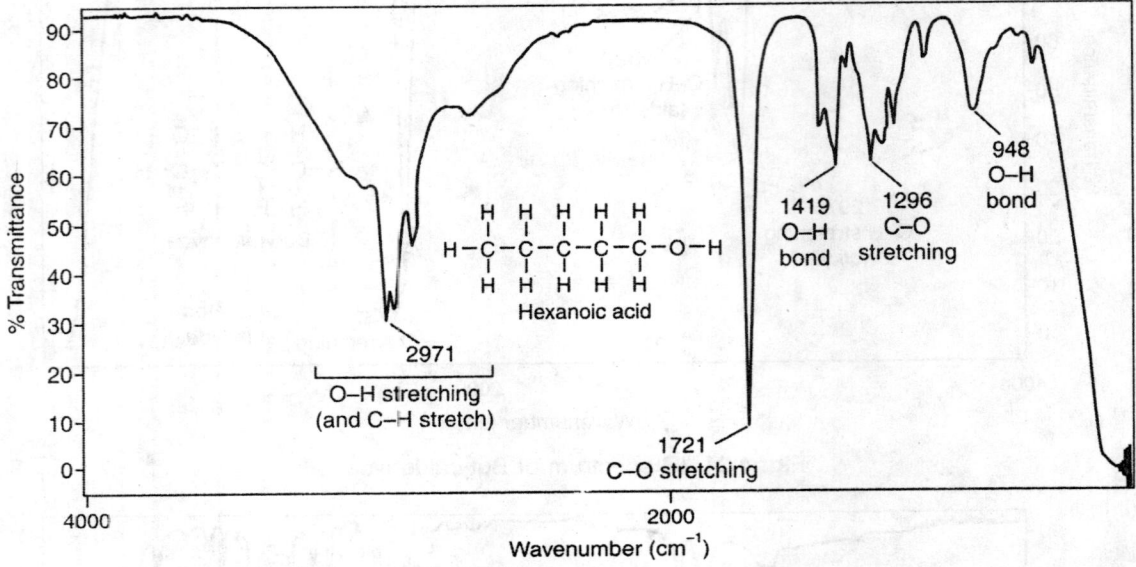

Fig. 4.23. IR Spectrum of Hexanoic acid.

Esters

The carbonyl stretch C=O of aliphatic esters appears from 1750–1735 cm^{-1}; that of α, β-unsaturated esters appears from 1730–1715 cm^{-1}. The C–O stretches appear as two or more bands in the region 1300–1000 cm^{-1}.

The spectra of ethyl acetate and ethyl benzoate are shown in Fig. 4.24 and 4.25 respectively. Note that the C=O stretch of ethyl acetate (1752 cm^{-1}) is at a higher wavelength than that of the α, β-unsaturated ester ethyl benzoate (1726 cm^{-1}). Also note the C–O stretches in the region 1300–1000 cm^{-1}.

Amines

The N–H stretches of amines are in the region 3300–3000 cm^{-1}. These bands are weaker and sharper than those of the alcohol O–H stretches which appear in the same region. In primary amines (RNH$_2$), there are two bands in this region, the asymmetrical N–H stretch and the symmetrical N–H stretch.

Asymmetric N–H stretch, higher wavenumber

Symmetric N–H stretch, lower wavenumber

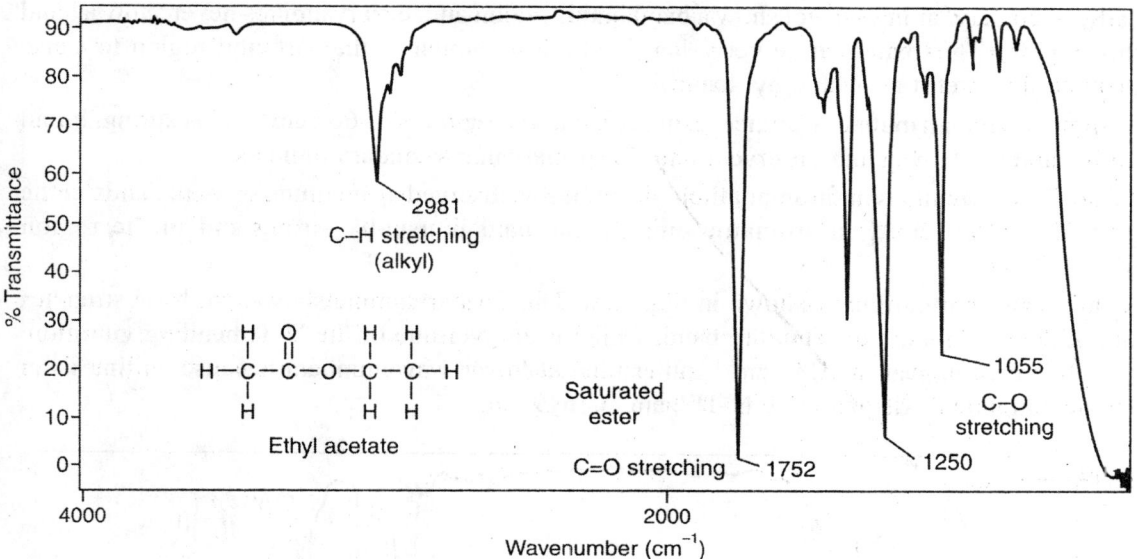

Fig. 4.24. IR spectrum of Ethyl acetate.

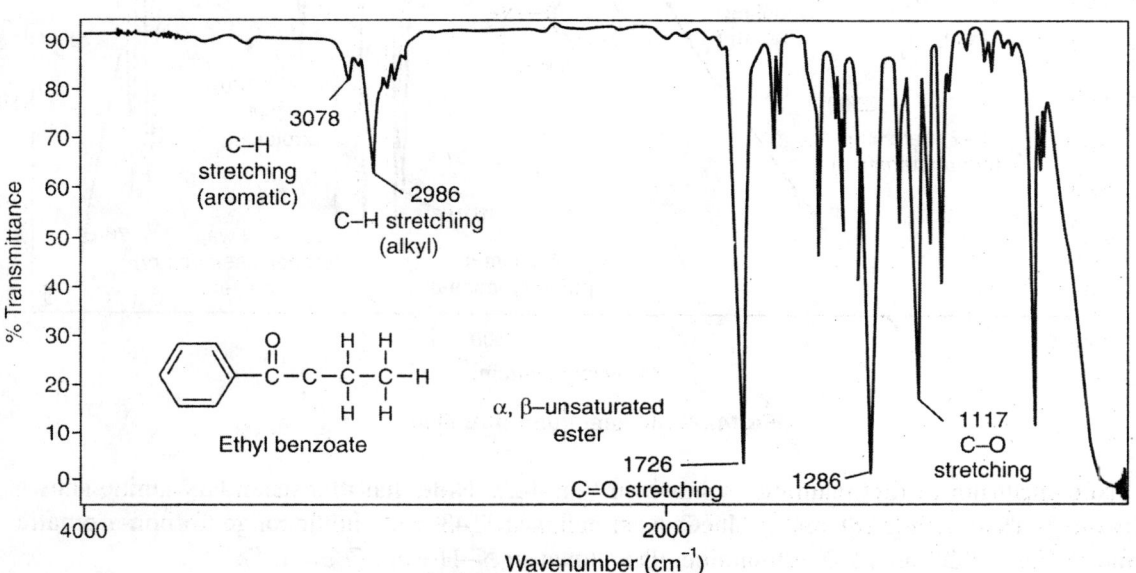

Fig. 4.25. IR spectrum of Ethyl benzoate.

Secondary amines (R_2NH) show only a single weak band in the 3300–3000 cm^{-1} region, since they have only one N–H bond. Tertiary amines (R_3N) do not show any band in this region since they do not have an N–H bond.

The N–H bending vibration of primary amines is observed in the region 1650–1580 cm^{-1}.

Usually, secondary amines do not show a band in this region and tertiary amines never show a band in this region. (This band can be very sharp and close enough to the carbonyl region to cause students to interpret it as a carbonyl band.)

Another band attributed to amines is observed in the region 910–665 cm^{-1}. This strong, broad band is due to N–H wag and observed only for primary and secondary amines.

The C–N stretching vibration of aliphatic amines is observed as medium or weak bands in the region 1250–1020 cm^{-1}. In aromatic amines, the band is usually strong and in the region 1335–1250 cm^{-1}.

The spectrum of aniline is shown in Fig. 4.26. This primary amine shows two N–H stretches (3442, 3360 cm^{-1}); note the shoulder band, which is an overtone of the N–H bending vibration. The C–N stretch appear at 1281 cm^{-1} rather than at lower wavenumbers because aniline is an aromatic compound. Also note the N–H bend at 1619 cm^{-1}.

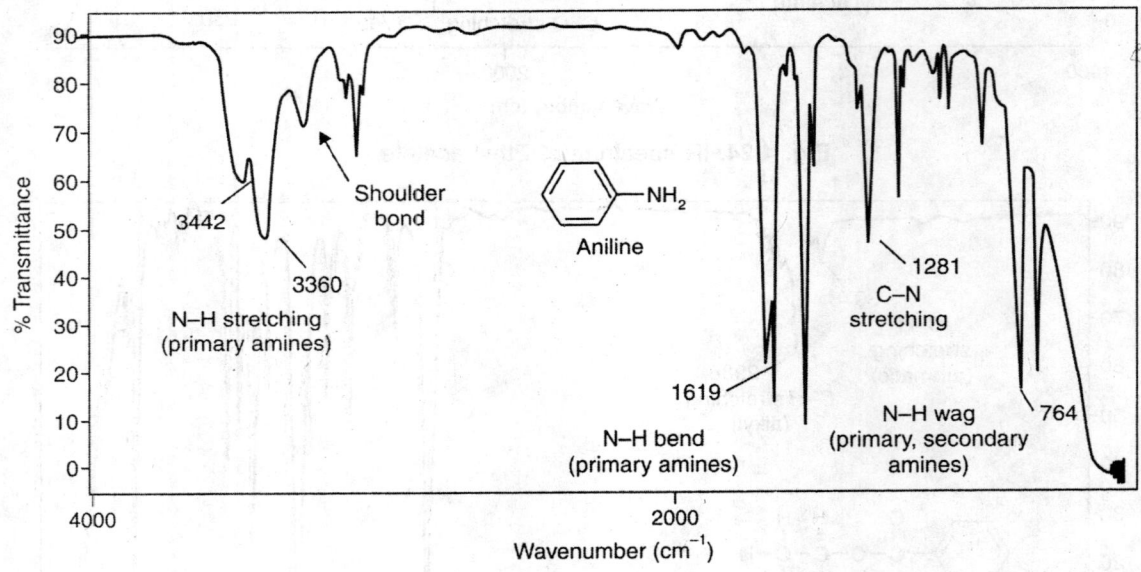

Fig. 4.26. IR spectrum of Aniline.

The spectrum of diethylamine is shown in Fig. 4.27. Note that this secondary amine shows only one N–H stretch (3288 cm^{-1}). The C–N stretch is at 1143 cm^{-1}, in the range for non-aromatic amines (1250–1020 cm^{-1}). Diethylamine also shows an N–H wag (733 cm^{-1}).

Trietylamine (Fig. 4.28) is a tertiary amine and does not have an N–H stretch, nor an N–H wag. The C–N stretch is at 1214 cm^{-1} (non-aromatic).

Nitro compounds

The N–O stretching vibrations In nitroalkanes occur near 1550 cm^{-1} (asymmetrical) and 1365 cm^{-1} (symmetrical), the band at 1550 cm^{-1} being the stronger of the two. If the nitro group is

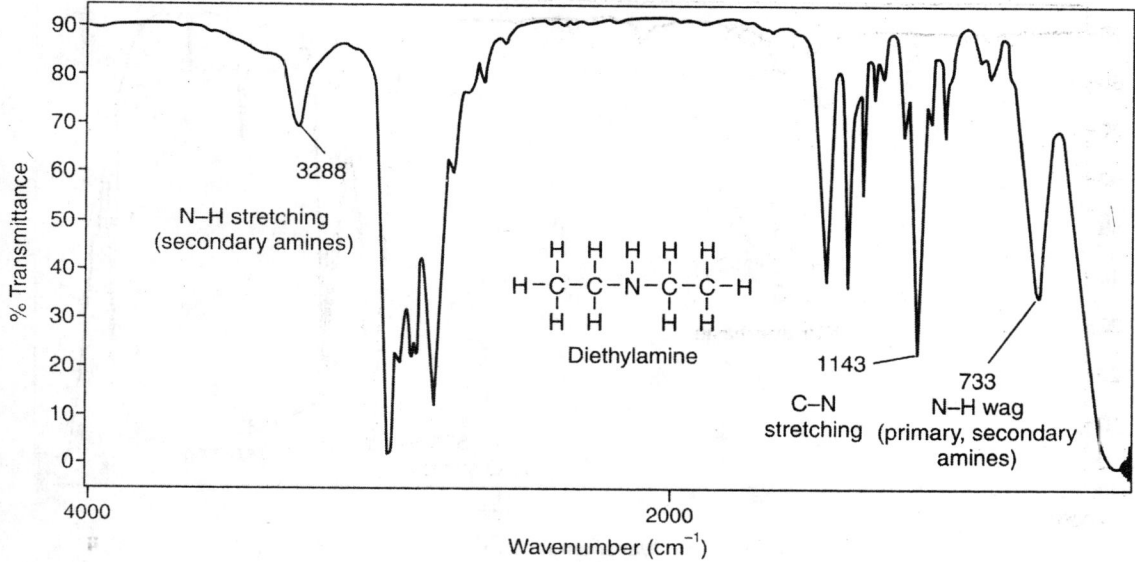

Fig. 4.27. IR spectrum of Diethylamine.

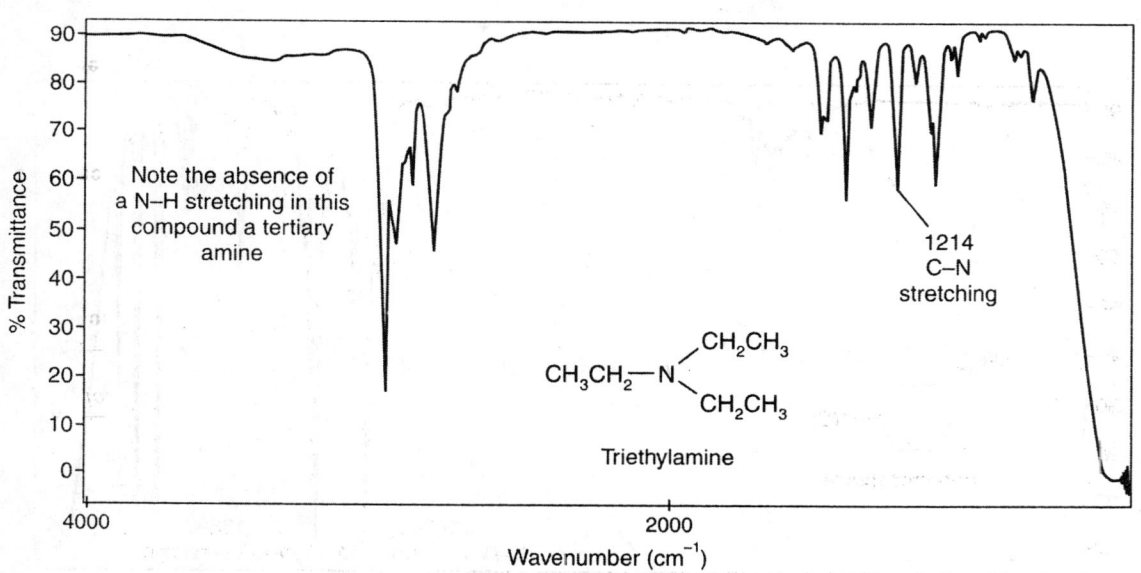

Fig. 4.28. IR spectrum of Triethylamine.

attached to an aromatic ring, the N–O stretching bands shift to down to slightly lower wavenumbers: 1550–1475 cm^{-1} and 1360–1290 cm^{-1}.

Compare the spectra of nitromethane (Fig. 4.29) and *m*-nitrotoluene (Fig. 4.30), below. In nitromethane, the N–O stretches are at 1573 and 1383 cm^{-1}, while in nitrotoluene, they are a little more to the right, at 1537 and 1358 cm^{-1}.

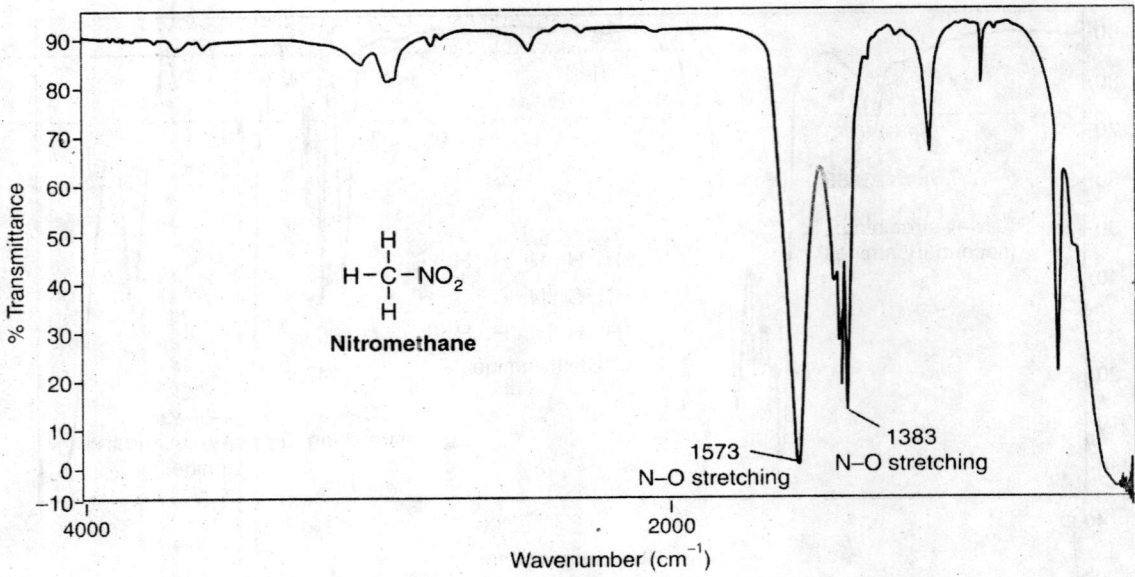

Fig. 4.29. IR spectrum of Nitromethane.

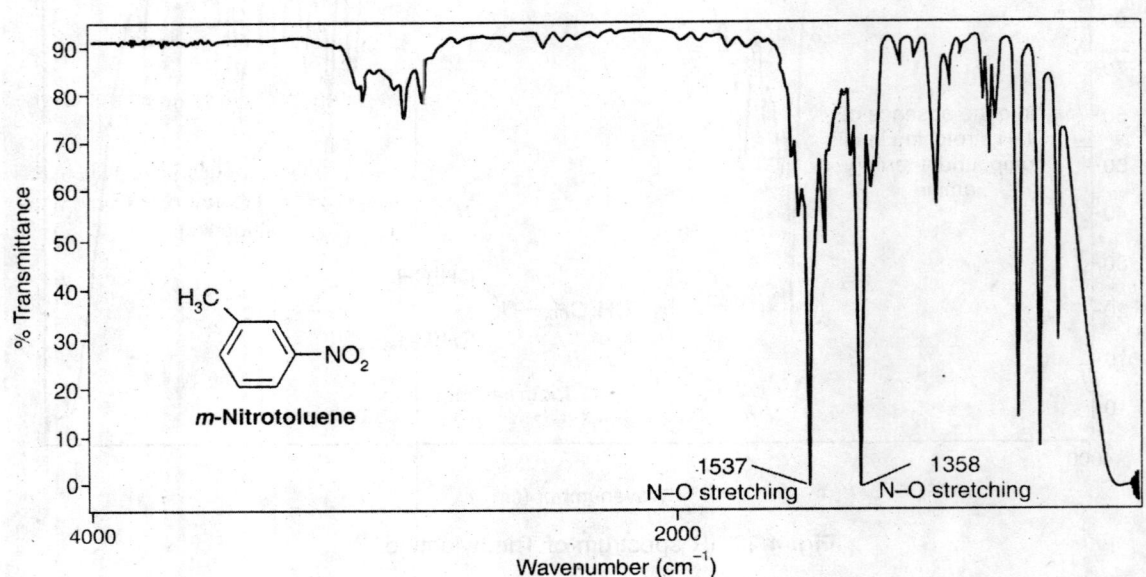

Fig. 4.30. IR spectrum of *m*-Nitrotoluene.

Table 4.1. Characteristic IR absorption frequencies of organic functional groups

Functional group	Types of vibration	Characteristic absorptions (cm^{-1})	Intensity
Alcohol			
O–H	Stretch, H-bonded	3200–3600	Strong, broad
O–H	Stretch, free	3500–3700	Strong, sharp
C–O	Stretch	1050–1150	Strong
Alkane			
C–H	Stretch	2850–3000	Strong
–C–H	Bending	1350–1480	Variable
Alkene			
=C–H	Stretch	3010–3100	Medium
=C–H	Bending	675–1000	Strong
C=C	Stretch	1620–1680	Variable
Alkyl halide			
C–F	Stretch	1000–1400	Strong
C–Cl	Stretch	600–800	Strong
C–Br	Stretch	500–600	Strong
C–I	Stretch	500	Strong
Alkyne			
C–H	Stretch	3300	Strong, sharp
–C≡C–	Stretch	2100–2260	Variable, not present in symmetrical alkynes
Amine			
N–H	Stretch	3300–3500	Medium (primary amines have two bands; secondary have one band, often very weak)
C–N	Stretch	1080–1360	Medium-weak
N–H	Bending	1600	Medium
Aromatic			
C–H	Stretch	3000–3100	Medium
C=C	Stretch	1400–1600	Medium-weak, multiple band
Analysis of C–H out-of-plane bending can often distinguish substitution patterns			
Ether			
C–O	Stretch	1000–1300 (1070–1150)	Strong
Nitrile			
CN	Stretch	2210–2260	Medium
Nitro			
N–O	Stretch	1515–1560 and 1345–1385	Strong, two bands

(Contd.)

IR Absorption frequencies of functional groups containing a carbonyl (C=O)

Functional group	Types of vibration	Characteristic absorptions (cm^{-1})	Intensity
Carbonyl			
C=O	Stretch	1670–1820	Strong
		(conjugation moves absorptions to lower wave numbers)	
Acid			
C=O	Stretch	1700–1725	Strong
O–H	Stretch	2500–3300	Strong, very broad
C–O	Stretch	1210–1320	Strong
Aldehyde			
C=O	Stretch	1740–1720	Strong
=C–H	Stretch	2820–2850 and 2720–2750	Medium, two peaks
Amide			
C=O	Stretch	1640–1690	Strong
N–H	Stretch	3100–3500	Unsubstituted have two bands
N–H	Bending	1550–1640	
Anhydride			
C=O	Stretch	1800–1830 and 1740–1775	Two bands
Ester			
C=O	Stretch	1735–1750	Strong
C–O	Stretch	1000–1300	Two bands or more
Ketone			
Acyclic	Stretch	1705–1725	Strong
		3-membered - 1850	
		4-membered - 1780	
		5-membered - 1745	Strong
		6-membered - 1715	
		7-membered - 1705	
α, β-unsaturated	Stretch	1665–1685	Strong
Aryl ketone	Stretch	1680–1700	Strong

CHAPTER 5

NMR Spectroscopy

INTRODUCTION

Over the past five decades, nuclear magnetic resonance spectroscopy, commonly referred to as NMR, has become the prominent technique for determining the structure of organic compounds. Of all the spectroscopic methods, it is the only one by which a complete analysis and interpretation of the entire spectrum is normally expected. Although larger amounts of sample are needed than for mass spectrometry, NMR technique is non-destructive, and with modern instruments, good data may be obtained from samples weighing less than few milligram. To be successful in using NMR as an analytical tool, it is necessary to understand the physical principles on which this method is based.

NUCLEAR SPIN AND THE SPLITTING OF ENERGY LEVELS IN A MAGNETIC FIELD

Subatomic particles (electrons, protons and neutrons) can be imagined as spinning on their axes. In many atoms (such as ^{12}C), these spins are paired against each other, such that the nucleus of the atom has no overall spin (I = 0). However, in some atoms (such as ^1H and ^{13}C) the nucleus does possess an overall spin. The rules for determining the net spin of a nucleus are as follows:

(a) If the number of neutrons and the number of protons are both even, then the nucleus has no spin.
(b) If the number of neutrons plus the number of protons is odd, then the nucleus has a half-integer spin (i.e. 1/2, 3/2, 5/2).
(c) If the number of neutrons and the number of protons are both odd, then the nucleus has an integer spin (i.e. 1, 2, 3).

The overall spin, I, is important. Quantum mechanics tells us that a nucleus of spin I will have $2I + 1$ possible orientations. A nucleus with spin 1/2 will have 2 possible orientations. In the absence of an external magnetic field, these orientations are of equal energy. If a magnetic field is applied, then the energy levels split. Each level is given a *magnetic quantum number, m*.

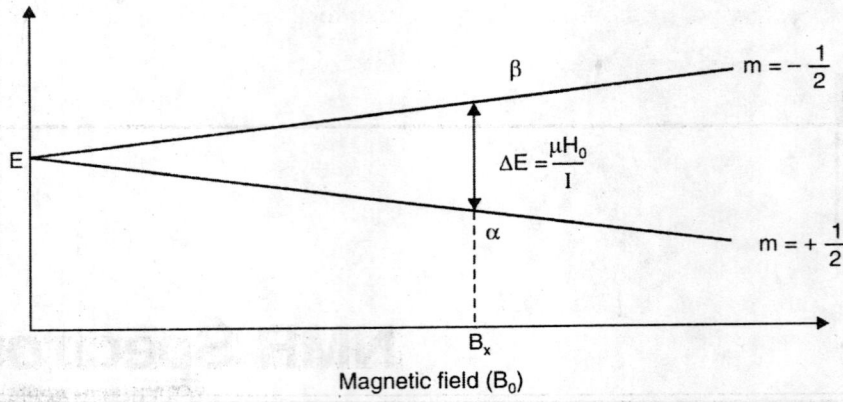

Fig. 5.1. Energy levels for a nucleus with spin quantum number ½.

The magnetic moment of the lower energy +1/2 state (often given the notation α) is aligned with the external field, but that of the higher energy −1/2 spin state (often given the notation β) is opposed to the external field. The difference in energy, ΔE between the two spin states is dependent on the external magnetic field strength, and is always very small. The Fig. 5.1 illustrates that the two spin states have the same energy when the external field is zero, but diverge as the field increases. It is possible to excite these nuclei into the higher level with electromagnetic radiation. The process of excitation is done in NMR spectroscopy. The frequency of radiation needed is determined by the difference in energy between the energy levels.

CALCULATION OF TRANSITION ENERGY

The nucleus has a positive charge and is spinning. This generates a small magnetic field. The nucleus therefore possesses a magnetic moment, μ, which is proportional to its spin, I.

$$\mu = \frac{\gamma I h}{2\pi} \quad ...(5.1)$$

h is Planks constant

The constant, γ, is called the *magnetogyric ratio* and is a fundamental nuclear constant which has a different value for every nucleus. Some characteristic properties of selected nuclei are given in the following Table 5.1.

The energy of a particular energy level is given by:

$$E = \frac{\gamma h}{2\pi} \times H_o \quad ...(5.2)$$

Table 5.1. Some characteristic properties of selected nuclei

Isotope	Natural % abundance	Spin (I)	Magnetic moment (μ)*	Magnetogyric ratio (γ)†
^{1}H	99.9844	1/2	2.7927	26.753
^{2}H	0.0156	1	0.8574	4.107
^{11}B	81.17	3/2	2.6880	–
^{13}C	1.108	1/2	0.7022	6.728
^{17}O	0.037	5/2	−1.8930	−3.628
^{19}F	100.0	1/2	2.6273	25.179
^{29}Si	4.700	1/2	−0.5555	−5.319
^{31}P	100.0	1/2	1.1305	10.840

* μ in unit of nuclear magnetons = $5.05078 \cdot 10^{-27}$ JT^{-1}
† γ is unit of 10^7 rad T^{-1} sec^{-1}

where H_o is the strength of the magnetic field at the nucleus.

The difference in energy between levels (the transition energy) can be found from

$$hv = \Delta E = \frac{\gamma h H_o}{2\pi} \qquad ...(5.3)$$

where v is the frequency.

This means that if the magnetic field, H_o is increased, so is ΔE. It also means that if a nucleus has a relatively large magnetogyric ratio, then ΔE is correspondingly large.

ABSORPTION OF RADIATION BY A NUCLEUS IN A MAGNETIC FIELD

Imagine a nucleus (of spin 1/2) in a magnetic field. This nucleus is in the lower energy level (i.e. its magnetic moment does not oppose the applied field). The nucleus is spinning on its axis (Fig. 5.2). In the presence of a magnetic field, the rotational axis of the spinning nucleus cannot be oriented exactly parallel (or antiparallel) with the direction of applied field, H_o but must precess around the magnetic field at the angle for protons about 54 (Fig. 5.2).

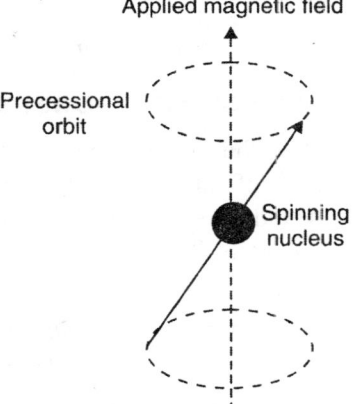

Fig. 5.2. Process of spinning nucleus.

The frequency of precession is termed the *Larmor frequency*, which is identical to the transition frequency.

The potential energy of the precessing nucleus is given by:

$$E = -\mu \, H_o \cos \theta$$

where q is the angle between the direction of the applied field and the axis of nuclear rotation.

If energy is absorbed by the nucleus, then the angle of precession, q, will change. For a nucleus of spin 1/2, absorption of radiation "flips" the magnetic moment so that it opposes the applied field (the higher energy state) (Fig. 5.3).

According to eq. 5.3, how much energy is needed to flip (excite) the proton depends on the strength of external fields, the stronger the field, the greater the tendency to aligned with it and the higher the frequency ($\Delta E = hv$) of the radiation to do the job.

It is important to realise that only a small proportion of "target" nuclei are in the lower energy state (and can absorb radiation). There is the possibility that by exciting these nuclei, the populations of the higher and lower energy levels will become equal. If this occurs, then there will

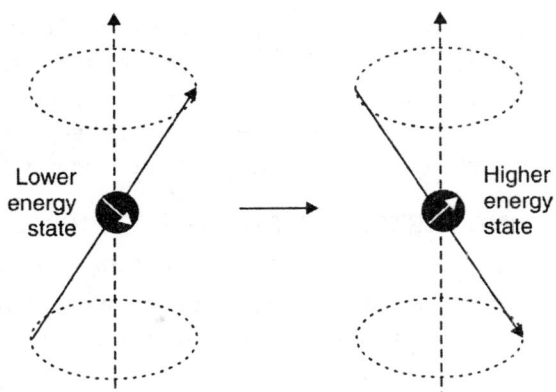

Fig. 5.3. Absorption of energy to change the state of spinning nucleus.

be no further absorption of radiation. The spin system is *saturated*. Then, excited nuclei return to the lower energy state through the relaxation process.

RELAXATION PROCESSES

How the nuclei return to the lower state from the higher energy state? Emission of radiation is insignificant because the probability of re-emission of photons varies with the cube of the frequency. At radio frequencies, re-emission is negligible. The excited nuclei return via non-radiative relaxation processes.

There are two major relaxation processes:
- Spin-lattice (longitudinal) relaxation.
- Spin-spin (transverse) relaxation.

Spin-lattice relaxation

Nuclei in an NMR experiment are in a sample. The sample in which the nuclei are held is called the *lattice*. Nuclei in the lattice are in vibrational and rotational motion, which creates a complex magnetic field. The magnetic field caused by motion of nuclei within the lattice is called the *lattice field*. This lattice field has many components. Some of these components will be equal in frequency and phase to the Larmor frequency of the nuclei of interest. These components of the lattice field can interact with nuclei in the higher energy state, and cause them to lose energy (returning to the lower state). The energy that a nucleus loses increases the amount of vibration and rotation within the lattice (resulting in a tiny rise in the temperature of the sample).

The relaxation time, T_1 (the average lifetime of nuclei in the higher energy state) is dependent on the magnetogyric ratio of the nucleus and the mobility of the lattice. As mobility increases, the vibrational and rotational frequencies increase, making it note likely for a component of the lattice field to be able to interact with excited nuclei. However, at extremely high mobilities, the probability of a component of the lattice field being able to interact with excited nuclei decreases.

Spin-spin relaxation

Spin-spin relaxation describes the interaction between neighbouring nuclei with identical precessional frequencies but differing magnetic quantum states. In this situation, the nuclei can exchange quantum states; a nucleus in the lower energy level will be excited, while the excited nucleus relaxes to the lower energy state. There is no net change in the populations of the energy states, but the average lifetime of a nucleus in the excited state will decrease. This can result in line-broadening.

NMR INSTRUMENTATION

There are two general types of NMR instruments (i) continuous wave and (ii) Fourier transform. Early experiments were conducted with continuous wave (C.W.) instruments, and in 1970 the first Fourier transform (F.T.) instruments became available. This type of NMR instrument now dominates the market.

(i) Continuous wave NMR instruments

Continuous wave NMR spectrometers are similar in principle to optical spectrometers. The sample

NMR Spectroscopy 115

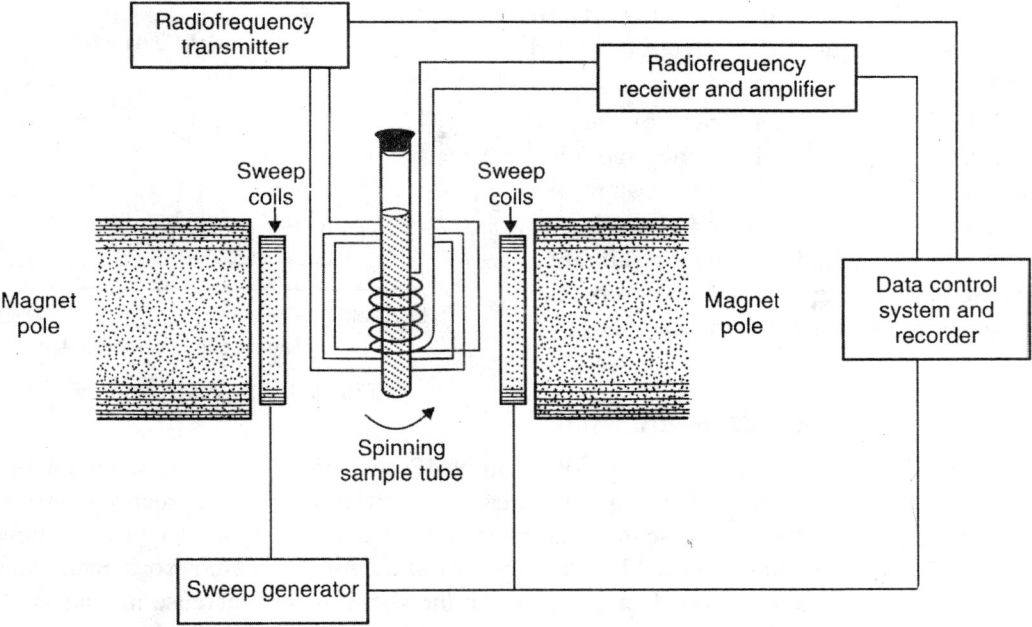

Fig. 5.4. NMR instrumentation.

(in a uniform 5 mm glass tube) is held in a strong magnetic field, and the frequency of the source is slowly scanned (in some instruments, the source frequency is held constant, and the field is scanned). Generally, the instrument (Fig. 5.4) consists of following part:

Magnet

Either a permanent magnet or electromagnet can be employed in NMR to supply magnetic field, H_o. Currently, superconducting magnets cooled in liquid helium are being used in instrument which require high magnetic strength. Since chemical shift is a function of magnetic strength, greater dispersion achieved at a higher magnetic field. In practice, the field is varied over a very small range (about a milligauss).

Radiofrequency oscillator (transmitter)

The rf field is provided by a transmitter coil whose magnetic vector component moves in a plane perpendicular to the direction of H_o. The rf field induces nuclear transition when its frequency equal to angular precessional velocity.

Radiofrequency receiver (detector)

The flipping of nuclei as a result of irradiation induces a voltage in receiving coil.

Recorder

The voltage from the receiving coil is amplified and observed in a recorder. The peaks of an NMR spectrum are result of plotting intensity of absorption vs frequency or strength (field strength).

An NMR spectrum is acquired by varying the frequency of the radiofrequency radiation while holding the external field constant. An equality effective technique is by varying or sweeping the magnetic field over a small range while holding frequency constant to observe the radiofrequency signal from the sample (Fig. 5.5).

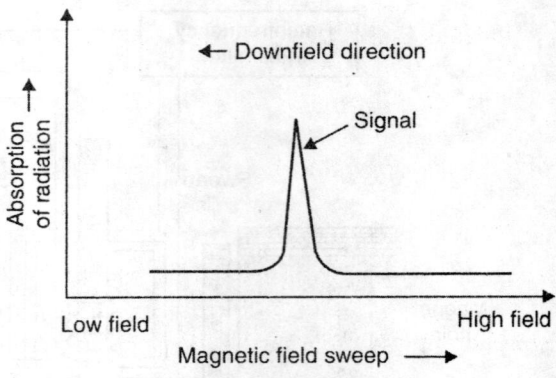

Fig. 5.5. The NMR spectrum.

(ii) Fourier transform NMR instruments

The magnitude of the energy changes involved in NMR spectroscopy is small. This means that sensitivity is a major limitation. One way to increase sensitivity would be to record many spectra, and then add them together; because noise is random, it adds as the square root of the number of spectra recorded. For example, if one hundred spectra of a compound are recorded and summed, then the noise would increase by a factor of ten, but the signal would increase in magnitude by a factor of one hundred - giving a large increase in sensitivity. However, if this is done using a continuous wave instrument, the time needed to collect the spectra is very large (one scan takes two to eight minutes).

In FT-NMR, all frequencies in a spectrum are irradiated simultaneously with a radiofrequency pulse. Following the pulse, the nuclei return to thermal equilibrium. A time domain emission signal is recorded by the instrument as the nuclei relax. A frequency domain spectrum is obtained by Fourier transformation.

NMR SPECTRUM

Theoretically, the situation is NMR spectroscopy looks very simple. All the proton in organic molecule are alike and should absorb at same field strength and the spectrum would consist of single signal. It would tell us little about the structure of the molecule. But the frequency at which proton absorb depend on the actual magnetic field which that proton feels and this effective field strength is not exactly the same as the applied field strength. It means, there is difference in the effective magnetic field and applied magnetic field. The effective field strength at each proton depends on the environment of that proton (the electron density at the proton and the presence of other, nearby protons). Each proton or more precisely, each set of equivalent proton will have a slightly different environment from other set of protons, and hence will require a slightly *different applied* field strength to produce the *same effective* field strength, the particular field strength at which absorption takes place.

In conclusion, *all protons absorb at the same effective field strength, but they absorb at different applied field strengths*. It is this applied field strength that is measured, and against which the absorption is plotted. This plot is called NMR spectrum (Fig. 5.5).

Various aspects of the NMR spectrum, useful to determine molecular structure are as follows:
(a) the *number of signals*
(b) the *position of the signals*
(c) the *intensities of the signals*
(d) the *splitting of a signals*

(a) Number of signals

In a given molecule, protons in the same environment (equivalent proton) absorb at the same (applied) field strength; protons with different environments (non-equivalent protons) absorb at different (applied) field strengths. The number of signals in the NMR spectrum tells us, therefore, how many sets of equivalent protons – how many "kinds" of protons – present in a molecule.

For example, in the undermentioned compound, equivalent protons designated with the same letter. In ethyl chloride, isopropyl chloride and n-propyl chloride, there are two, two and three types of protons respectively; hence two, two and three NMR signals appear in the NMR spectrum:

$$CH_3-CH_2-Cl \qquad CH_3-CHCl-CH_3 \qquad CH_3-CH_2-CH_2-Cl$$
$$a b \qquad a b a \qquad a b c$$

2 NMR signals   2 NMR signals   3 NMR signals
Ethyl chloride   Isopropyl chloride   n-Propyl chloride

In case of ethyl chloride, all the protons of methyl group are equivalent and so give one signal. Similarly, methylene protons gives one signal. The same features are present in isopropyl and n-propyl chloride.

The protons must also be *stereo*-chemically equivalent to show one signal.

```
    a            b           a             b
   H₃C          H           H₃C           H
      \       /                \        /
       C = C                    C = C
      /      \                 /       \
    Br        H              Br         H
              c                          c

  3 NMR signals           3 NMR signals
  2-Bromopropene          Vinyl chloride
```

In 2-bromopropene and and vinyl chloride, these signals are obtained because in both the cases, the protons 'b' and 'c' are not stereochemically equivalent.

Similarly, 1,2-Dichloropropane (optically active or optically inactive) gives four NMR signals.

```
              c
         Cl   H
      3   2|  |1
     CH₃—CH—C—Cl
      a   b  |
             H
             d
```

The environments of the two protons on C-1 position are not the same. These protons are not stereochemistry equivalent, and so absorb at different field strength.

(b) Position of signals (Chemical shift)

The *position of the signals* indicates the kinds of proton. They may be aromatic, aliphatic, primary, secondary, tertiary, benzylic, vinylic, acetylenic, adjacent to halogen or to other atoms or groups. These different kinds of protons have different electronic environments, and it is the electronic environment that determines where a proton absorbs or shows its signal in NMR spectrum.

When a molecule is placed in a magnetic field, its electrons are also caused to circulate and, in circulating, they generate secondary magnetic fields; called *induced* magnetic fields which may either (i) opposes the applied field; the field felt by the proton is thus diminished, and the proton is said to be *shielded*, or (ii) reinforces the applied field, then the field felt by the proton is augmented, and the proton is said to be *deshielded*.

Compared with a naked proton, a shielded proton requires a higher applied field strength and a deshielded proton requires a slower applied field strength to provide the particular effective field strength at which absorption occurs. Shielding thus shifts the absorption upfield, and deshielding shifts the absorption downfield (Fig. 5.6). Such shifts in the position of NMR absorption, arising from shielding and deshielding by electrons, are called *chemical shifts*.

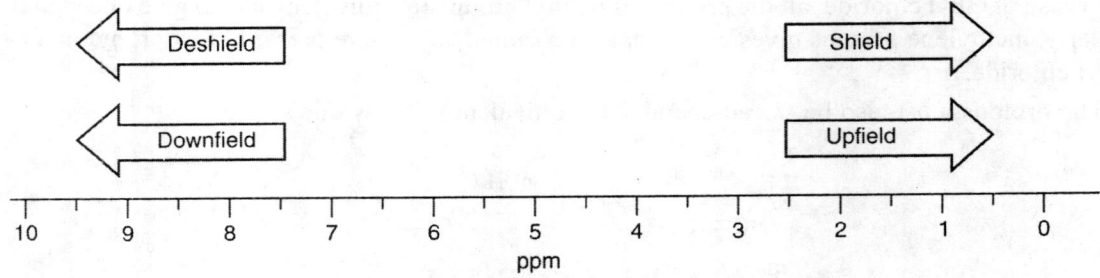

Fig. 5.6. Deshielding and sheilding effect.

Since shielding and deshielding arise from induced secondary fields, the magnitude of a chemical shift is proportional to the strength of the applied field.

The *reference point* from which chemical shifts are measured is, for practical reason, not the signal from a naked proton, but the signal from the actual compound; usually tetramethylsilane (TMS), $(CH_3)_4Si$. Because of the low electronegativity of silicon, the shielding of the protons in the silane is greater than in most other organic molecules; as a result, most NMR signals appear in the same direction from the tetramethylsilane signal: *downfield*. TMS is chemically inert and has a low boiling point and so it can be easily removed from a recoverable sample of valuable organic compound. It is soluble in most organic solvent and can be added to the sample solution (0.01–1.0%) as an internal standard. TMS is not soluble in H_2O or D_2O; for solution in these solvents, the sodium salt of 3-(trimethyl silyl) propane sulphonic acid is used.

The most commonly used scale is the δ (delta) scale. The position of the tetramethylsilane signal is taken as 0 delta value (0.0 ppm). Most of the chemical shifts have δ values between 0 and 10 (minus 10, actually). A small δ value represents a small downfield shift, and a large δ value represents a large downfield shift.

There is another scale, the τ (tau), on which the tetramethyl-silane signal is taken as 10.0 ppm. Most τ values lie between 0 and 10. The two scales are related by the expression τ = 10 − δ. *The chemical shift in absolute terms is defined by the frequency of the resonance expressed with reference to a standard compound which is defined to be at 0 ppm. The scale is made more manageable by expressing it in parts per million (ppm) and is independent of the spectrometer frequency.*

$$\text{Chemical shift, } a = \frac{\text{Frequency of signal} - \text{Frequency of reference}}{\text{Spectrometer frequency}} \times 10^6$$

It is often convenient to describe the relative positions of the resonances in an NMR spectrum. For example, a peak at a chemical shift, δ, of 10 ppm is said to be *downfield* or *deshielded* with respect to a peak at 5 ppm, or if you prefer, the peak at 5 ppm is *upfield* or *shielded* with respect to the peak at 10 ppm. Typical δ/ppm values for protons in different chemical environments are shown in the Table 5.2.

Table 5.2. Characteristic proton chemical shifts

Types of protons		Chemical shift, δ
Cyclopropane	△	0.2
Primary	RCH_3	0.9
Secondary	R_2CH_2	1.3
Tertiary	R_3CH	1.5
Vinylic	C = C–H	4.6–5.9
Acetylenic	C = C–H	2–3
Aromatic	Ar–H	6–8.5
Benzylic	Ar–CH_3 or CH_2	2.2–3
Allylic	C = C–CH_3	1.7
Fluorides	H_3C–F	4–4.5
Chlorides	H_3C–Cl	3–4
Bromides	H_3C–Br	2.5–4
Iodides	H_3C–I	2–4
Alcohols	H_3C–OH	3.4–4
Ethers	H_3C–OR	3.3–4
Esters	RCOO–CH_3	3.7–4.1
Esters	H_3C–COOR	2–2.6
Acids	H_3C–COOH	2–2.2
Carbonyl compounds	$(H_3C)_2$–C = O	2–2.7
Aldehydic	RCHO	9–10

(Contd.)

Types of protons		Chemical shift, δ
Hydroxylic	ROH	1–5.5
Phenolic	ArOH	4–12
Enolic	$H_2C=C-OH$	15–17
Carboxylic	RCOOH	10.5–12
Amino	RNH_2	1–5

Factors affecting the chemical shift

The chemical shift is influenced by the following undermentioned factors:

1. Electronegativity

The electrons around the proton create a magnetic field that opposes the applied field. Since this reduces the field experienced at the nucleus, the electrons are said to shield the proton. It can be useful to think of this in terms of vectors.

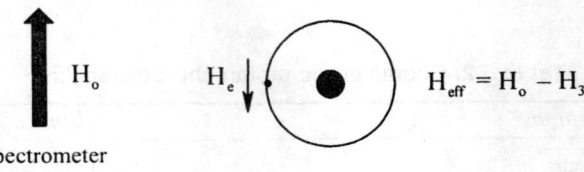

Spectrometer field

Since the field experienced by the proton defines the energy difference between the two spin states, the frequency and hence the chemical shift, δ/ppm, will change depending on the electron density around the proton. Electronegative groups attached to the C–H system decrease the electron density around the proton, and there is less shielding (i.e. deshielding) so the chemical shift increases. This is reflected by the data shown in Table 5.3.

Table 5.3. Effect of electronegativity on chemical shift

Compound CH_3X	CH_3F	CH_3OH	CH_3Cl	CH_3Br	CH_3I	CH_4	$(CH_3)_4Si$
X	F	O	Cl	Br	I	H	Si
Electronegativity of X	4.0	3.5	3.1	2.8	2.5	2.1	1.8
Chemical shift, δ/ppm	4.26	3.4	3.05	2.68	2.16	0.23	0

These effects are cumulative, so the presence of more electronegative groups produce more deshielding and therefore, larger chemical shifts.

Compound	CH_4	CH_3Cl	CH_2Cl_2	$CHCl_3$
δ/ppm	0.23	3.05	5.30	7.27

The effect of electronegativity on chemical shift fade rapidly as position of proton move away from the electronegative group. This effect is illustrated in the example of a primary bromide.

H signal	$-CH_2-CH_2-CH_2Br$		
d/ppm	1.25	1.69	3.30

2. Magnetic Anisotropy

The word "anisotropic" means "non-uniform". Magnetic anisotropy means that there is a "non-uniform magnetic field". Electrons in π systems (e.g. aromatics, alkenes, alkynes, carbonyls etc.) interact with the applied field which induces a magnetic field that causes the anisotropy. As a result, the nearby protons will experience 3 fields: the applied field, the shielding field of the valence electrons and the field due to the π system (Fig. 5.7). Depending on the position of the proton in this third field, it can be either shielded (smaller δ) or deshielded (larger δ), which implies that the energy required for, and the frequency of the absorption will change.

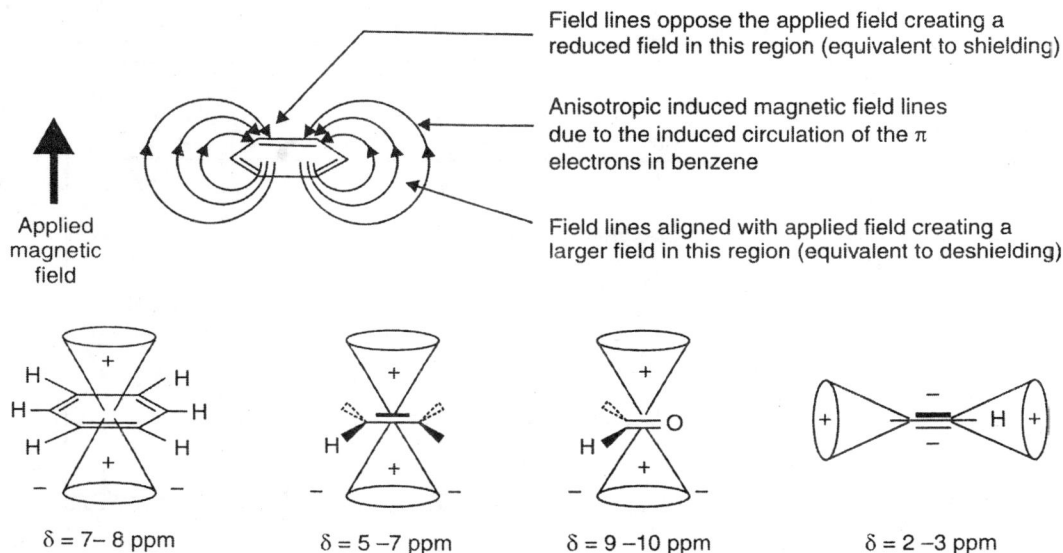

Fig. 5.7. Schematic diagram of shielding comes for common π systems. The + denotes shielding areas and − denotes deshielding areas. Remember shielding lowers the chemical shift, δ and deshielding increases δ. Typical H δ values are also shown.

3. Hydrogen bonding

Protons that are involved in hydrogen bonding (this usually means −OH or −NH) are typically observed over a large range of chemical shift values. The more hydrogen bonding there is, the more the proton is deshielded (due to decrease of electron density around the proton) and the higher its chemical shift will be. However, since the amount of hydrogen bonding is susceptible to factors such as solvation, acidity, concentration and temperature, it can often be difficult to predict.

(c) Intensities of the signal (peak area and proton counting)

Consider a NMR spectra (Fig. 5.8) of toluene and p-xylene.

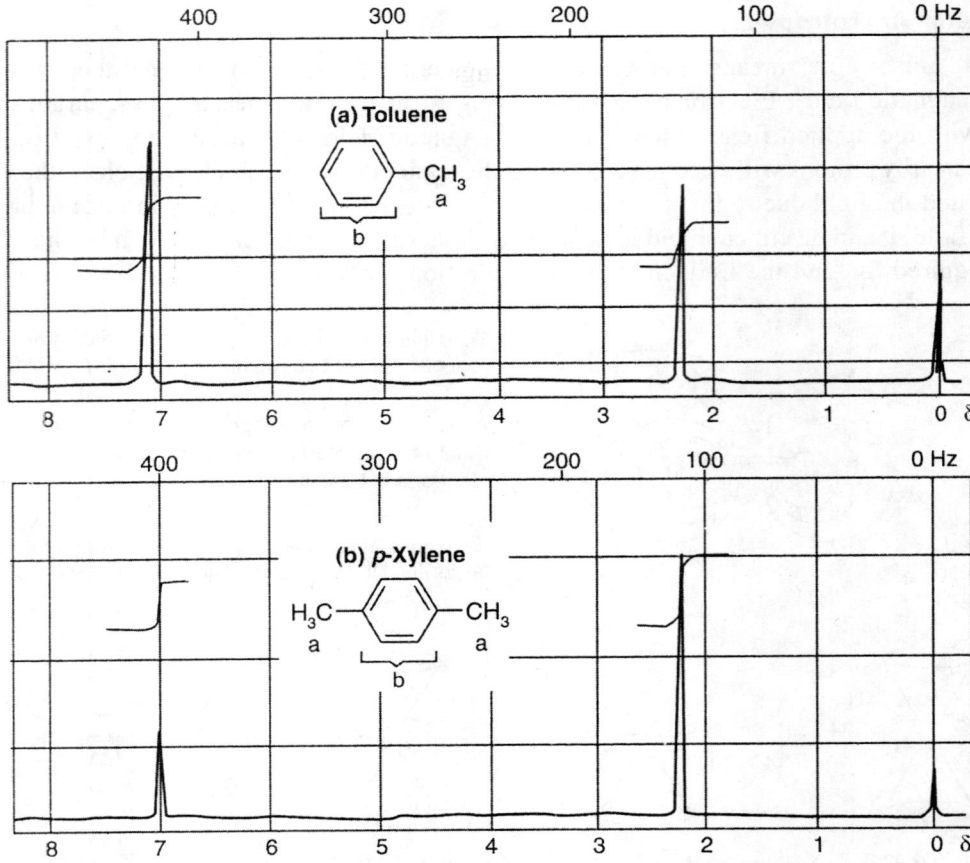

Fig. 5.8. NMR spectra: Intensities of methyl and aromatic protons signal (a) Toluene, (b) p-xylene.

Each compound possess two types of protons – methyl and aromatic protons, hence shows two signals in NMR spectra at nearly d 2.9 and d 7.2 values. Intensities of methyl proton and aromatic protons signal varies in each NMR spectra on comparison. Most exact comparison, based on the areas under the peaks shows that methyl proton and aromatic protons have the peak in the ratio of 3:5 for NMR spectrum of toluene while it is the ratio of 6:4 (3:2) in p-xylene.

Areas under NMR signals are measured by an electronic integrator and are usually given on the spectrum chart in the form of stipped curve.

(d) Splitting of signals (spin-spin coupling)

In 1,1,2-tribromoethane, there is a secondary protons and a tertiary proton, and consider first the absorption by one of the secondary protons:

$$-CH-CH_2-$$

The magnetic field that a secondary proton feels at a particular instant is slightly increased or slightly decreased by the spin of the neighbouring tertiary proton: increased if the tertiary proton happens at that instant to the aligned with the applied field; or decreased if the tertiary proton happens to be aligned against the applied field (Fig. 5.9).

For half the molecules, then, absorption by a secondary proton is shifted slightly downfield, and for the other half of the molecules the absorption is shifted slightly upfield. The signal is split into two peaks: a doublet, with equal peak intensities.

Similarly, absorption of tertiary proton is affected by the spin of the neighbouring secondary protons. But now there are two protons whose alignments in the applied field we must consider. There are four equally probable combinations (Fig. 5.10) of spin alignments for these two protons, of

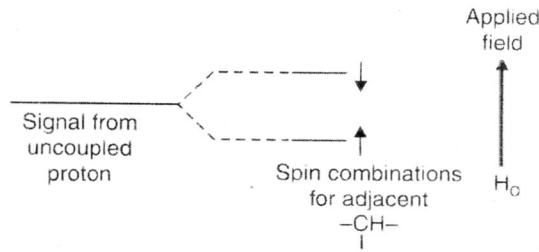

Fig. 5.9. Spin-spin coupling. Coupling with one proton gives a 1:1.

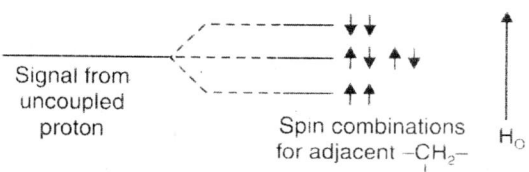

Fig. 5.10. Spin-spin coupling. Coupling with two protons given a 1:2:1 triplet.

which two are equivalent. At any instant, therefore, the tertiary proton feels any one of three fields, and its signal is split into three equally spaced peaks: a triplet, with relative peak intensities 1:2:1 (Fig. 5.11), reflecting the combined (double) probability of the two equivalent combinations.

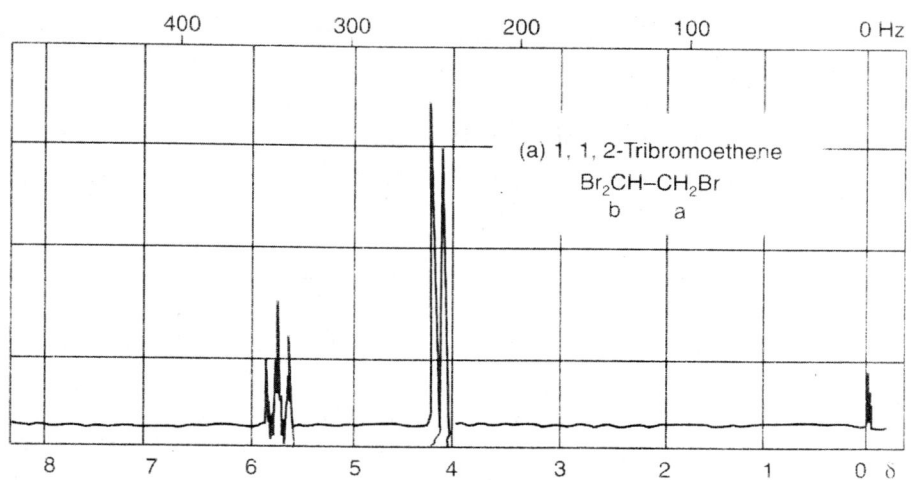

Fig. 5.11. NMR spectrum of 1,1,2-Tribromoethane.

Fig. 5.11 shows an idealized NMR spectrum due to the grouping $-CH-CH_2-$. We see a 1:1 doublet (from the $-CH_2-$) and a 1:2:1 triplet (from the $-CH-$). The total area (both peaks) under

124 Pharmaceutical Analysis

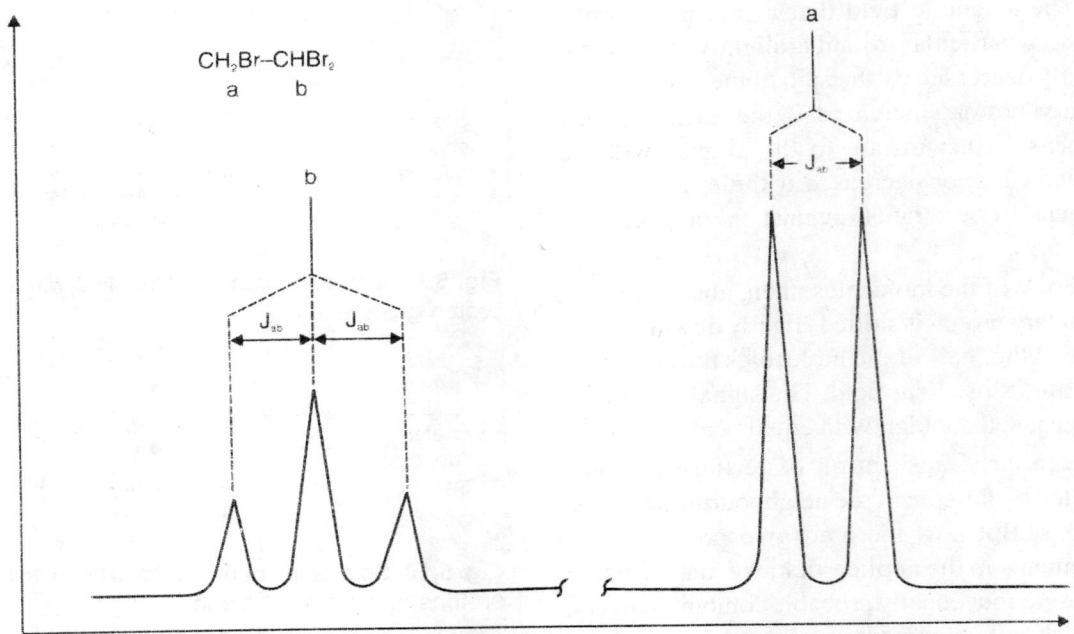

Fig. 5.12. Spin-spin splitting. Signal a is split into a doublet by coupling with one proton; signal b is split into a triplet by two protons. Spacings in both sets the same (J_{ab}).

the doublet is twice as big as the total area (all three peaks) of the triplet, since the doublet is due to absorption by twice as many protons as the triplet.

A little measuring shows us that the separation of peaks (coupling constant, discussed in the later section) in the doublet is exactly the same as the separation of peaks in the triplet. Spin-spin coupling is a reciprocal affair, and the effect of the secondary protons on the tertiary proton must be identical (Fig. 5.12) with the effect of the tertiary proton on the secondary protons.

In a spectrum, an NMR signal is split into a doublet by one nearby proton, and into a triplet by two (equivalent) nearby protons.

Downfield triplet   Downfield doublet
Area: 1   Area: 2

$$-\underset{\underset{H}{|}}{\overset{|}{C}}-CH_2- \quad\quad -\underset{\underset{H}{|}}{\overset{|}{C}}-CH_2-$$

Similarly, in 1,1-dibromoethane, the NMR signal (Fig. 5.13) due to tertiary proton is shifted into four peaks (greatest) due to 3 protons of methyl group (four spin combinations) (Fig. 5.14).

In each spectrum, peak area reflects the number of *absorbing* protons, and the multiplicity of splitting reflects the number of *neighbouring* protons in each spectrum just what we would expect.

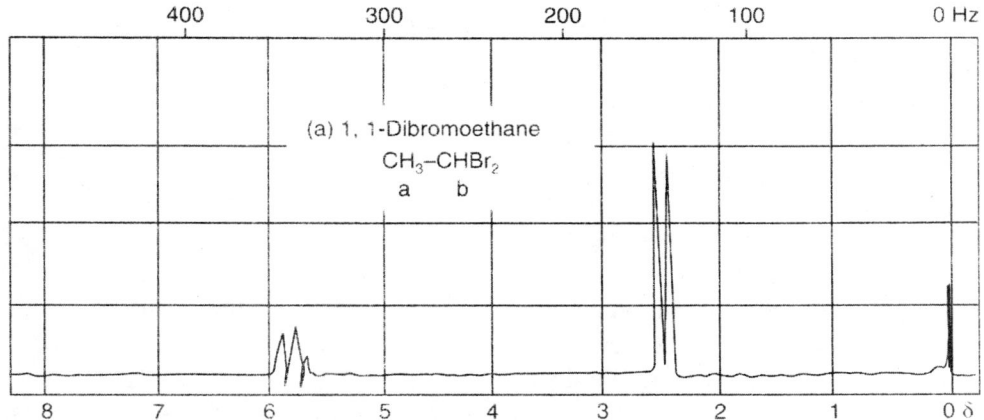

Fig. 5.13. Spin-spin coupling. Coupling with three protons gives a 1:3:3:1 quartet.

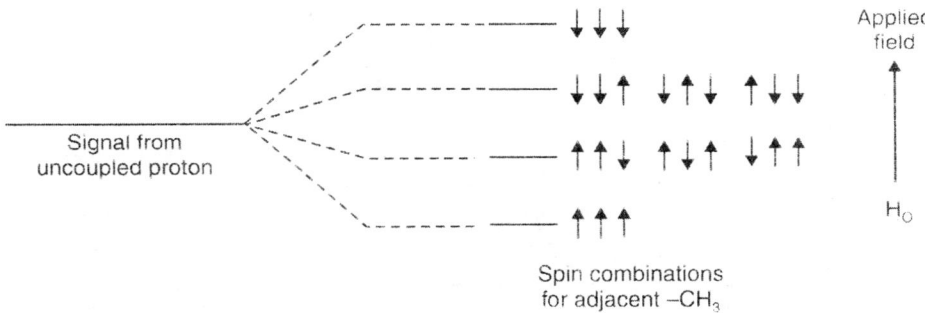

Fig. 5.14. Spin-spin coupling (four ways of coupling to 1:3:3:1 quartet).

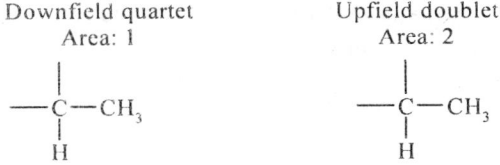

In the NMR spectrum of CH_3CHBr_2, there is downfield quartet and upfield doublet.

In each spectrum, we see that the spacing of the peaks within one multiplet is the same within the other, so that even in a spectrum with many other peaks, we could pick out these two multiplets as being coupled.

Pascal's Triangle

The relative intensities of the lines in a coupling pattern is given by a binomial expansion or more conveniently by Pascal's triangle (Fig. 5.15).

To derive Pascal's triangle, start at the apex, and generate each lower row by creating each number by adding the two numbers above and to either side in the row above together. The first six rows are shown in Fig. 5.15.

Hence, H–NMR spectrum, a proton with zero neighbours, n = 0, appears as a single line, a proton with one neighbours, n = 1 as two lines of equal intensity, a proton with two neighbours, n = 2, as three lines of intensities 1 : 2 : 1, etc.

We don't observe splitting due to coupling between the protons making up the same –CH$_3$ group, since they are equivalent. We do not observe splitting due to coupling between the protons on C-1 and C-2 of 1,2-dichloroethane since, although on different carbons, they, too, are equivalent.

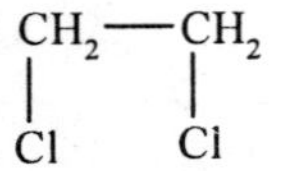

n = 0				1				Singlet
n = 1			1		1			Doublet
n = 2			1	2	1			Triplet
n = 3		1	3		3	1		Quartet
n = 4		1	4	6	4	1		Quintet
n = 5	1	5	10		10	5	1	Sextet

Fig. 5.15. Pascal triangle.

$$\underset{\text{Cl}}{\text{CH}_2} - \underset{\text{Cl}}{\text{CH}_2}$$

1,2-Dichloroethane

$$\underset{\text{H}_3\text{C}}{\overset{\text{H}_3\text{C}}{>}} \text{C}=\text{C} \underset{\text{H}}{\overset{\text{H}}{<}}$$

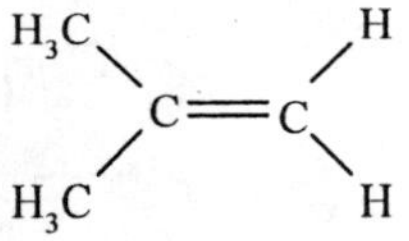

Isobutylene

In isobutylene, we don't observe any splitting because methylenic protons and vinylinic protons are equivalent.

On the other hand, we may observe splitting between the two vinyl protons on the same carbon if, as in 2-bromopropene, they are non-equivalent.

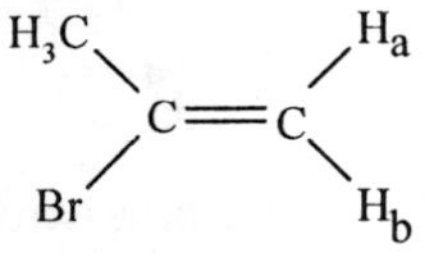

$$\underset{\text{Br}}{\overset{\text{H}_3\text{C}}{>}} \text{C}=\text{C} \underset{\text{H}_b}{\overset{\text{H}_a}{<}}$$

2-Bromopropene

Similarly, in the spectrum of 1,2-dibromo-2-methylpropane,

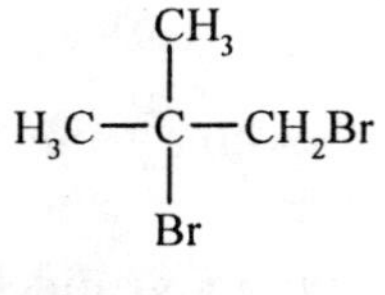

$$\text{H}_3\text{C} - \underset{\underset{\text{Br}}{|}}{\overset{\overset{\text{CH}_3}{|}}{\text{C}}} - \text{CH}_2\text{Br}$$

1,2-Dibromo-2-methylpropane

we don't observe splitting between the six methyl protons, on the one hand, and also with the two $-CH_2-$ protons on the other hand. The methyl and methylenic protons are non-equivalent, and so give two signals at different position in the NMR spectrum. The methyl and methylenic protons are not present on adjacent carbons and so their spins don't (noticeably) affect each other. Due to this reason, the NMR spectrum contains two singlets (one for CH_3 and other for CH_2), with a peak area ratio of 3:1 (or 6:2).

NMR coupling constant

Spin-spin coupling is the coupling through the bonding electrons. It results in the multiple peaks observed in the NMR spectra. The distance (in Hz) between peaks in a multiplet is a measure of the effectiveness of spin-spin coupling, and is called the **coupling constant (J)**. Coupling (unlike chemical shift) is not a matter of induced magnetic fields. The value of the coupling constant – as measured, in Hz, remains the same, whatever the applied magnetic field (that is, whatever the radiofrequency used). In this respect, spin-spin splitting differs from chemical shift, and, when necessary, the two can be distinguished on this basis. The size of a coupling constant depends markedly on the structural relationship between the coupled protons. For example, in any substituted ethylene, or in any pair of geometric isomers, J is always larger between *trans* protons than between *cis* protons. Aromatic coupling depends on whether the coupling protons are ortho, meta or para to each other and in simple cases, the coupling constant is valuable tool in deciding orientation, thus J_{ortho}, 7–10 Hz, J_{meta}, 2–3 Hz, J_{para}, 0–1 Hz. Furthermore, the size of J varies in a regular way with the electronegativity of substituents, so that one can often assign configuration without having both isomers in hand.

Gauche J = 2–6 Hz

Anti J = 5–14 Hz

Vicinal protons
J varies with dihedral angle
J = 2–15 Hz

J = 10–21 Hz

J = 0–7 Hz

J = 2–13 Hz

Vinyl proton

Examples of coupling constants J are shown in Table 5.4.

Table 5.4. Examples of proton-proton coupling constant (J) as a function of structure

Structural type	J (Hz)	Structural type	J (Hz)
H–C–(C)$_n$–C–H	0 (unless in a rigid ideal orientation)	H_b\C=C/H_a (cis/trans)	12 to 18
H_3C–CH_2–X (vicinal)	6 to 8	H_b\C=C/H_a	7 to 12
(H_3C)$_2$CH–X	5 to 7	\C=C/H_a with H_b	0.5 to 3
H–C(X)–C(Y)–H	2 to 12 (depends on dihedral angle and the nature of X and Y)	C=C–C–H	3 to 11 (depends on dihedral angle)
–C–C(=O)–H_a with H_b	0.5 to 3	–C(H)–C≡C–H	2 to 3
\C(/H_a)(\H_b) (geminal)	12 to 15 (must be diastereotopic)	aromatic H_a/H_b	o 7 to 10 m 2 to 3 p 0 to 1
		R,R$_1$–C(H_a)–O–H_b	0 to 7

DEUTERIUM EXCHANGE

The technique of deuterium is widely used to detect the presence of OH, SH, NH, groups etc. specially in the complex spectra. The NMR spectrum is first recorded conventionally in a solvent other than D_2O and then few drops of D_2O are shaken with a sample and spectra is re-run. Peak diminish disappear for OH, NH signals etc. as D_2O exchanges with the labile proton present in these groups.

$$R-OH + D-O-D \longrightarrow ROD + H-O-D$$

Peak corresponding to H–O–D appear at δ5. This method can also be extended to detect methylene groups, such as those flanked by carboxyl groups.

$$\underset{\text{H H}}{-\overset{\overset{\displaystyle O}{\|}}{C}-\overset{}{C}-\overset{\overset{\displaystyle O}{\|}}{C}-} \xrightarrow{D_2O} \underset{\text{D D}}{\overset{\overset{\displaystyle O}{\|}}{C}-\overset{}{C}-\overset{\overset{\displaystyle O}{\|}}{C}-}$$

SAMPLE HANDLING

Until recently, high-resolution NMR studies have been restricted to samples that could be converted to a non-viscous liquid state. Most often, solutions of the sample (2 to 15%) are used, although liquid samples can also be examined neat if they are sufficiently non-viscous.

The solvents for proton NMR spectroscopy should not contain any protons; for this reason, halogenated or deuterated compounds are commonly used as solvent. Deuterated chloroform ($CDCl_3$) and deuterated benzene (C_6D_6), D_2O, d_6-DMSO (dimethyl sulphoxide), CD_3COCD_3 (acetone-d_6) are usually used as solvents to dissolve the sample for recording spectra. Because some of these solvents have π-electron function and/or may serve as hydrogen bonding partners, the chemical shift of different groups of protons may change depending on the solvent used.

APPLICATIONS OF NMR SPECTROSCOPY

Unquestionably, the most important applications of proton NMR spectroscopy are related to the *identification and structural elucidation of organic, metal-organic, and biochemical molecules*. In addition, however, the method often proves useful for *quantitative determination of absorbing species*.

Identification of compounds

An NMR spectrum, like an infrared spectrum, seldom is a valuable tool for the identification of an organic compound. However, in conjunction with other observations such as elemental analysis, as well as ultraviolet, infrared, and mass spectra, NMR is a major tool for the characterization of pure compounds. The simple examples that follow give some idea of the kinds of information that can be extracted from NMR spectra.

Example 1

Compound I contain C, H, and O. Analytical data were obtained (62.6% C, 10.3% H) and shows the NMR spectrum as fiven in Fig. 5.16. Deduce the structure of the compound.

The below given NMR spectrum (Fig. 5.16) shows the four types of protons indicated by four signals. The signal of 1.2 is more intense and shows the 2 × CH_3 group in the same environment. The signal at δ 2.2 shows the presence of CH_3 proton, present in the more electronegatively may be attached to keto group. The signal at δ 2.6 shows the CH_2 protons with increasing deshielding. The signal at δ 3.9 appears due to hydroxy group. On the basis of above facts, the structure of the compound is:

$$H_3C-CO-CH_2-\underset{\underset{\displaystyle OH}{|}}{\overset{\overset{\displaystyle CH_3}{|}}{C}}-CH_3$$

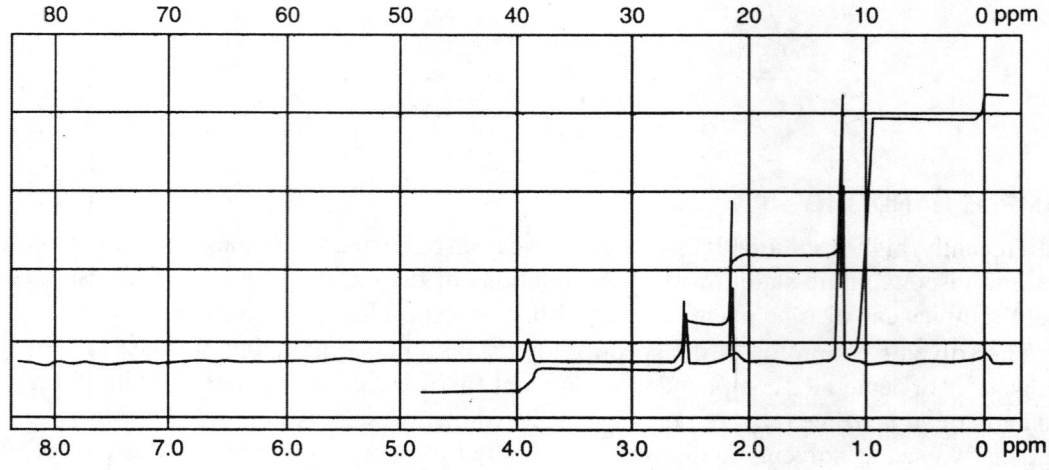

Fig. 5.16. NMR spectrum of compound, I.

Example 2

The spectrum shown in Fig. 5.17 is for colorless liquid, containing only carbon and hydrogen. Identify the unknown compound.

The single peak at about d 7.2 indicates the aromatic structure. The relative area under integration corresponds to 5 protons. The seven peak at d 2.9 for one proton doublet at d 1.2 can only be explained by the structure:

$$\begin{array}{c} CH_3 \\ | \\ -C-CH_3 \\ | \\ H \end{array}$$

Thus, on the basis of NMR data we can conclude that this compound is cumene.

Application of NMR to quantitative analysis

A unique aspect of NMR spectra is the direct proportionality between peak areas and the number of nuclei responsible for the peak. As a consequence, a quantitative determination of a specific compound does not require pure samples for calibration. Thus, if an identifiable peak for one of the constituents of a sample does not overlap the peaks of the other constituents, the area of this peak can be employed to establish the concentration of the species directly, provided only that the signal area per proton is known. The latter parameter can be obtained conveniently from a known

NMR Spectroscopy   131

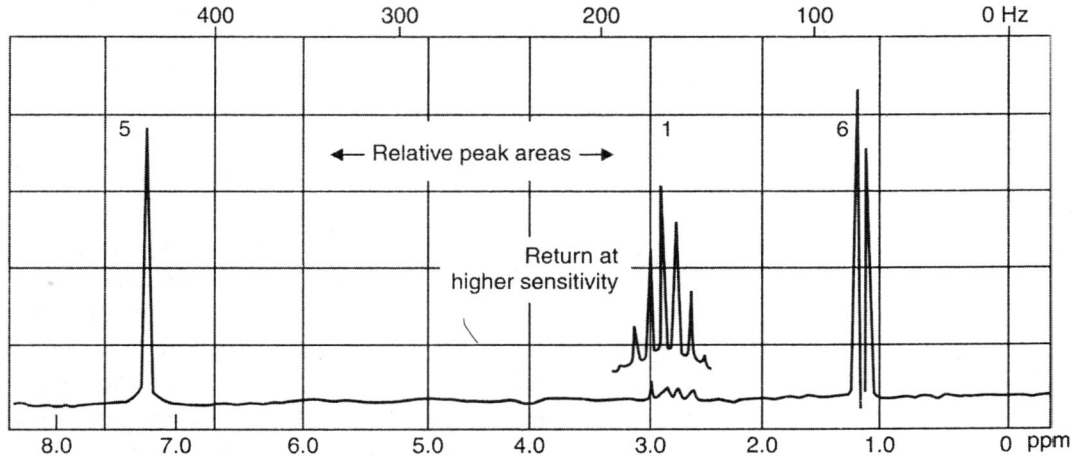

Fig. 5.17. NMR spectrum of unknown compound.

concentration of an internal standard. For example, if the solvent present in a known amount is benzene, cyclohexane, or water, the areas of the single proton peak for these compounds could be used to give the desired information; of course, the peak of the internal standard should not overlap with any of the sample peaks. Organic silicon derivatives are uniquely attractive for calibration purposes, owing to the high upfield location of their proton peaks.

The widespread use of NMR spectroscopy for quantitative work has been inhibited by the cost of the instruments. In addition, the probability that resonance peaks will overlap becomes greater as the complexity of the sample increases. Often, too, analyses that are possible by the NMR method can be conveniently accomplished by other techniques.

Analysis of multicomponent mixtures

Methods for the analysis of many multicomponent mixtures have been reported. For example, Hollis described a method for the determination of aspirin, phenacetin, and caffeine in commercial analgesic preparations. The procedure requires about 20 min., and the relative errors are in the range of 1 to 3%. Chamberlain describes a procedure for the rapid analysis of benzene, heptane, ethylene glycol, and water in mixtures. A wide range of these mixtures was analyzed with a precision of 0.5%.

Quantitative organic functional group analysis

One of the useful applications of the NMR has been to the determination of functional groups, such as hydroxyl groups in alcohols and phenols, aldehydes, carboxylic acids, olefins, acetylenic hydrogens, amines, and amides. Relative errors in the 1 to 5% range are reported.

Elemental analysis

NMR spectroscopy can be employed to determine the total concentration of a given kind of magnetic nucleus in a sample. For example, Jungnickel and Forbes have investigated the integrated NMR intensities of the proton peaks for numerous organic compounds and have concluded that accurate quantitative determinations of total hydrogen atoms in organic mixtures are possible. Paulsen and Cook have shown that the resonance of fluorine-19 can be used for the quantitative analysis of that element in an organic compound – an analysis that is difficult to carry out by classical methods. For quantitative work, a low-resolution or wide-line spectrometer can be employed.

C-13 NMR SPECTROSCOPY

The ^{12}C isotope of carbon – which accounts for up about 99% of the carbons in organic molecules, does not have a nuclear magnetic moment, and thus is NMR-inactive. Fortunately for organic chemists, however, the ^{13}C isotope, which accounts for most of the remaining 1% of carbon atoms in nature, has a magnetic moment just like protons. Most of what we have learned about ^1H-NMR spectroscopy also applies to ^{13}C-NMR, although there are several important differences.

The magnetic moment of a ^{13}C nucleus is much weaker than that of a proton, meaning that NMR signals from ^{13}C nuclei are inherently much weaker than proton signals. This, combined with the low natural abundance of ^{13}C, means that it is much more difficult to observe ^{13}C carbon signals: more sample is required, and often the data from hundreds of scans must be averaged in order to bring the signal-to-noise ratio down to acceptable levels.

Unlike ^1H-NMR signals, the area under a ^{13}C-NMR signal cannot be used to determine the number of carbons to which it corresponds. This is because the signals for some types of carbons are inherently weaker than for other types – peaks corresponding to carbonyl carbons, for example, are much smaller than those for methyl or methylene (CH_2) peaks. Peak integration is generally not useful in ^{13}C-NMR spectroscopy, except when investigating molecules that have been enriched with ^{13}C isotope.

The resonance frequencies of ^{13}C nuclei are lower than those of protons in the same applied field. In a 7.05 Tesla instrument, protons resonate at about 300 MHz, while carbons resonate at about 75 MHz. This is fortunate, as it allows us to look at ^{13}C signals using a completely separate 'windows' of radio frequencies. Just like in ^1H-NMR, the standard used in ^{13}C-NMR experiments to define the 0 ppm point is tetramethylsilane (TMS), although of course in ^{13}C-NMR it is the signal from the four equivalent *carbons* in TMS that serves as the standard. Chemical shifts for ^{13}C nuclei in organic molecules are spread out over a much wider range than for protons – up to 200 ppm for ^{13}C compared to 12 ppm for protons (see Table 5.5 for a list of typical ^{13}C-NMR chemical shifts). This is also fortunate, because it means that the signal from each carbon in a compound can almost always be seen as a distinct peak, without the overlapping that often plagues ^1H-NMR spectra. The chemical shift of a ^{13}C nucleus is influenced by essentially the same factors that influence a proton's chemical shift: bonds to electronegative atoms and diamagnetic anisotropy effects tend to shift signals downfield (higher resonance frequency). In addition, sp^2 hybridization results in a large downfield shift. The ^{13}C-NMR signals for carbonyl carbons are generally the furthest downfield (170–220 ppm), due to both sp^2 hybridization and to the double bond to oxygen.

Because of the low natural abundance of ^{13}C nuclei, it is very unlikely to find two ^{13}C atoms near each other in the same molecule, and thus *we do not see spin-spin coupling between neighbouring carbons in a ^{13}C-NMR spectrum*. There is, however, **heteronuclear coupling** between ^{13}C carbons and the hydrogens to which they are bound. Carbon-proton coupling constants are

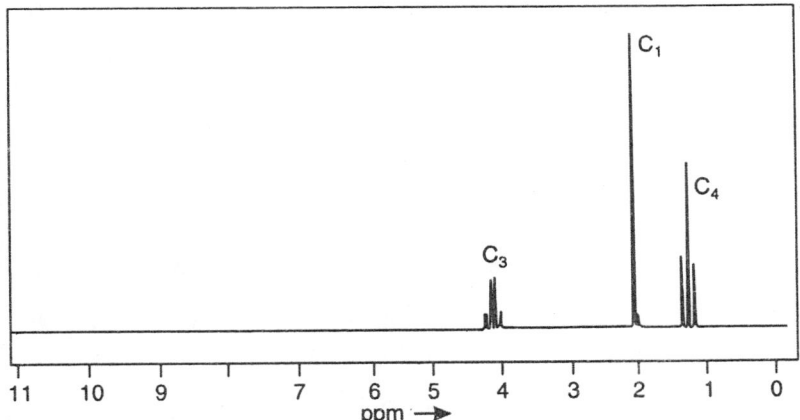

Fig. 5.18(a). ^{1}H-NMR spectrum of Ethyl acetate.

very large, on the order of 100–250 Hz. For clarity, chemists generally use a technique called **broadband decoupling**, which essentially 'turns off' C–H coupling, resulting in a spectrum in which all carbon signals are singlets. The Fig. 5.18b shows the proton-decoupled ^{13}C-NMR spectrum of ethyl acetate, showing the expected four signals, one for each of the carbons. Two methyl carbon (C-4 and C-1) atoms appear at 16 and 21 ppm respectively depending on electronic environment. The C-3 appear at 61 ppm. The carbonyl carbon appear at 170 ppm. The carboxyl carbon appear in a downfield position at 171 ppm. For comparison, ^{1}H-NMR spectrum of Ethyl acetate, ^{1}H-NMR spectrum (Fig. 5.18a) is also given here for comparison purpose. In the proton decoupled spectrum, all the four carbons appears as singlet in the spectrum at position depending on their chemical shift.

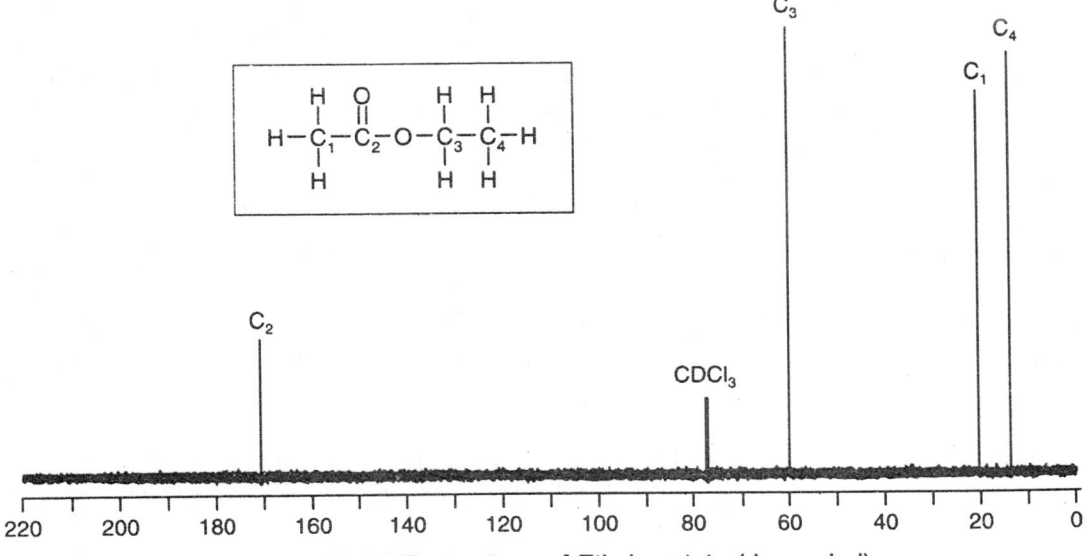

Fig. 5.18(b). NMR spectrum of Ethyl acetate (decoupled).

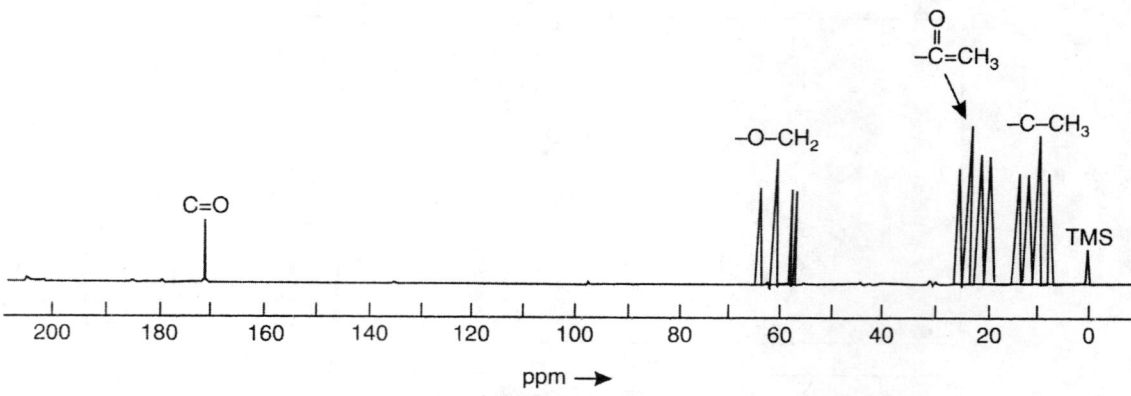

Fig. 5.18(c). Coupled ^{13}C-NMR spectrum of Ethyl acetate.

The broadband decoupling technique gives simpler spectrum but useful information about the presence of neighbouring protons is lost. However, another modern NMR technique called DEPT (Distortionless Enhancement by Polarization Transfer) allows us to determine how many hydrogens are bound to each carbon. For example, in DEPT spectrum of Ethyl acetate (Fig. 5.18c), that the signal at 171 ppm in the ethyl acetate spectrum is a quaternary carbon (no hydrogens bound, in this case a carbonyl carbon) due to presence of singlet. The triplet signal at 60 ppm is due to methylene (CH_2, two hydrogen atoms) carbon, and quartet signal at 21 ppm and 16 ppm signals are due to both methyl (CH_3, three hydrogen atoms) carbons.

Another comparison is illustrated for ethyl phenyl acetate. The Fig. 5.19 shows the decoupled spectrum, signal appears at δ 18, 41, 60, 110 and 171 due to presence of CH_3, CH_2CO, OCH_2, aromatic carbon and carbonyl carbon atoms respectively. All the signals appear as discrete pack. The same signal in ^{13}C-NMR spectrum coupled with protons appears a quartet, triplet, multiplet and singlet depending on the basis of number of hydrogen atoms attached on it.

The carbonyl group appear as singlet as there is no hydrogen atom attached to it. In the aromatic region, only C-1 position appear as singlet slightly away from the other carbon atoms as it also do not contain hydrogen atom.

Table 5.5. ^{13}C-NMR chemical shifts

Carbon environment	Chemical shift (ppm)	Carbon environment	Chemical shift (ppm)
C=O (in ketones)	205–220	RCH_2Cl	40–45
C=O (in aldehydes)	190–200	RCH_2NH_2	37–45
C=O (in acids and esters)	170–185	R_3CH	25–35
C in aromatic rings	125–150	CH_3CO-	20–30
C=C (in alkenes)	115–140	R_2CH_2	16–25
RCH_2OH	50–65	RCH_3	10–15

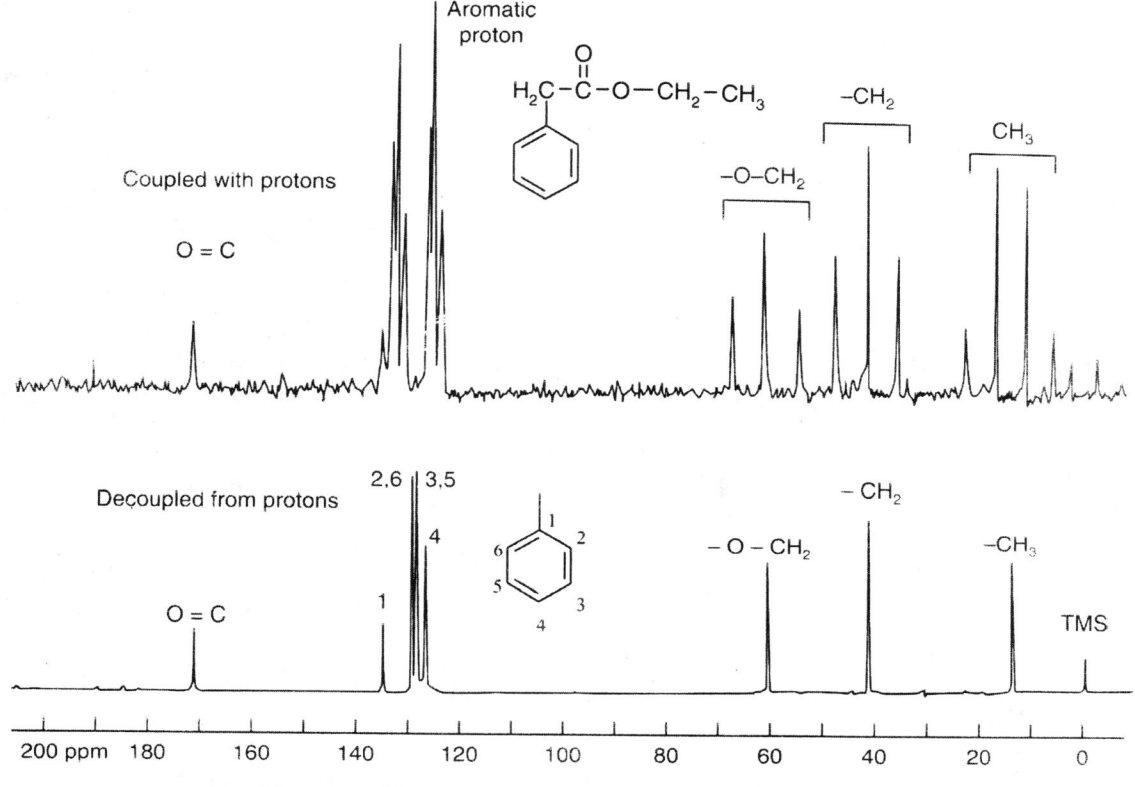

Fig. 5.19. ^{13}C-NMR spectrum of phenyl ethyl acetate.

Nuclear Overhauser Enhancement (NOE)

Under conditions of broad band decoupling - found that the area of the C-13 are enhanced by a factor that is significantly greater than that which is expected from the collapse of multiplets into single lines. This is a manifestation of *nuclear overhauser enhancement*. It arises from direct magnetic coupling between a decoupled proton and a neighbouring 13C nucleus that results in an increase in the population of the lower energy state of the 13C nucleus than that predicted by the Boltzmann relation. C-13 signal may be enhanced by as much as a factor of 3x. The disadvantage is the loss of proportionality between peak areas and the number of nuclei of that type of ^{13}C.

2D-NMR SPECTROSCOPY

So far the NMR spectral methods we have discussed have been one dimensional (since they have a single chemical shift x coordinate axis). With the development of more advanced spectroscopic methods as computational power has increased, it has become possible to obtain two dimensional spectra. In two dimensional experiments, both the x and the y axes have chemical shift scales and the 2D spectra are plotted as a grid like a map. Information is obtained from the spectra by looking at the peaks in the grid and matching them to the x and y axes.

136 Pharmaceutical Analysis

Types of 2D NMR

Two dimensional (2D) NMR spectroscopy is of two types:

1. Homonuclear correlation
- Through bond: COSY, TOCSY
- Through space: NOESY, ROESY

2. Heteronuclear correlation
- One-bond correlation HSQC, HMQC
- Long-range correlation HMBC

1. Homonuclear correlation spectroscopy

COSY - Correlation Spectroscopy

Special features

- Both axes correspond to the proton NMR spectra.
- The COSY spectra indicates which H atoms are coupling with each other.
- Examples of a COSY is provided in Figs. 5.20 and 5.21.

COSY spectra

Example 1

- The information on the 'H' that are coupling with each other is obtained by looking at the peaks inside the grid. These peaks are usually shown in a contour type format, like height intervals on a map.
- In order to see where this information comes from, let us consider an example shown in Fig. 5.20 the COSY spectrum of ethyl 2-butenoate.

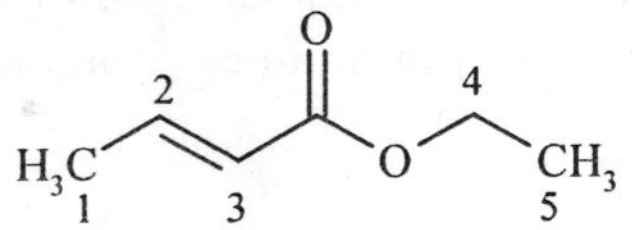

$$H_3C - \overset{2}{CH} = \overset{3}{CH} - \overset{O}{C} - O - \overset{4}{CH_2} - \overset{5}{CH_3}$$

- First look at the peak marked A in the top left corner. This peak indicates a coupling interaction between the H at 6.9 ppm and the H at 1.8 ppm. This corresponds to the coupling of the CH_3 group and the adjacent H on the alkene.
- Similarly, the peak marked B indicates a coupling interaction between the H at 4.15 ppm and the H and 1.25 ppm. This corresponds to the coupling of the CH_2 with methyl protons in the ethyl group.

- Notice that for each pair of coupled protons or groups, the cross peak always appears in pair, equidistance on either side of the diagonal, and that the overall pattern is symmetrical.

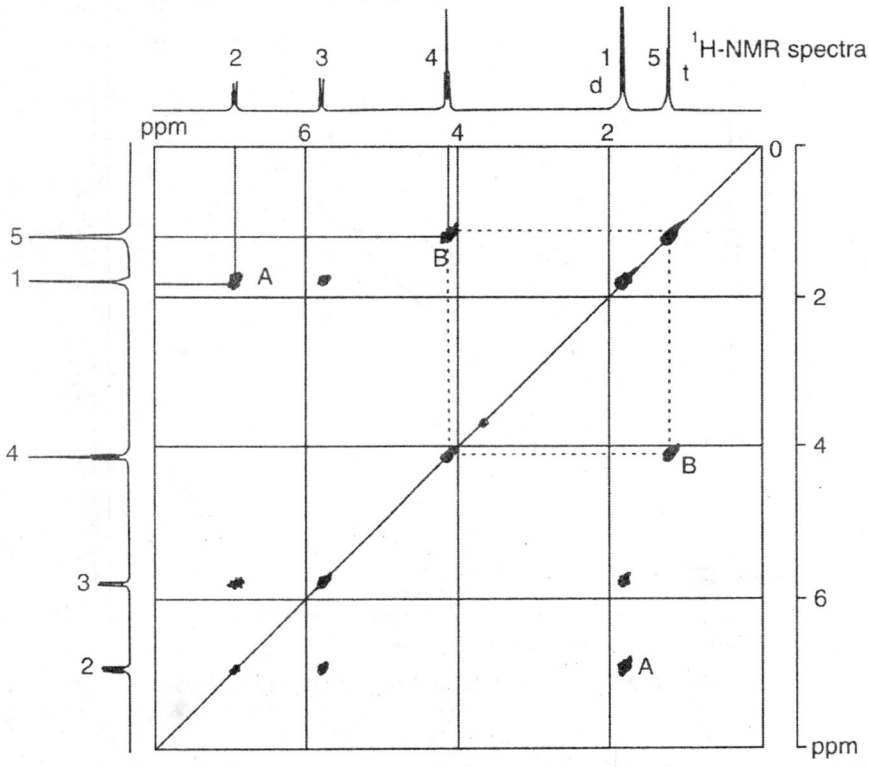

Fig. 5.20. Cosy spectrum of Ethyl butenoate.

Example 2

In the homonuclear COSY spectrum of Ethylbenzene (Fig. 5.21), the ^1H signal at 1.4 ppm correlates with the ^1H signal at 2.8 ppm because there are cross-peaks but they do not correlate with the signals at 7.3 ppm.

TOCSY: Total Correlation SpectroscopY, same as **COSY**, but also able to generate cross peaks via intermediate spins (mix).

NOESY: Nuclear Overhauser Effect SpectroscopY, allows one to see through-space effects, useful for investigating conformtion and for determination proximity of adjacent spin systems. Not so useful for MWs in the 1 kDa range due to problems arising from the NMR correlation time.

ROESY: Rotational Overhauser Effect SpectroscopY, same as **NOESY**, but works for all molecular weights.

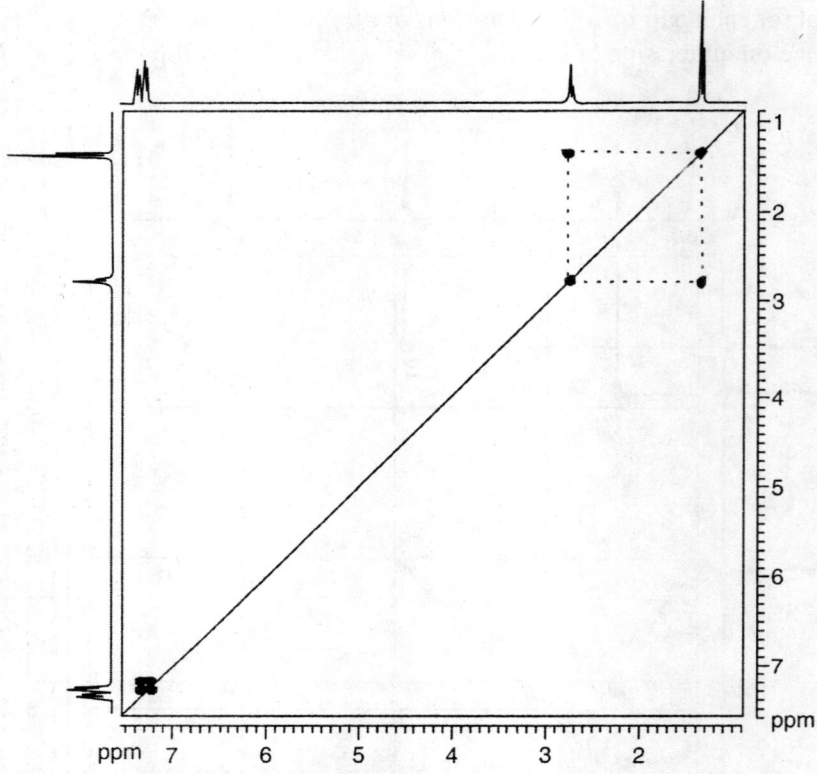

Fig. 5.21. 2D COSY spectrum of ethylbenzene.

2. Heteronuclear Correlation Spectroscopy

Special features

- Proton NMR spectra on one axis and the ^{13}C nmr spectra on the other.
- The HETCOR spectra matches the H to the appropriate C.
- An example of HSQC spectrum is given in Fig. 5.22 and 5.23.

Example 1

- The information on how the H and C are matched is obtained by looking at the peaks inside the grid. Again, these peaks are usually shown in a contour type format, like height intervals on a map.
- In Fig. 5.22 the HETCOR spectrum of ethyl 2-butenoate.
- First look at the peak marked A near the middle of the grid. This peak indicates that the H at 4.1 ppm is attached to the C at 60 ppm. This corresponds to the $-OCH_2-$group.

- Similarly, the peak marked B towards the top right in the grid indicates that the H at 1.85 ppm is attached to the C at 17 ppm. Since the H is a singlet, we know that this corresponds to the CH_3-group attached to the carbonyl in the acid part of the ester and not the CH_3-group attached to the $-CH_2$ in the alcohol part of the ester.
- Notice that the carbonyl group from the ester has no "match" since it has no H attached in this example.

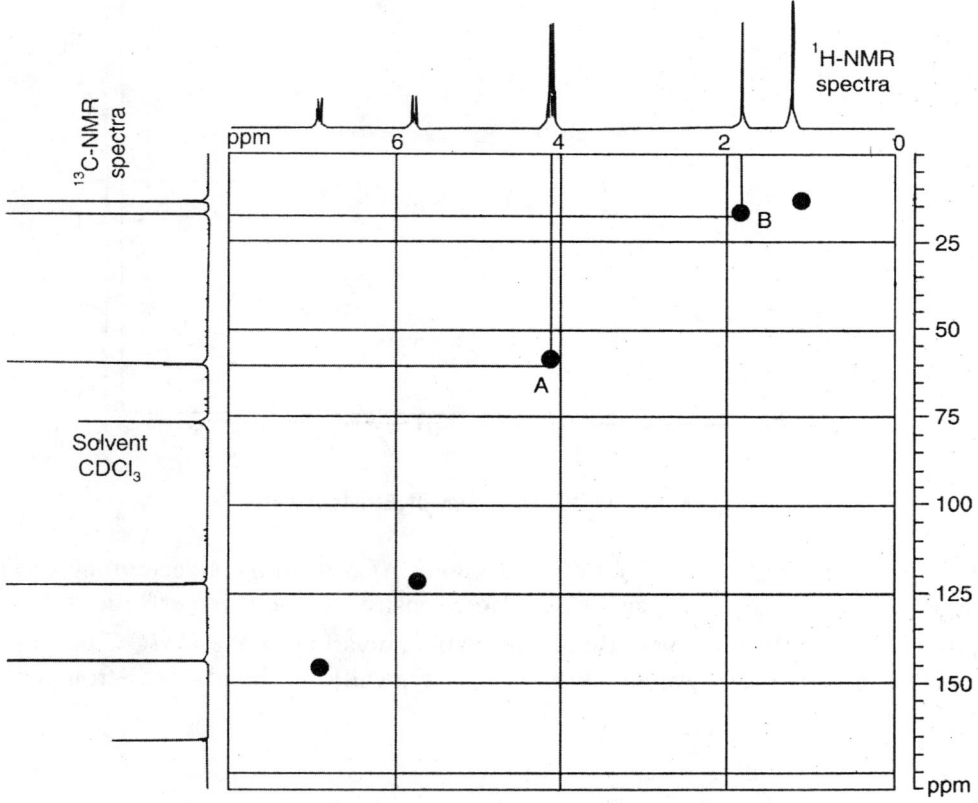

Fig. 5.22. HSQC spectrum of Ethyl 2-butenoate.

● The cross peaks obtained by vertical line from proton axis and horizontal line from C-axis indicates coupling of that particular 'H' to the carbon.

Example 2

The heteronuclear HSQC spectrum of ethyl benzene in Fig. 5.22, the ^1H signal at 1.4 ppm correlates with the ^{13}C signal at 15.7 ppm, the ^1H signal at 2.8 ppm correlates with the ^{13}C signal at 29.0 ppm, etc.

HMQC: Heteronuclear Multiple Quantum Correlation, allows one to pair NH or CH resonance.
HSQC: Heteronuclear Single Quantum Correlation, provides the same information as **HMQC**,

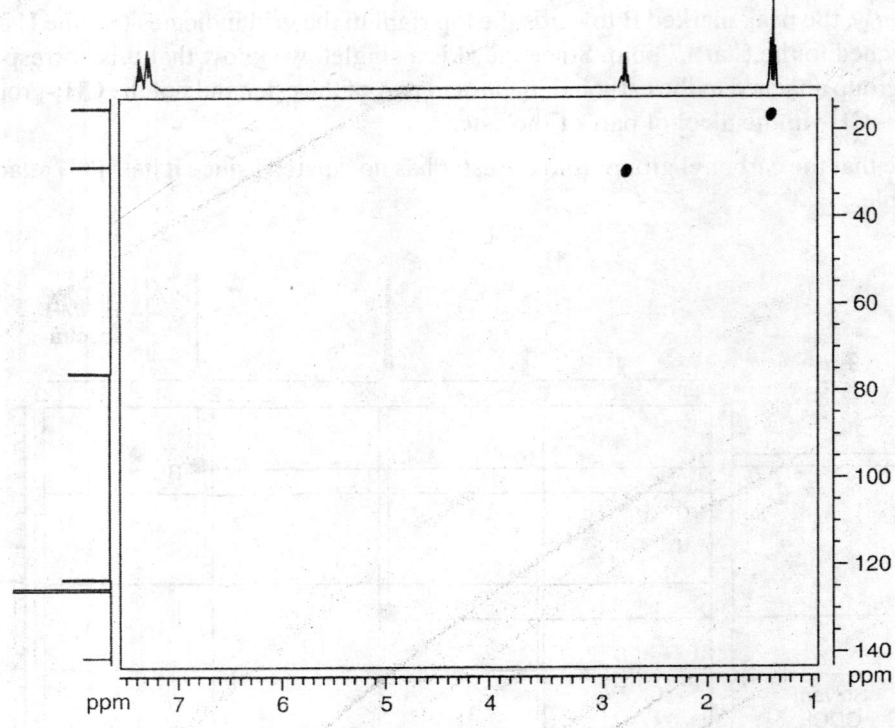

Fig. 5.23. HSQC spectrum of Ethylbenzene.

but gives narrower resonances for ^1H–^{13}C correlations. Also requires X-decoupling and hence a large number of steady state scans and is also more sensitive to pulse imperfections.

HMBC: **H**eteronuclear **M**ultiple **B**ond **C**orrelation, a variant of the **HMQC** pulse sequence that allows one to correlate X-nucleus shifts that are typically 2–4 bonds away from a proton.

CHAPTER 6

Atomic Absorption Spectroscopy

The science of atomic spectroscopy has given us three analytical techniques (i) Atomic emission, (ii) Atomic absorption, and (iii) Atomic fluorescence. In order to understand relationship of these techniques to each other, it is necessary to have an understanding of atom itself and of atomic process involved in each technique.

The atom consists of a nucleus surrounded by electrons. Every element has specific number of electrons, which are associated with the atomic nucleus in orbital structure. The number of electrons and their arrangement are unique to each element. The electrons occupy orbital positions in an orderly and predictable way. The lowest energy, most stable electronic configuration of an atom, known as the ground state, is normal orbital configuration for an atom. If the energy of right magnitude is applied to an atom, the energy will be absorbed by an atom, and an outer electron will be promoted to a less stable configuration or 'excited state' (Fig. 6.1). As this state is unstable, the atom will immediately and spontaneously return to its ground state configuration. The electron returns to its initial, stable orbital position, and radiant energy equivalent to the amount of energy

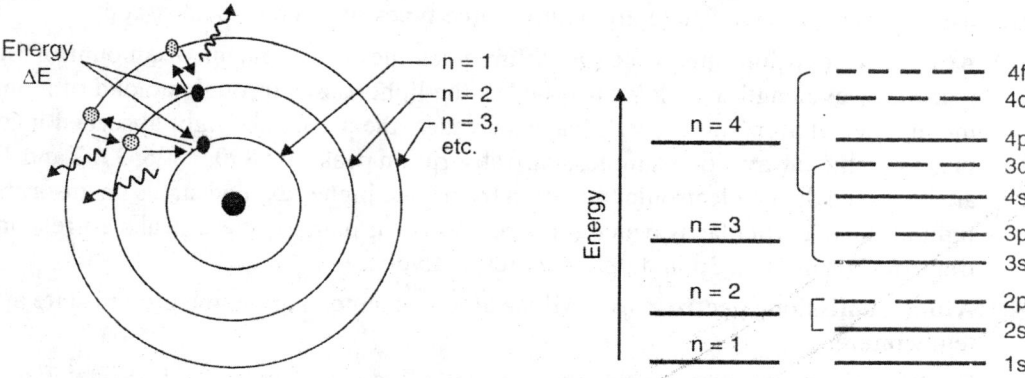

Fig. 6.1. Atomic structure associated with arrangement of electrons.

142 Pharmaceutical Analysis

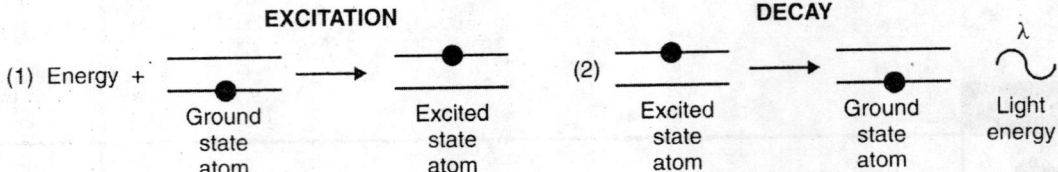

Fig. 6.2. Excitation and decay process.

initially absorbed in the excitation process will be emitted out. The process is illustrated in Fig. 6.2. In the step 1 of the process, the excitation is forced by supplying energy. The step 2 is the decay process in which light is emitted out. The wavelength of emitted light is directly related to the electronic transition from excited level to ground level which has occurred. Since every element has a unique electronic structure, the wavelength of emitted light is unique property of each individual element. The orbital configuration of a large atom may be complex and so many transitions can occur. Each transition can cause emission of a characteristic wavelength of light, as shown in Fig. 6.3.

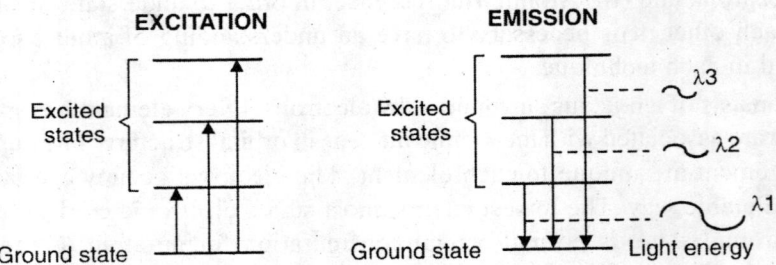

Fig. 6.3. Energy transitions.

The process of absorption, excitation and decay process (emission of radiant energy on returning to ground state) is involved in each types of atomic spectroscopy. Either the energy absorbed in excitation process or the energy emitted in the decay process is measured and used for analytical purposes as shown in Fig. 6.4. There are mainly three types of atomic spectroscopy:

(a) **Atomic absorption spectroscopy:** It involves the measurement of amount of light at resonant wavelength which is absorbed as the light passes through a cloud of atoms. As the number of atoms in the light path increases, the amount of light absorbed increases in a predictable way. For example, sharp absorption peaks at 5890, 5896, 3302 and 3303Å are observed due to electronic transition from 3s to higher excited states on absorption of light at these particular wavelength. Each adjacent pairs of these peaks corresponds to transition from 3s to 3p and 4p levels respectively.

(b) **Atomic emission spectroscopy:** All the atoms of a metal are in the ground state at room temperature.

For example, the single outer electron of metallic sodium occupies the 3s orbital. Excitation of this electron to higher orbital can be brought out by the heat of the flame or by electric

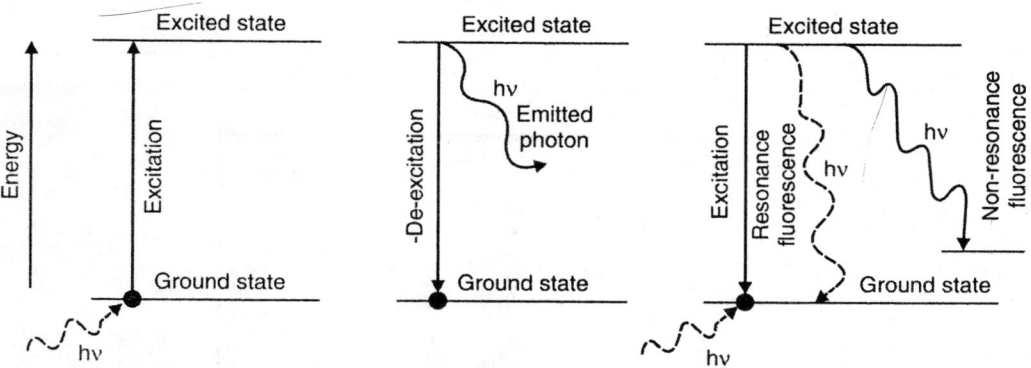

Fig. 6.4. Schematic representation of the transitions in atomic (a) absorption, (b) emission, and (c) fluorescence (resonance and nonresonance) emission.

arc or spark. The life time of the excited atom is brief, however, and its return to the ground state is accompanied by the emission of photon of radiation. The intense radiation of the wavelength 5890 and 5896 Å is emitted out which are responsible for the yellow color when sodium salts are introduced into a flame. It is due to return of electron from 3p to 3s. The resolving power of the monochromator used is insufficient to separate the peak. The much smaller peak at about 5700 Å is in fact two unresolved peaks that arise due to return of electron from 3d to 3p level.

(c) **Atomic fluorescence spectroscopy:** Atoms in a flame can be made to fluorescence by irradiation with an intense source containing wavelength that are absorbed by the element. For example, magnesium atoms are exposed to an ultraviolet source, radiation of wavelength 2852 Å is absorbed as electrons are promoted from 3s to the 3p level. The resonance fluorescence emitted at this same length may be used for analysis. The resulting fluorescence spectra are most conveniently measured at an angle of 90° to light path.

BASIC PRINCIPLE OF ATOMIC ABSORPTION SPECTROSCOPY

In atomic absorption spectroscopy specially flame atomic absorption spectroscopy (FAAS), liquid sample is aspirated, aerosolized and mixed with combustible gases, such as acetylene and air or acetylene and nitrous oxide. Then, this mixture is ignited in a flame whose temperature ranges from 2100 to 2800°C.

During combustion, elements of interest in the sample are reduced to free, unexcited ground state atoms (Fig. 6.5) which absorb light as specific wavelength, as shown in Fig. 6.6 and excited. The wavelength of absorbed light is element specific and accurate to 0.01–0.1 nm. To provide element specific wavelength, a light beam from lamp whose cathode is made of the element being determined is passed through the flame. The detector, photomultiplier detects the reduction of light intensity due to absorption by the element (analyte) and this can be directly related to amount of the element (analyte) present in the sample. This technique is very reliable and simple to use to determine various metals. The Fig. 6.7 shows the list of elements which can be analysed by this technique.

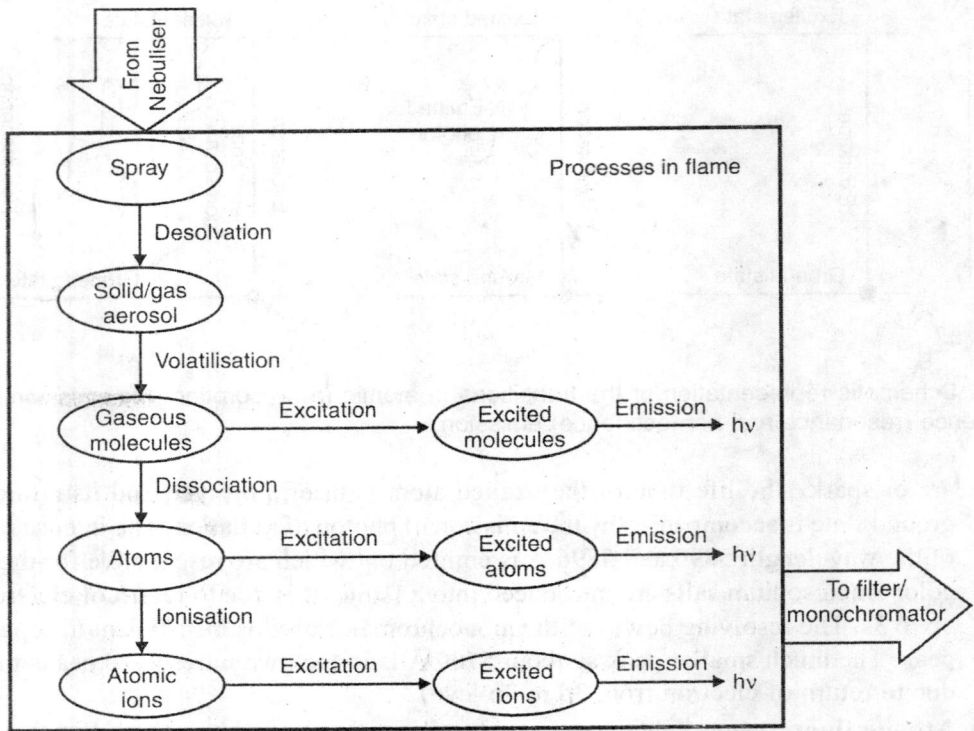

Fig. 6.5. Diagrammatic representation of various steps occurring during atomization in flame obtained from any hydrogen flame.

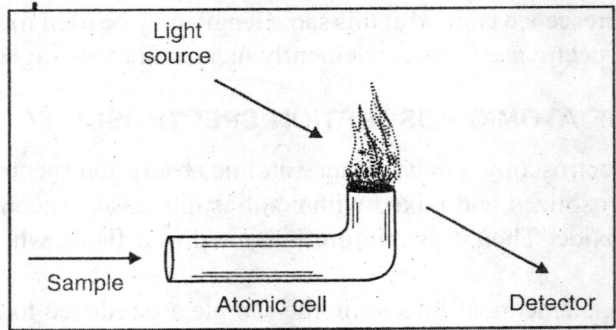

Fig. 6.6. Absorption of energy by sample.

ATOMIC ABSORPTION SPECTROPHOTOMETER

Each type of absorption spectrometer must have basic components like (i) light source, (ii) a sample cell, (iii) device for light measurement as shown in Fig. 6.8. In atomic absorption spectrophotometer (Fig. 6.9), there is light source, which is referred as line source as it emits the sharp atomic absorption lines of element which is to be analysed. The most widely used source is the **hollow cathode lamp**.

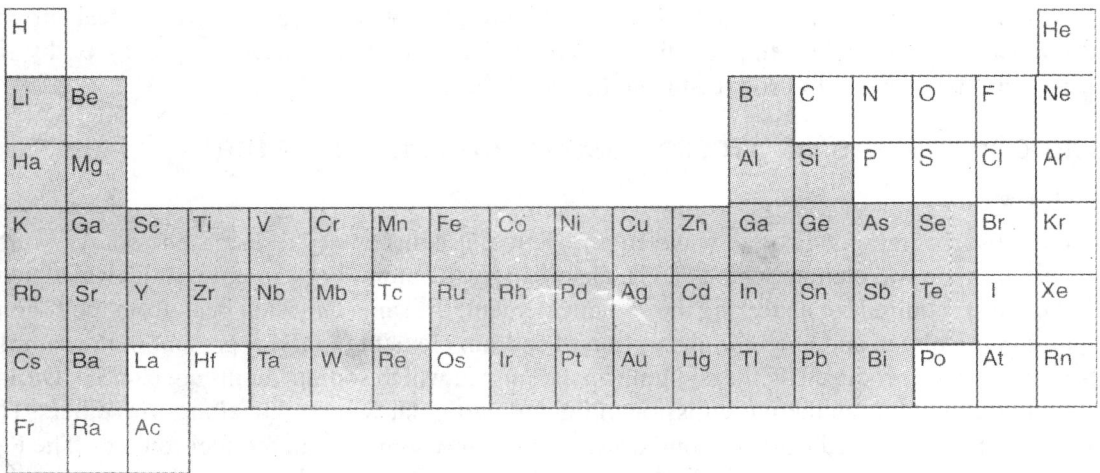

Fig. 6.7. Elements detectable by AAS are highlighted.

These lamps are designed to emit the atomic spectrum of particular element and so specific lamps are selected for use depending on the element to be analysed.

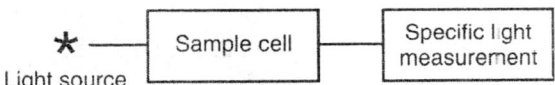

Fig. 6.8. Requirements for a spectrometer.

It is also required that the source radiation be modulated (switched on and off rapidly) to provide a means of selectively amplifying light emitted from the source and ignoring emission from the flame. Source modulation can be accompanied with the rotating chopper located between the source and the sample cell or pulsing the power to the source. Special consideration is also required for a sample cell for atomic absorption. An atomic vapour must be generated in the light beam from the source. This is generally obtained from introducing or atomizing the sample into a burner system of electrically heated furnace aligned in the optical path of spectrophotometer.

Several components are required for specific light measurement. A monochromator is used to disperse the various wavelength of light which are emitted from the source and to isolate the particular wavelength of interest. The selection of particular wavelength allows the determination of selected elements in present of others. The light of particular wavelength coming out from the sample cell

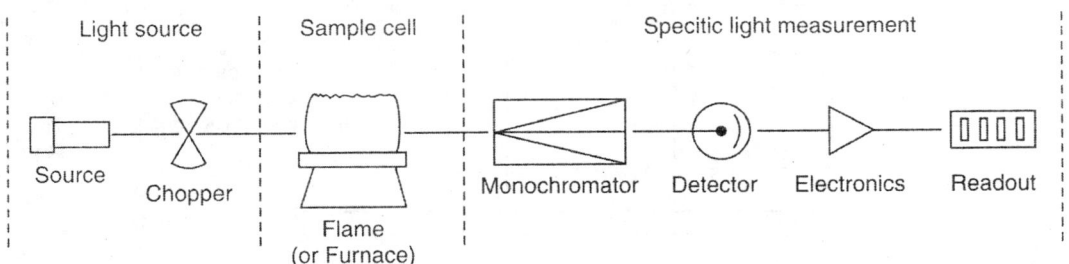

Fig. 6.9. Schematic of atomic absorption spectrometer.

146 Pharmaceutical Analysis

is directed onto the detector. It is normally the photomultiplier which produces an electrical current. The intensity of current depends on light intensity. The electrical current is processed by the instrumental data system to produce the signal.

BASIC COMPONENTS OF ATOMIC ABSORPTION SPECTROMETER

1. Light source

An atom absorbs light as discrete wavelength. Hence, it is necessary to use a line source which emits the specific wavelength which can be absorbed by the atom. For example, if the wavelength of 589.6 nm is required for analyzing the sodium element, the same emission peak from the sodium line source is isolated and used for absorption of sodium element (analyte) present in the sample. This means, line is produced by the sodium vapour lamp in which sodium atoms are excited. During the return to ground level, there is emission of light of particular wavelength along with others. The other sodium lines emitted from the source are removed by using filter or monochromator. The Fig. 6.10 shows the emission of typical line source which consists of four narrow lines. On passing

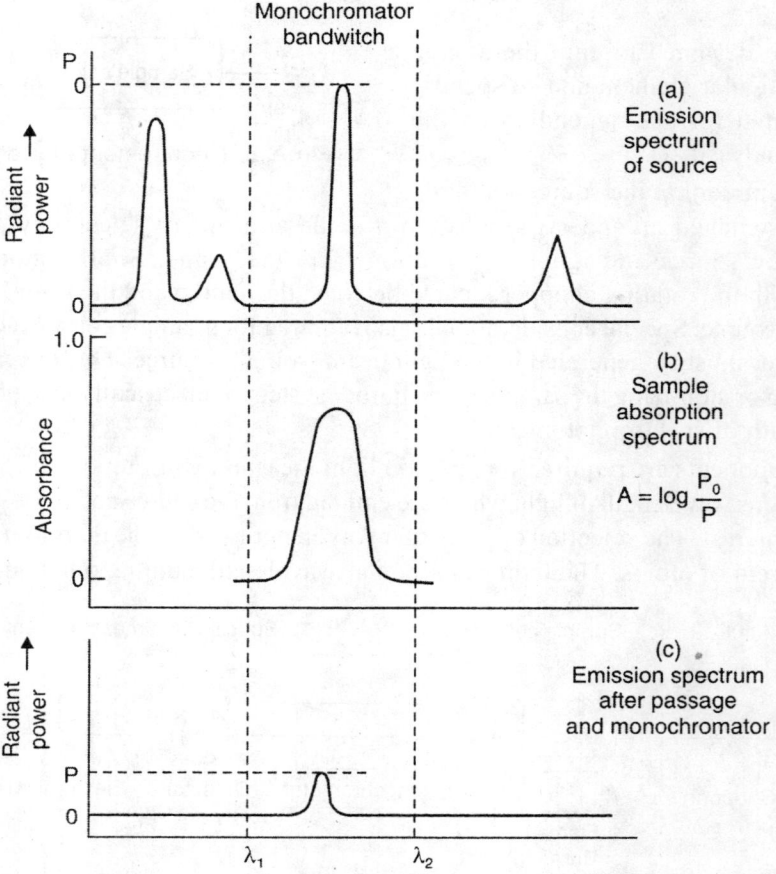

Fig. 6.10. Absorption of a resonance line by atoms.

through filter or monochromator, all except one (desirable one) are removed. Narrow line sources not only provide high sensitivity but also make accurate analytical technique with minimum spectral interferences. A disadvantage of this procedure that separate lamp source is needed for each element or sometimes group of elements. The two most common line sources used are hollow cathode lamp (HCL) and the electrodeless discharge lamp (EDL).

(i) Hollow cathode lamp

It consists of hollow glass envelope with a cathode inside made of element being analysed and a suitable anode (Fig. 6.11). The glass envelope is filled with either neon or argon at low pressure. At the end of the glass cylinder is a window transparent to the emitted radiation. The emission process is illustrated in Fig. 6.12. When an electrical potential is applied between the anode and cathode, some of filled gas atoms are ionized. The positively charged filled gas ions accelerate through the electrical field to collide the negatively charged cathode and dislodge individual metal atoms in a process called 'sputtering'. The sputtered metal atoms are then excited to emission state through a kinetic energy transfer by impact with filled gas ions. On returning to ground state, light of specific wavelength (λ) is emitted out. Hollow cathode lamps have a finite lifetime. Adsorption of filled gas atoms onto the inner surfaces of the lamp is the primary cause for lamp failure. As filled gas pressure decreases, the efficiency of sputtering and excitation of sputtered metal atoms

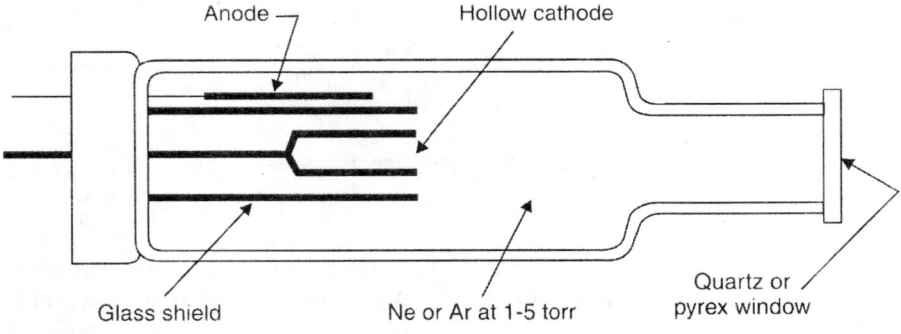

Fig. 6.11. Hollow cathode lamp.

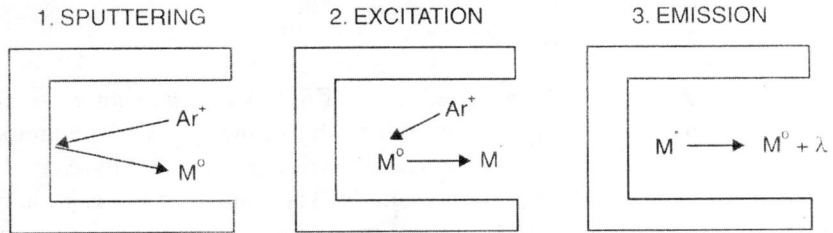

Fig. 6.12. Hollow cathode lamp process where Ar^+ is a positively charged argon ion, M^0 is a sputtered, ground state metal atom, M^* is an excited state metal atom and λ is emitted radiation at a wavelength characteristic for the sputtered metal.

also decreases, thus reducing the intensity of lamp emission. To prolong hollow cathode lamp life, some manufacturers produce lamps with larger internal volumes to accommodate more gas pressure.

(ii) Electrodeless discharge lamp

Electrodeless discharge lamps (EDL) (Fig. 6.13) contains a inert gas (e.g. argon) and metal or its salt (whose spectrum is to be determined) in a quartz bulb. The bulb is inserted into a coil that generates intense field of radiofrequency. The lamp don't contain any electrode. Ionization of argon gas occurs by the intense radiofrequency field to give ions that are accelerated by the high frequency component of the field until they gain sufficient energy to excite the atoms of metal whose spectrum is sought. The emission from an EDL is higher than that from an HCL, and the line width is frequently narrower, but EDL need a separate power supply and need a longer time to stabilize.

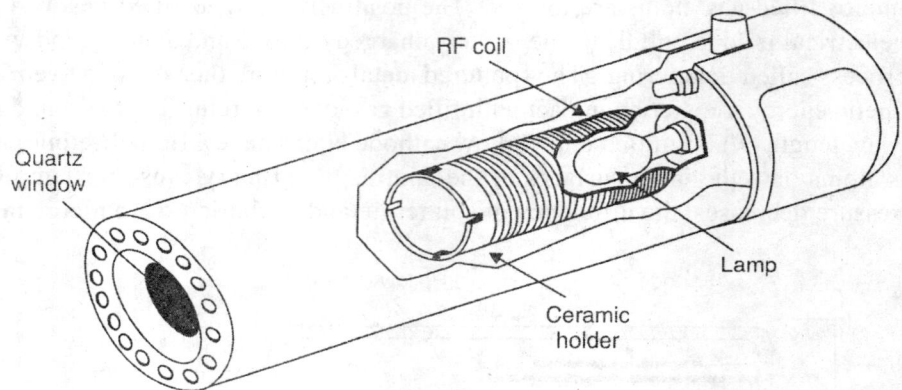

Fig. 6.13. Electrodeless discharge lamp.

2. Atomizers

The most important difference between spectrophotometer for atomic absorption and one for molecular absorption is the requirement to convert the analyte into a free atom. The process of converting an analyte in solid, liquid or solution form to a free gaseous atom is called atomization. In most of the cases, the sample containing the analyte undergoes some form of sample preparation in an organic or aqueous solution. Two types of atomizers are used: (a) Flame atomizers, and (b) Electrothermal atomizers.

(a) Flame atomizers

In flame atomizer, the sample is first converted into a fine mist consisting of small droplets of solution. It is accomplished using a nebulizer assembly as shown in Fig. 6.14. The sample is aspirated into a spray chamber by passing a high pressure steam consisting of one or more combustion gases, part the end of a capillary tube immersed in the sample. The impact of the sample with the glass impact head produces an aerosol mist. The aerosol mist mixes with the combustion gases in the spray chamber before passing to flame which desolvates the aerosol mist to a dry aerosol of small solid particles. Subsequently, flame thermal energy volatizes the particles, producing a vapour consisting of molecular species, ionic species and free atoms.

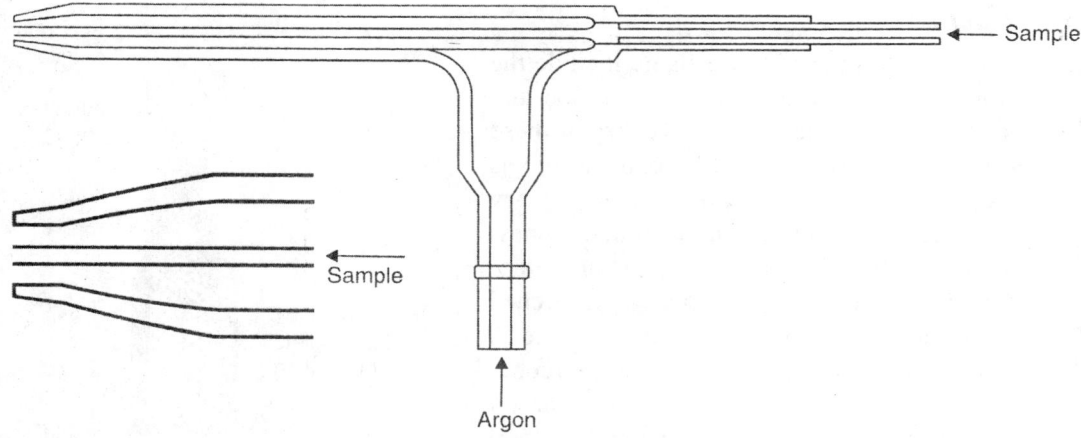

Fig. 6.14. A concentric tube nebulizer.

Thermal energy in flame atomization is provided by the combustion of a fuel-oxidant mixture. Common fuels and oxidants and their normal temperature ranges are listed in Table 6.1.

Table 6.1. List of common fuels and oxidants used in flame atomic absorption spectroscopy

Fuel	Oxidant	Temperature (^{0}°C)	Maximum burning velocity (cm s^{-1})
Natural gas	Air	1700–1900	39–43
Natural gas	Oxygen	2700–2800	370–390
Hydrogen	Air	2000–2100	300–400
Hydrogen	Oxygen	2550–2700	900–1400
Acetylene	Air	2100–2400	158–266
Acetylene	Oxygen	3055–3150	1100–2480
Acetylene	Nitrous oxide	2600–2800	285

Temperature of 1700 to 2400°C is obtained with the various fuels when air serves as the oxidant. At these temperature, only easily excitable species such as the alkali and alkaline earth metals can be analysed. For heavy metal species which are less readily excited, oxygen or nitrous oxide must be employed as oxidant.

The burning velocities listed in Table 6.1 are of considerable importance because flames are stable in certain ranges of flow rates only. If the flow rate does not exceed the burning velocity, the fmale propagates itself back into the burner, giving flashback. As the flow rate increases, the flame rises until it reaches a point above the burner where the flow velocity and the burning velocity are equal. This region is where the flame is stable. At higher flow rates, the flame rises and eventually reaches a point where it blows off the burner. Clearly, the flow rate of the fuel/oxidant mixture is an important variable that has to be closely controlled and this rate is highly dependent on type of fuel and oxidant being used.

Flame structure

Important regions (Fig. 6.15) of a flame include the primary combustion zone, the interconal region and outer cone. The appearance and relative size of these region vary considerably with fuel to oxidant ratio as well as the type of fuel and oxidant. The primary combustion zone is recognizable by its blue luminescence arising from band spectra of C_2, CH and other radicals. Thermal equilibrium is ordinarily not reached in this region and so primary combustion zone is seldom used for flame spectroscopy. The interconal zone which is narrow in stoichiometric hydrocarbon flames, may reach several centimeter in height in fuel rich acetylene/oxygen or acetylene/NO_2 sources. This zone is often rich in free atoms and is the most widely part of flame for spectroscopy.

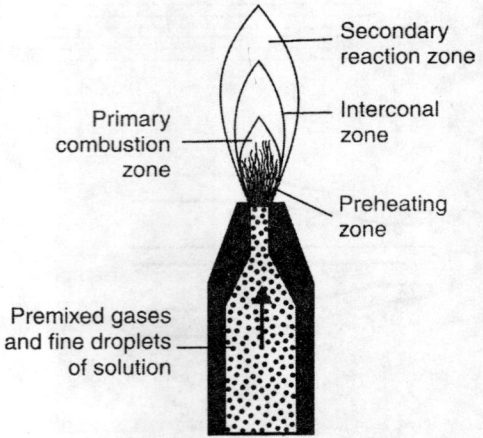

Fig. 6.15. Schematic structure of a flame showing various zones.

The outer cone is secondary reaction combustion zone where the products of the inner cone are converted to stable molecular oxides.

Temperature profiles

The maximum temperature is located somewhat above the primary combustion zone. Hence, this part of flame is focussed for calibration and analytical measurements.

Flame absorbance profiles

Magnesium exhibits a maximum in absorbance at about the middle of the flame (Fig. 6.16) because of two opposing effects. The initial increase in absorbance as the distance from base become larger, results an increased number of magnesium atom produced by the longer exposure to the heat of the flame. As the outerzone is approached, appreciable oxidation of magnesium begins. This process leads to decrease in absorbance because the oxide particles are non-absorbing at the wavelength used. To obtain maximum analytical sensitivity, the flame must be adjusted with respect to beam until a maximum absorbance is obtained.

Silver does not form oxide so absorbance is increased continuously from the base to periphery Chromium shows continuous decrease due to formation of stable oxide. Clearly, a different portion of the flame should be used for the analysis of each of these elements.

Flame atomizer are of two types – continuous and discrete. In continuous type, the sample is fed into

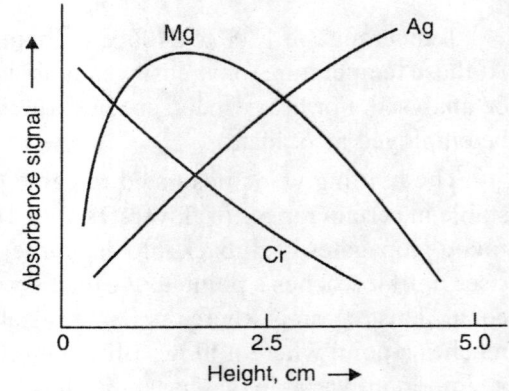

Fig. 6.16. Flame absorbance profile.

atomizer at a constant rate. The spectral line is then constant with time. It requires 2–5 ml of the sample. Continuous type of atomizer is not used for the sample containing high concentration of dissolved solids, such as sea water. It may result in the build up of solid deposits on the burner head. These deposits partially obstruct the flame, lowering the absorbance. With discrete atomizer, a measured quantity of the sample is introduced as a plug of liquid or solid. The spectral signal in this case rises to a maximum and then decreases to zero as the atomic vapour is carried out of the heated region. It is useful when the volume of sample is limited.

Advantages of flame atomizers

The principle advantage of flame atomization is the reproducibility of result.

Disadvantages of flame atomizers

The efficiency of flame atomizers is very poor. This may occur for two reasons. First, the majority of the aerosol may be produced during nebulization consists of droplets that are too large to be carried to the flame by the combustion gases. Consequently, as much as 95% of the sample never reaches the flame. A second reason for poor atomization efficiency is that the large volume of the combustion gases significantly dilutes the sample. Together, these contributions to the efficiency of atomization reduce sensitivity since the analyte's concentration in the flame may be only 2.5×10^{-6} of that in solution.

(b) Electrothermal atomizers

A significant improvement in sensitivity is achieved by using resistive heating in place of a flame. The electrothermal atomization involves the heating of sample to a temperature (2000–3000°C) to produce volatilization and atomization. Flame atomizer can only analyse the solution but electrothermal atomizers like graphite tube furnance can accept the very small quantities of solution, slurry or solid samples. The graphite tube furnace, consist of a cylindrical graphite tube approximately 1–3 cm in length and 3–8 mm in diameter (Fig. 6.17).

The graphite tube is housed in an assembly that seals the ends of the tube with optically transparent windows. The assembly also allows for the passage of a continuous stream of inert gas, protecting the graphite tube from oxidation, and removing the gaseous products produced during atomization. A power supply is used to pass a current through the graphite tube, resulting in resistive heating.

Samples between 5 and 50 µl are injected into the graphite tube through a small-diameter hole located at the top of the tube. Atomization is achieved in three stages. In the first stage, the sample is **dried** using a current that raises the temperature of the graphite tube to about 110°C. Desolvation leaves the sample as a solid residue. In the second stage, which is called **ashing**, the temperature is increased to 350–1200°C. At these temperatures, any organic material in the sample is converted to CO_2 and H_2O, and volatile inorganic materials are vaporized. These gases are removed by the inert gas flow. In the final stage, the sample is **atomized** by rapidly increasing the temperature to 2000–3000°C. The result is a transient absorbance peak whose height or area is proportional to the absolute amount of analyte injected into the graphite tube. The three stages are complete in approximately 45–90 seconds, with most of this time used for drying and ashing the sample.

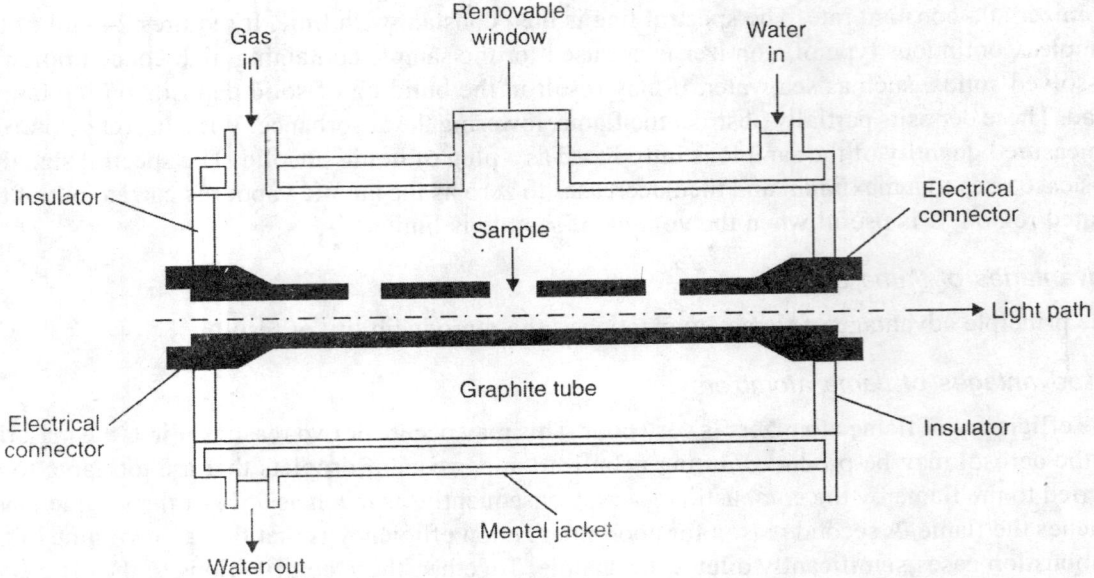

Fig. 6.17. Graphite tube furnace.

Electrothermal atomization provides a significant improvement in sensitivity by trapping the gaseous analyte in the small volume of the graphite tube. The analyte's concentration in the resulting vapour phase may be as much as 1000 times greater than that produced by flame atomization. Flame atomization can only analyse the solution, but graphite furnace can accept very small quantities of solution, slurry or solids samples. The improvement in sensitivity, and the resulting improvement in detection limits, is offset by a significant decrease in precision. Atomization efficiency is strongly influenced by the sample's contact with the graphite tube, which is difficult to control reproducibly.

Disadvantages

- Background absorption effects.
- Analyte may be lost at the ashing stage.
- The sample may not be completely atomised.
- The precision is poor than the flame method.

(c) Carbon rod analyser

This device can be used to convert a powdered sample into atomic vapour. A current is applied to a very thin, heated carbon rod that contains the solid sample in order to vaporise it.

(d) Tantalum boat analyser

This is another technique that produces an atomic vapour from a solid sample. A Tantalum boat is electrically heated in a manner similar to the carbon rod system, within an inert atmosphere.

(e) Miscellaneous atomization method

A few elements may be atomized by a chemical reactions that produce a volatile product. Elements such as As, Se, Sb, Bi, Ge, Sn, Te and Ps form volatile hydrides when reacted with $NaBH_4$ in acid. An inert gas carries the volatile hydrides to either a flame or to a heated quartz observation tube situated in the optical path.

$$As(v) \text{ (Sol.)} \xrightarrow{NaBH_4} AsH_3 \xrightarrow{\text{Heat in flame}} As° + H_2 \text{ gas}$$

Mercury is determined by the cold-vapour method in which it is reduced to elemental mercury with $SnCl_2$. The volatile Hg is carried by an inert gas to an unheated observation tube situation in the instrument's optical path.

$$Hg^{2+} + SnCl_2 + 2Cl^- \longrightarrow Hg° + SnCl_4$$

3. Filter/Monochromator

Similar to UV, but inexpensive filter/monochromator is used to isolate the narrow hand width of wavelength that are absorbed by the metals.

4. Source Modulation in Atomic Absorption Spectrometer

In atomic absorption instrument, it is necessary to eliminate interferences caused by emission of radiation by the flame. For these, output of the radiation source is modulated so that the intensity fluctuates at a constant frequency. The detector then receives two types of signals, an alternating one from the source and a continuous one from flame. These signals are then converted to the corresponding types of electrical response. A simple and entirely easy way of modulating the emission from the source is to interpose a circular metal disk or chopper in the beam between the source and the flame. The chopper is motor driven that has open and solid (mirror in some cases) alternating regions as given below. Alternate quadrant of this disk permits the passage of light. Rotation of the disk to the desired speed provides a beam that is chopped to the desired frequency. As an alternative, the power supply for the source can be designed for the intermittant operation.

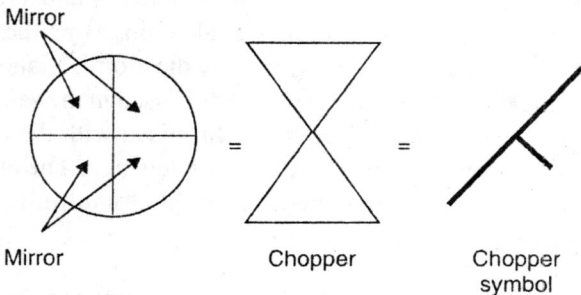

Mirror — Chopper — Chopper symbol

5. Detector

The photomultiplier is used to detect the light absorbed by the analyte. It is the same as described in UV/mass spectrometer. The light energy is converted to electrical energy leading the generation of current the strength of current measured to measure the intensity of light.

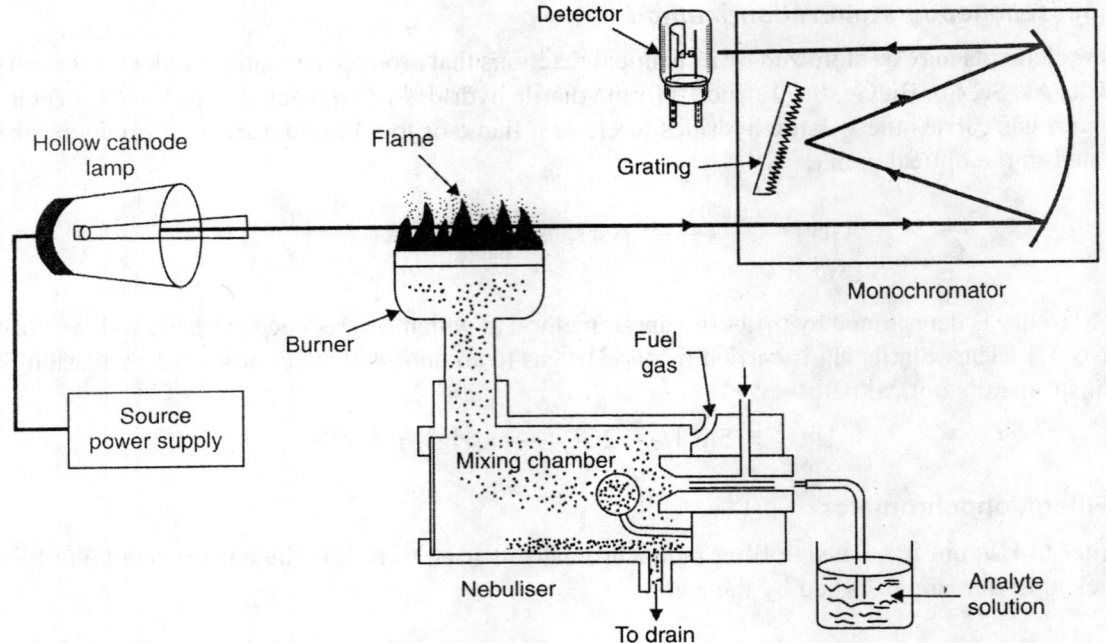

Fig. 6.18. Schematic diagram of a single beam flame atomic absorption spectrophotometer.

TYPES OF ATOMIC ABSORPTION SPECTROPHOTOMETER

Single beam atomic absorption spectrophotometer

A simplified sketch of a single beam flame atomic absorption spectrophotometer is shown in Fig. 6.18. It consists of hollow cathode lamp (HCL), a radiation source, flame as a atomisation device, a monochromator, a photomultilier detector and a recording system. The HCL radiation is chopped to eliminate the background signal arising from the radiation emitted by the sample itself, focussed on the atomic vapour produced by the atomiser and then directed to the monochromator where the atomic line of interest is isolated. It is used in the same way as UV/IR single beam spectrophotometer. The electronic amplifier is synchronised with the chopper so that the signal component generated by emission from the sample is not detected. The attenuation of the source radiation by the analyte atomic vapour is detected by the photomultiplier. A blank is aspirated into the flame and the transmittance is adjusted to 100%.

Double beam atomic absorption spectrophotometer

In this instrument, the beam from the HCL is split by a mirrored chopper, one half passing through the atomiser and the other half around it, as schematically shown in Fig. 6.19. The two beams are then recombined by a half-silvered mirror and passed through the monochromator. The ratio between the reference and sample signal is then amplified and fed to the readout display and recorder. These instruments correct the fluctuations in the intensity of radiation coming from the radiation source and for changes in the sensitivity of the detector. It must be noted that reference beam in double

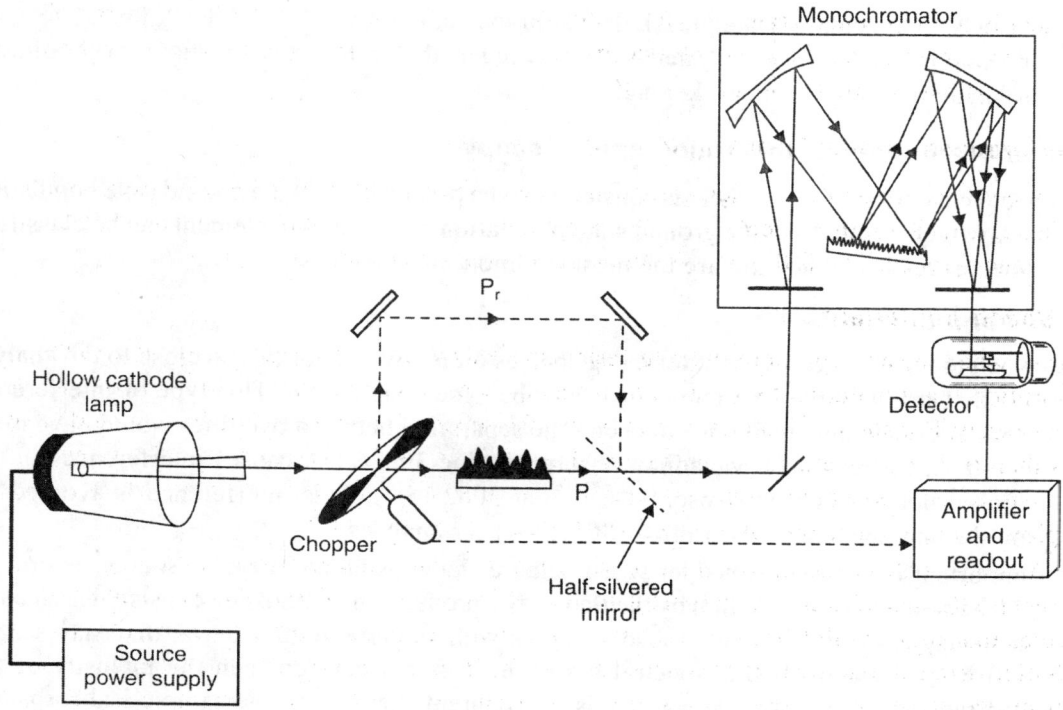

Fig. 6.19. Schematic diagram of a double beam atomic absorption spectrophotometer.

beam instruments does not pass through the flame and thus corrects for the loss of radiant power due to absorption or scattering by the flame itself. The beam from hollow cathode source (Fig. 6.19) is split by mirror chopper so that one half passed through the flame and the other half around it. The two beam are then recombined by a half silver mirror and passed into grating monochromator. The photomultiplier tube serves as detector. The output from the latter is fed to a lock in amplifier that is synchronized with the chopper drive. The ratio between the reference and sample signal is then amplified and fed to the data acquisition system.

Preparation of sample

Flame and electrothermal atomization require the sample in a liquid or solution form for atomization. Sample in solid form are prepared for analysis by dissolving in an appropriate solvent. When the sample is not soluble, it may be digested, either on a hot plate or by microwave, using HNO_3, H_2SO_4, or $HClO_4$. Alternatively, the analyte may be extracted via Soxhlet extraction. Liquid samples may be analyzed directly or may be diluted or extracted if the matrix is incompatible with the method of atomization. Serum samples, for instance, may be difficult to aspirate when using flame atomization and may produce unacceptably high background absorbances when using electrothermal atomization. A liquid-liquid extraction using an organic solvent containing a chelating agent is frequently used to concentrate analytes. Dilute solutions of Cd^{2+}, Co^{2+}, Cu^{2+}, Fe^{3+}, Pb^{2+}, Ni^{2+}, and Zn^{2+}, for example, can be concentrated by extracting with a solution of ammonium pyrolidine dithiocarbamate in methyl isobutyl ketone.

Interferences in atomic absorption spectroscopy

Since the concentration of the element is considered to be proportional to the ground state population in flame. Any factor that affect the ground state population of the analyte element can be classified as an interference. The following are the most common interferences:

A. Spectral interferences

It arise when the absorption of the interfering species either overlap or lies so close to the analyte absorption that resolution by the monochromator becomes impossible. This type of interference occur rarely. For such an interference to occur, the separation between two lines would have to be less than 0–1 Å. For example, vanadium absorption line 3082.11 Å causes interferences in the analysis based upon aluminium absorption line at 3082.15 Å. This interference is avoided by employing the another line of absorption (3092.7 Å) for analysis.

An important question to consider when using a flame as an atomization source, is how to correct for the absorption of radiation by the flame. The products of combustion consist of molecular species that may exhibit broad-band absorption, as well as particulate material that may scatter radiation from the source. If this spectral interference is not correct, then the intensity of the transmitted radiation decreases. The result is an apparent increase in the sample's absorbance. Fortunately, absorption and scattering by the flame are corrected by analyzing blank.

B. Chemical interference: Formation of compounds of lower volatility

It result from various chemical processes occurring during atomization that alter the absorption characteristics of the analyte. There are different types. Some examples are given here.

Cation-anion interference

Anions which forms compound of low volatility with the analyte and thus reduce the rate at which it is atomized low results are consequence. *Decrease in calcium absorbance is observed with increasing concentration of sulphate or phosphate.* This can be avoided by adding EDTA solution which can chelate the calcium ion preferentially. This chelate can be subjected for analysis.

$$3Ca^{2+} + 2PO_4^{3-} \longrightarrow Ca_3(PO_4)_2$$

Alternatively releasing agent (cations mostly) that react preferentially with the interference and prevent its interaction with analyte, can be employed. For example, addition of excess of Sr or Lanthanum chloride minimizes the interference of phosphate in the determination.

Addition of a chelating agent for the analysis of calcium:

$$Ca_3(PO_4)_2 + 3EDTA \longrightarrow 3Ca(EDTA) + 2PO_4^{3-}$$

Addition of a release agent for the determination of calcium:

$$Ca_3(PO_4)_2 + 2LaCl_3 \longrightarrow 3CaCl_2 + 2LaPO_4$$

Interference due to oxide formation

This type of interference arises due to formation of stable metal oxide if oxygen is present in the flame, resulting in reduced signal intensity. The alkaline earth metals are subject to this type of interference. This type of interference can be eliminated by either using very high flame temperature to dissociate the oxides or by using oxygen deficient environment to produce excited atoms.

Cation-cation interference

Aluminium is found to cause low results in the determination of magnesium due to formation of heat stable aluminium/magnesium compound (perhaps an oxide). It can be minimised by using higher temperature.

C. Ionization interference

There is a third major interference, however, which is often encountered in hot flames. As illustrated in Fig. 6.5, the dissociation process does not necessarily stop at the ground state atom. If additional energy is applied, the ground state atom can be thermally raised to the excited state or an electron may be totally removed from the atom, creating an ion. As these electronic rearrangements deplete the number of ground state atoms available for light absorption, atomic absorption at the resonance wavelength is reduced. When an excess of energy reduces the population of ground state atoms, an ionization interference exists. Ionization interferences are most common with the hotter nitrous oxide-acetylene flame. In an air-acetylene flame, ionization interferences are normally encountered only with the more easily ionized elements, notably the alkali metals and alkaline earths.

$$M(g) \longrightarrow M^+(g) + e^- \quad \text{Problem}$$

Example: 2450°C, p = 0.1 Pa $\longrightarrow$ Na 5% ionised
$\longrightarrow$ K 33% ionised

Ionisation leads to reduced signal intensity, as energy levels of ions are different from those of the parent ions.

Ionization interference can be eliminated by adding an excess of an element which is very easily ionized, creating a large number of free electrons in the flame and suppressing the ionization of the analyte. Rubidium, and cesium salts are commonly used as ionization suppressants. Addition of 1000 ppm CsCl is done for analysing Na or K element. Fig. 6.20 shows ionization suppression for the determination of barium in a nitrous oxide-acetylene flame. The increase in absorption at the barium resonance line, and the corresponding decrease in absorption at the barium ion line as a function of added potassium, illustrate the enhancement of the ground state species as the ion form is suppressed. By adding 1000 mg/L to 5000 mg/L potassium to all blanks, standards and samples, the effects of ionization can usually be eliminated.

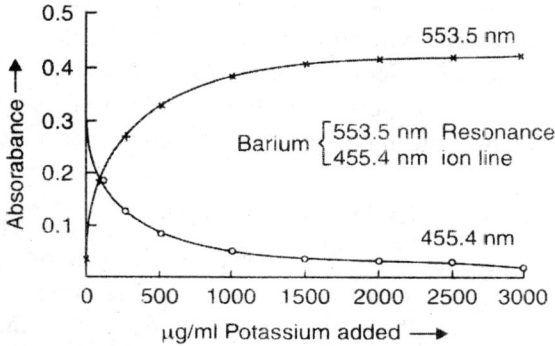

Fig. 6.20. Effect of added potassium on ionization.

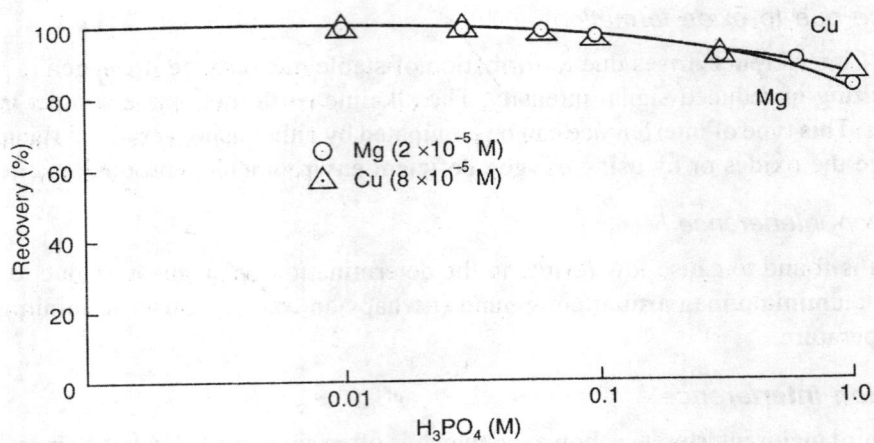

Fig. 6.21. Matrix interference from viscosity effects.

D. Matrix Interference

The first place in the flame atomization process subject to interference is the very first step, the nebulization. If the sample is more viscous or has considerably different surface tension characteristics than the standard, the sample uptake rate or nebulization efficiently may be different between sample and standard. If samples and standards are not introduced into the process at the same rate, it is obvious that the number of atoms in the light beam and, therefore the absorbance, will not correlate between the two (sample and standard solution). Thus, a matrix interference will exist. An example of this type of interference is the effect of acid concentration on absorbance. From Fig. 6.21, it can be seen that as phosphoric acid concentration increases (and the sample viscosity increases), the sample introduction rate and the sample absorbance decrease. Increased acid or dissolved solids concentration normally will lead to a negative error is not recognized and corrected. Matrix interferences can also cause positive error. The presence of an organic solvent in a sample will produce an enhanced nebulization efficiency, resulting in an increased absorption. One way of compensating for this type of interference is to match as closely as possible the major matrix components of the standard to those of the sample. Any acid or other reagent added to the sample during preparation should also be added to the standards and blank in similar concentrations.

E. Broadening of a spectral line

The lines are generally symmetric around the λ_{max} (here indicated as λ_0), the wavelength at which the intensity of emitted radiation is maximum. The absorption is also the maximum at the same wavelength. The **line width** is defined as the width of the signal measured at one half the height of the maximum signal. It is expressed as λ ½ and is measured in the units of wavelength. This full width is measured at one half of the maximum (FWHM) is also called as **effective line width**. Fig. 6.22 shows the schematic diagram defining the atomic line width. The line width resulting from a transition of an electron between two discrete, single valued energy states is expected to be zero. The width of atomic lines are of considerable importance in AAS. Narrow lines reduces the possibility of interferences due to overlapping spectra. Broadening of lines can occur due to a number of factors. The most common line width broadening factors are:

(i) Doppler effect

This effect arises because atoms will have different components of velocity along the line of observation.

(ii) Lorentz effect

This effect occurs as a result of the concentration of foreign atoms present in the environment of the emitting or absorbing atoms. The magnitude of the broadening varies with the pressure of the foreign gases and their physical properties.

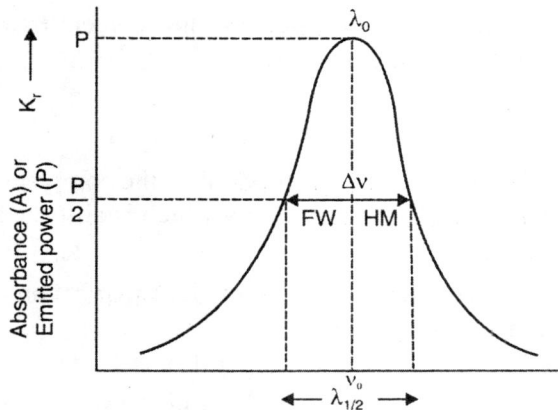

Fig. 6.22. Schematic diagram defining the atomic line width.

(iii) Quenching effect

In a low-pressure spectral source, quenching collision can occur in flames as the result of the presence of foreign gas molecules with vibrational levels very close to the excited state of the resonance line.

(iv) Self absorption or self-reversal effect

The atoms of the same kind as that emitting radiation will absorb maximum radiation at the centre of the line than at the wings, resulting in the change of shape of the line as well as its intensity. This effect becomes serious if the vapour which is absorbing radiation is considerably cooler than that which is emitting radiation.

QUANTITATIVE ATOMIC ABSORPTION SPECTROSCOPY

The atomic absorption process is illustrated in Fig. 6.5. Light at the resonance wavelength of initial intensity, I_o, is focussed on the flame cell containing ground state atoms. The initial light intensity is decreased by an amount determined by the atom concentration in the flame cell. The light is then directed onto the detector where the reduced intensity, I, is measured. The amount of light absorbed is determined by comparing I to I_o. Several related terms are used to define the amount of light absorption which has taken place. The "transmittance" is defined as the ratio of the final intensity to the initial intensity.

$$T = \frac{I}{I_o}$$

Transmittance is an indication of the fraction of initial light which passes through the flame cell to fall on the detector. The "percent transmission" is simply the transmittance expressed in percentage terms.

$$\%T = 100 \times \frac{I}{I_o}$$

The "percent absorption" is the complement of percent transmission defining the percentage of the initial light intensity which is absorbed in the flame.

$$\%A = 100 - \%T$$

These terms are easy to visualize on a physical basis. The fourth term, "absorbance", is purely a mathematical quantity.

$$A = \log\left(\frac{I}{I_o}\right)$$

Absorbance in the most convenient term for characterizing light absorption in absorption spectrophotometry, as this quantity follows a linear relationship with concentration.

Beer's law defines this relationship:

$$A = abc$$

where "A" is the absorbance; "a" is the absorption coefficient, a constant which is characteristic of

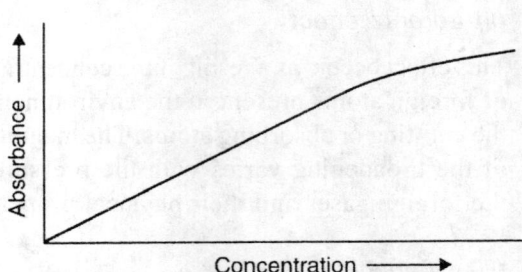

Fig. 6.23. Concentration versus absorbance.

the absorbing species at a specific wavelength; "b" is the length of the light path intercepted by the absorption species in the absorption cell; and "c" is the concentration of the absorbing species. This equation simply states that the absorbance is directly proportional to the concentration of the absorbing species for a given set of instrumental conditions. This directly proportional behaviour between absorbance and concentration is observed in atomic absorption. When the absorbances of standard solutions containing known concentrations of analyte are measured and the absorbance data are plotted against concentration, a calibration relationship similar to that in Fig. 6.23 is established.

Over the region where the Beer's law relationship is observed, the calibration yields a straight line. As the concentration and absorbance increase, non ideal behaviour in the absorption process can cause a deviation from linearity.

After such calibration is established, the absorbance of solutions of unknown concentrations may be measured and the concentration determined from the calibration curve. In modern instrumentation, the calibration can be made within the instrument to provide a direct readout of unknown concentrations. Since the advent of microcomputers, accurate calibration, even in the nonlinear region, is simple.

If the sample concentration is too high to permit accurate analysis in linearity response range, there are three alternatives that may help to bring the absorbance into the optimum working range:
(a) sample dilution,
(b) using an alternative wavelength having a lower absorptivity,
(c) reducing the path length by rotating the burner hand.

Applications of atomic absorption spectroscopy

Atomic absorption spectroscopy is a sensitive means for the quantitative determination of more than 60 metals or metalloid elements.

Columns two and three of Table 6.2 provide information on detection limit for a number of common elements by flame and electrothermal atomic absorption. For comparison purpose, limits for some of the other atomic procedures are also included.

For many elements, detection limits for atomic absorption spectroscopy with flame atomization lie in the range of 1 to 20 ng/ml or 0.001 to 0.020 ppm; for electrothermal atomization, the corresponding figures are 0.002 to 0.01 ng/ml or 2×10^{-6} to 1×10^{-5} ppm. In a few cases, detection limits outside these ranges are encountered.

Table 6.2. Detection limits (ng/ml)* for selected elements

Element	AAS flame	AAS electrothermal	AES flame	AES ICP	AFS flame
Al	30	0.005	5	2	5
As	100	0.02	0.0005	40	100
Ca	1	0.02	0.1	0.02	0.001
Cd	1	0.0001	800	2	0.01
Cr	3	0.01	4	0.3	4
Cu	2	0.002	10	0.1	1
Fe	5	0.005	30	0.3	8
Hg	500	0.1	0.0004	1	20
Mg	0.1	0.00002	5	0.05	1
Mn	2	0.0002	5	0.06	2
Mo	30	0.005	100	0.2	60
Na	2	0.0002	0.1	0.2	–
Ni	5	0.02	20	0.4	3
Pb	10	0.002	100	2	10
Sn	20	0.1	300	30	50
V	20	0.1	10	0.2	70
Zn	2	0.00005	0.0005	2	0.02

* Nanogram/milliliter = 10^{-3} mg/ml = 10^{-3} ppm.

AAS = Atomic absorption spectroscopy; AES = Atomic emission spectroscopy; AFS = Atomic fluorescence spectroscopy; ICP = Inductively coupled plasma

Accuracy

Under usual conditions, the relative error associated with a flame absorption analysis is of the order of 1 to 2%. With special precautions, this figure can be lowered to a few tenths of one per cent. Errors encountered with electrothermal atomization usually exceed those for flame atomization by a factor of 5 to 10.

CHAPTER 7

Fluorimetry

Molecules, A* are excited from its ground state, E_1 to an excited state, E_2 on absorbing energy in the UV or visible region. Molecules in excited state, are short lived and so return to ground level with the release of energy.

$$E = E_2 - E_1$$

The energy release can take place via (i) relaxation process, (ii) photochemical reaction, and (iii) emission of photons. In the first process (i), called vibrational deactivation or nonradiative relaxation, the excess energy is released as heat.

$$A^* \longrightarrow A + \text{heat}$$

Energy release by photochemical reaction involves the decomposition of A

$$A^* \longrightarrow X + Y$$

or reaction between A* and another species.

$$A^* + Z \longrightarrow X + Y$$

In either case, the excess energy is used up or released as heat. In the third (iii) process, energy is released as emission of photons. The emission of photons after absorption of photons is called *photoluminescence*. In most of the cases of photoluminescence, emitted light is of longer wavelength than radiation light used for its excitation. In photoluminescence, light s produced at low temperatures. Therefore, the light produced by this process is regarded as "light without heat" or "cold light".

Photoluminescence is of two types:

(a) **Fluorescence:** In this process, excess of energy is released in the form of fluorescent light in UV-visible region. They emit visible light or radiations. This phenomenon is known as fluorescence and the substance showing this phenomenon are known as fluorescent substances. The phenomenon of fluorescence is instantaneous and starts immediately after the absorption of light and stops as soon as the incident light is cut off.

(b) **Phosphorescence:** When light radiation is incident on certain substances, they emit light continuously even after the incident light is cut off. This type of delayed fluorescence is called phosphorescence and the substances are called phosphorescent substances. Materials exhibiting fluorescence generally reemit excess of radiation within 10^{-8} to 10^{-4} second of absorption. On the other hand, materials exhibiting phosphorescence reemit excess radiation within 10^{-4} to 20 seconds or longer. The life time of phosphorescence is much longer than fluorescence. The measurement of intensity of emitted light in the form of fluorescent light constitutes the analytical technique, designated as *fluorimetry*. The emission of fluorescent light takes place due to presence of fluorophore. For example, aromatic compounds, benzfused heterocyclic compounds, etc. show the fluorescence. It is a very sensitive method, useful for quantitative estimation of variety of inorganic/organic drugs, even present in trace amounts. However, fluorimetric methods are only applicable to the limited number of chemical system. The compounds containing fluorophoric group (conjugated system) can be estimated by this technique owing to their property of producing fluorescence.

Difference between fluorescence and phosphorescence

The electronic transition state responsible for fluorescence does not involve a change in electron spin. Hence, fluorescence is short lived, ceased almost immediately (<10^{-5} seconds). In phosphorescence, there is delayed fluorescence because there is a change in electronic spin. Therefore, emission of radiation can be detected after transmission of source of light often several seconds of longer. Overall, the life span of phosphorescence is much larger than fluorescence.

THEORY OF FLUORESCENCE/PHOSPHORESCENCE

To understand the theoretical aspect of fluorescence/phosphorescence, it is necessary to understand the concept of electron spin, singlet and triplet states.

Electron spin

According to the Pauli exclusion principle, only two electron can be occupied in one orbital. These two electrons must possess opposite spin. Under this condition, the spin are said to be paired. Due to pairing of spin, there is no magnetic field in the molecule and so-called 'Diamagnetic'. In contrast, free radical contain unpaired electron. They have a magnetic moment and so they are called 'Paramagnetic'.

Singlet/Triplet excited states

A molecular electronic state in which all electron spins are paired, is called *singlet state*. The net value of spin (S) for such molecules is zero ($+1/2 - 1/2$) hence multiplicity of a molecular energy is 1 ($2s + 1$, where $s = 0$). Therefore, there is no splitting of energy level in a molecule on exposing in a magnetic field. In a free radical, odd electron can assume two orientation in a magnetic field. Hence, there are two slightly different energy level, accordingly it is called doublet state. In a triplet state, there is a unpairing of electron. The total value of spin will be one (either $+1/2 + 1/2$ or $-1/2 - 1/2$) and accordingly, multiplicity of energy level will be three. ($2s + 1$, where $s = 1$).

In conclusion, the multiplicity of energy level in singlet, doublet and triplet state level is 1, 2 and 3 respectively.

The ground electronic state, on excitation goes to either excited singlet or triplet state. In an excited singlet state, the spin of the promoted electron is still paired with the ground state electron. In the excited triplet state, the spins of the two electrons are unpaired and therefore parallel (Fig. 7.1).

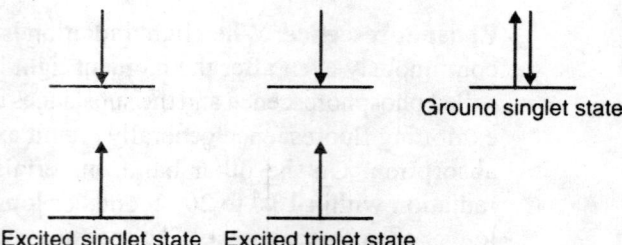

Fig. 7.1. Ground singlet state, excited singlet and triplet state.

In a excitation process, there is a transition of an electron from the highest occupied orbital to the lowest unoccupied orbital. The lowest triplet state is usually at slightly lower energy than the lowest excited singlet state.

A molecule in excited singlet state can return to the ground singlet by emitting light. Light emitted by a singlet-singlet transition give the fluorescence. As it is allowed transition, so the life time of excited singlet is quite short (less than 10^{-5} seconds). This means that fluorescence ceases as soon as excitation source is removed. If a molecule in an excited singlet state goes to triplet by radiation less transition, then further transition to the ground state is forbidden. The radiation emitted in this process is phosphorescence. Due to this forbidden transition, the life time of triplet state may be quite long. Thus, phosphorescence may persist after the excitation source is removed.

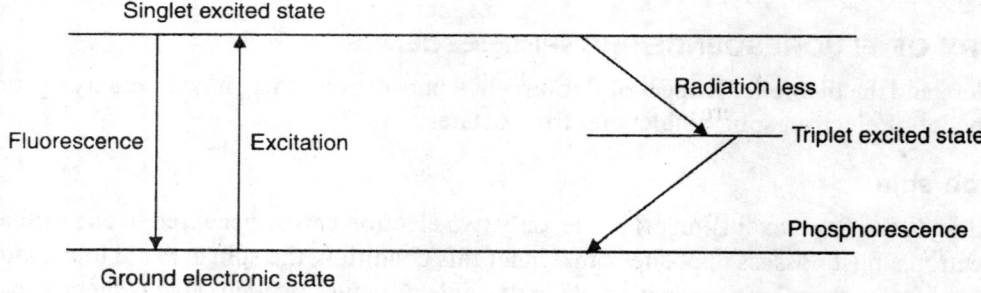

Fig. 7.2.

Deactivation process

Processes which occur between the absorption and emission of light are usually illustrated by a Jablonski diagram. *Note: The diagram is named after Professor Alexander Jablonski who is regarded as father of fluorimetry.* A typical Jablonski diagram is shown in Fig. 7.3. The ground, first and second electronic states are depicted by S_0, S_1 and S_2 respectively. At each of these electronic energy levels the fluorophores can exist in a number of vibrational energy levels (denoted by 0, 1, 2 etc.). Transitions between states are depicted as vertical lines to illustrate the instantaneous nature of light absorption. Transitions occur in about 10–15 seconds, a time too short for significant displacement of nuclei (Franck-Condon principle).

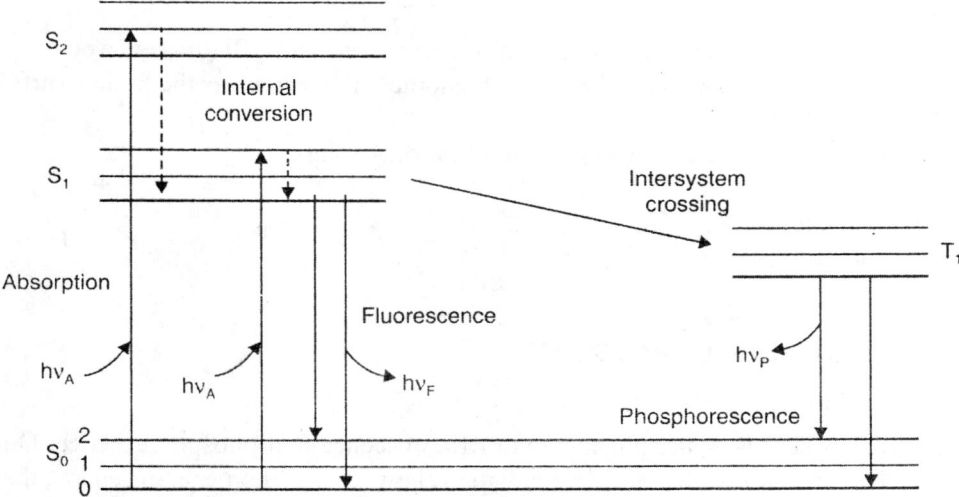

Fig. 7.3. A simplified Jablonski diagram with absorbance, internal conversion, fluorescence, intersystem crossing and phosphorescence.

Following light absorption, several processes usually occur:

(i) **Fluorescence:** A fluorophore is usually excited to some higher vibrational level of either S_1 or S_2. With a few rare exceptions, molecules in condensed phases rapidly relax to the lowest vibrational level of S_1. This process, called *internal conversion*, is non-radiative and takes place in 10–12 seconds or less. Since fluorescence life times are typically near 10^{-8} second, internal conversion complete prior to emission. Return to the ground state occurs to a higher excited vibrational ground-state level, which then quickly reaches thermal equilibrium. An interesting consequence of emission to a higher vibrational ground state is that the emission spectrum is typically a mirror image of the absorption spectrum of the $S_0 \rightarrow S_1$ transition.

(ii) **Intersystem crossing:** Molecules in the S_1 state can also undergo a spin conversion to the first triplet state, T_1. Emission from T_1 is termed phosphorescence and is generally shifted to longer wavelengths (lower energy) relative to fluorescence. Transition from the T_1 to the singlet ground state is forbidden, and as a result, the rate constants for triplet emission are several orders of magnitude smaller than those for fluorescence. Molecules containing heavy atoms such as bromine and iodine are frequently phosphorescent. The heavy atoms facilitate intersystem crossing and thus enhance phosphorescence quantum yields.

Excited molecules releases the energy to return to its ground state by releasing the photons of radiation (fluorescence and phosphorescence). The other process of deactivation are radiation less. These also compete with the above process. Thus, if deactivation by release of photons is rapid is comparison to radiation less processes, such fluorescence is observed. In contrast if radiationless process dominates, then fluorescence is either absent or of less intense radiation. The less radiation processes include vibrational relaxation, internal conversion, external conversion and inter system crossing.

Stokes' shift

The energy of emission is typically less than that of absorption. Thus, fluorescence occurs at lower energies or longer wavelengths, $hvF < hvA$. The phenomenon is known as the Stokes shift and can be caused by:
  (a) Energy losses due to relaxation to ground vibrational states
  (b) Solvent effects
  (c) Excited state reactions
  (d) Complex formation
  (e) Energy transfer

FACTORS AFFECTING FLUORESCENCE

1. Nature of molecules

All the molecules donot show the phenomena of fluorescence and phosphorescence. Only such molecules which absorb ultraviolet or visible radiation shows this phenomena. In general, the greater the absorbancy of a molecule, the more intense its luminescence. This requirement means that molecules having conjugated double (π-bonds) are particularly suitable for this study. On the other hand, aliphatic and saturated cyclic organic compounds are not suitable. Organic compounds possessing aromatic system in their structure produce fluorescence. Compounds containing aliphatic carbonyl structure or highly conjugated double bond structure may also exhibit fluorescence and their number is small compared with the number of aromatic compounds. The simple heterocycles (pyridine, furan, thiophene and pyrrole) do not exhibit fluorescence while benzfused heterocycles (qunazoline, isoquinazoline, indole) show the fluorescence.

2. Nature of substituents

Substituents often exhibit a marked effect on the fluorescence and phosphorescence of molecules. There are no rigid rules but a generalities may be useful. These are as follows:
  (a) Electron-donating groups like $-NH_2$ and $-OH$ often enhance fluorescence. On the other hand, groups like $-SO_3H$, NH_4^+ and alkyl groups do not have much effect on both phosphorescence and fluorescence.
  (b) Electron-withdrawing group like $-COOH$, $-NO_2$, $-N=N-$ and halides decrease or even destroy fluorescence.

3. Effect of concentration

It is already stated that the fluorescence is proportional to concentration but it must be emphasized that the equation applies only to small values of fluorescence and hence low concentrations of sample. Thus, it is true to about 5% when the extinction of a solution of the sample is about 0.05. Under these conditions, the amount of light absorbed by the test solution is very small, and for a linear calibration curve the extinction should not be greater than about 0.02. The fluorescence of a given analyte increases linearly with increasing concentration at low level (only when absorbance in 1 cm cell is < 0.02). At high concentration of analyte, negative deviation occurs and fluorescence reaches a limiting value and even decreases by increase in concentration (Fig. 7.4).

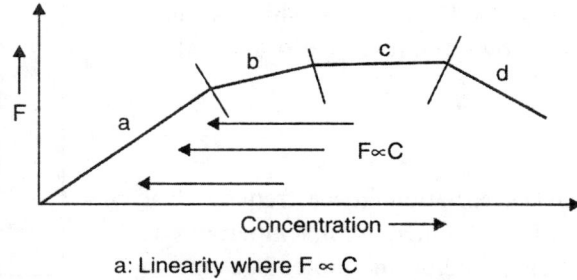

a: Linearity where $F \propto C$
b: Negative deviation of linearity
c: F is independent of concentration
d: Reabsorption of F (inner filter effect)

Fig. 7.4. Effect of concentration on fluorescent intensity (F).

4. Rigidity of structure

Most of the fluorescent organic molecules have highly rigid planar structures. For example, fluorene, due to presence of methylene group is a rigid molecule, hence exhibit the fluorescence. In contrast, biphenyl due to lack of rigidity do not show fluorescence. A steric hinderance of rings or substituents decreases fluorescence intensity as it facilitates the internal dissipation of energy in the excited state of the molecule.

Fluorene   Biphenyl

5. Adsorption

The extreme sensitiveness of the method requires very dilute solutions, 10–100 times weaker than those employed in spectrophotometry. Adsorption of the fluorescent substance on the container walls may therefore present a serious problem, and strong stock solutions must be kept and diluted as required. Quinine is a typical example of a substance which is absorbed on container/cuvette walls.

6. Light

Monochromatic light is essential for the excitation of molecules to cause fluorescence in quantitative work because the intensity will vary with wavelength. The purity of the irradiating beam especially if obtained via filters should, therefore, be checked by examination of the light scattered by a slightly turbid solution. The spectrum obtained should show one peak only, corresponding in wavelength to that expected.

7. pH

The fluorescence of an aromatic compound containing acidic or basic functional group is usually pH dependent. For example, phenol is fluorescent compound but phenolate ion is non-fluorescent in nature, α-naphthol does not exhibit fluorescence while its anion does. Similarly, aniline only shows fluorescence in neutral or alkaline solution.

8. Temperature

Variation in temperature causes variation in the frequency of collision between molecules. Thus, an increase in temperature is likely to decrease fluorescence by increasing molecular motion and collision (Fig. 7.5). This effect varies from one compound to another. Similarly, many substances not normally fluorescent at room temperature are capable of emitting light when excited at a low temperature.

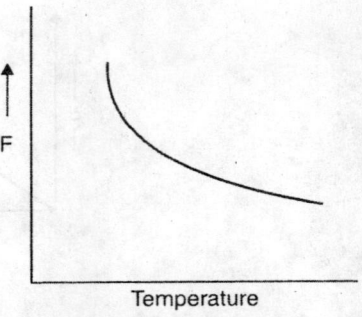

Fig. 7.5. Effect of temperature on fluorescent intensity (F).

9. Oxygen

The presence of oxygen may interfere in two ways: By direct oxidation of the fluorescent substance to non-fluorescent substance or nonfluorescent products, or by quenching of fluorescence. It is a useful precaution, therefore, to check the deaerated solution and compare the result obtained with that from the oxygen-containing solution. Anthracence is well known to be susceptible to the presence of oxygen.

10. Solvent effect

(a) *Viscosity*: Fluorescence increases by increase in the viscosity of the solvent, energy lost by molecular collision is decreased as viscosity increases.

(b) *Polarity*: Polar solvents decreases energy of π–π* transition and increase energy of n–π*. This enhances fluorescence.

(c) *Type of solvent*: Solvents containing heavy atoms (e.g. Br^- and I^-) decreases fluorescence (heavy atom effect). This effect promotes orbital spin changes. Therefore, phosphorescence is enhanced (triplet formation increases).

11. Quenching

'Quenching' decrease the intensity of fluorescence. Fluorescence quenching refers to any process that decreases the fluorescence intensity of a sample. There are a wide variety of quenching processes that include excited state reactions, molecular rearrangements, ground state complex formation, and energy transfer. Quenching experiments can be used to determine the accessibility of quencher to a fluorophore, monitor conformational changes, monitor association reactions of the fluorescence of one of the reactants changes upon binding. There are two basic types of quenching: *static* and *dynamic* (collisional). Both types require an interaction between the fluorophore and quencher. In the case of *dynamic* quenching, the quencher must diffuse to the fluorophore during the lifetime of the excited state. Upon contact the fluorophore returns to the ground state without emission of a photon. In the case of *static* quenching, quencher forms a complex with the flurophore. This complex is non-fluorescent. The formation of this complex does not rely upon population of the excited state.

QUANTITATIVE FLUORESCENCE ANALYSIS

The intensity of fluorescence intensity (F) is proportional to the concentration of fluorescent substances. For analytical purpose, concentration of fluorescent entities is always kept to a very low ($< 10^{-5}$ M). In concentrated solution, most of the incident light may be absorbed by first layer of solution and very little light goes to distant portion of the sample solution, hence fluorescence will not be proportional to concentration of the solution. It is valid when all the absorbed light is emitted in the form of fluorescence. But it does not happen, part of absorbed light is lost in other ways (e.g. vibrational relaxation, internal conversion etc.). Therefore, for quantitative estimation, we take the quantum efficiency (ϕ), which is defined as the number of quanta emitted by the fluorescence process (F, Fluorescence intensity) to the number of quanta absorbed (I_{ab}) in per unit time.

$$\phi = \frac{F}{I_{ab}} \qquad ...(7.1)$$

Number of quanta absorbed (I_{ab}) is equal to the intensity of incident radiation (I_o) minus the intensity of transmitted radiation (I). The value of ϕ may vary from 0 to 1.

$$I_{ab} = I_o - I_o^{-2.3abc} \qquad ...(7.2)$$

where
a = molar absorptivity
b = path length (thickness of sample solution through which incident light passes)
c = molar concentration

Note: The value of I is already derived from Beer Lambert law as $I = I_o e^{-kbc} = I_o 10^{-abc}$. If c is very small, eq. (7.2) can be adjusted in the approximate form.

$$I_{ab} = \frac{2.3abcI_o}{1 + 2.3abc} = 2.3abcI_o \qquad ...(7.3)$$

Note: $e^x = 1 + x$.

On combining the eq. 7.1 and eq. 7.3,

$$F = 2.3\, I_o\, \phi\, abc \qquad ...(7.4)$$

According to equation 7.4, fluorescent intensity is directly proportional to concentration. This equation also shows that F is proportional to I_o, so increased sensitivity can be achieved for a given concentration by increasing the incident excitation radiation. This is fundamental difference between fluorimetry and spectrometry; in the later technique, absorbance is independent of incident radiation.

To determine unknown concentrations from the amount of fluorescence that a sample emits, it is necessary to calibrate the fluorimeter with a standard (to determine quantum efficiency) or to prepare a working curve.

EXCITATION VERSUS EMISSION SPECTRA

The photoluminescence spectra are recorded by measuring the luminescence (emitted radiation) as function of either excitation wavelength or emission wavelength. The excitation spectrum (dotted line in Fig. 7.6) is a plot of the luminiscence vs. excitation wavelength with a constant emission wavelength. It is used to determine the best excitation wavelength for analysis and is related to the absorption spectrum of the analyte. This spectrum is similar to absorption spectrum provided other variable like source like intensity and detector response remain same. A plot of the luminescence signal vs. emission wavelength with a constant excitation wavelength is denoted an emission spectrum.

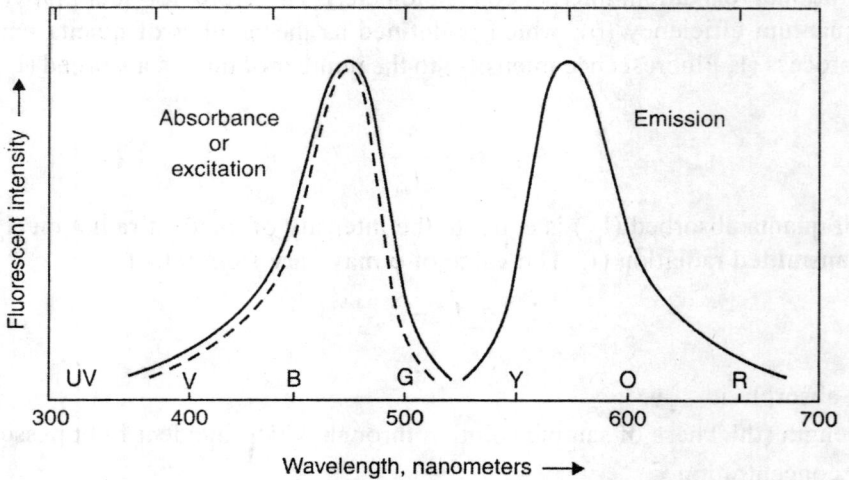

Fig. 7.6. Example of excitation and emission spectrum.

Instrumentation

The basic components of instruments, diagrammatically shown in the Fig. 7.7, are as follows:

Light source

It is more intense and stable in comparison to instruments required to measure absorption. Mercury arc lamps and xenon arc lamps are commonly used light source. These emit the light in the visible and UV region. The xenon lamp emission is uniformly distributed from about 300 to 1300 nm while the emission of mercury lamp is concentrated at several intense line for example, 254, 366, 405, 436, 546, 577, 691 and 773 nm.

Primary (excitation) filter

To achieve specificity in the excitation, a narrow band width of radiation emitted from light source is selected. This narrow band width is selected by using either filter or monochromator.

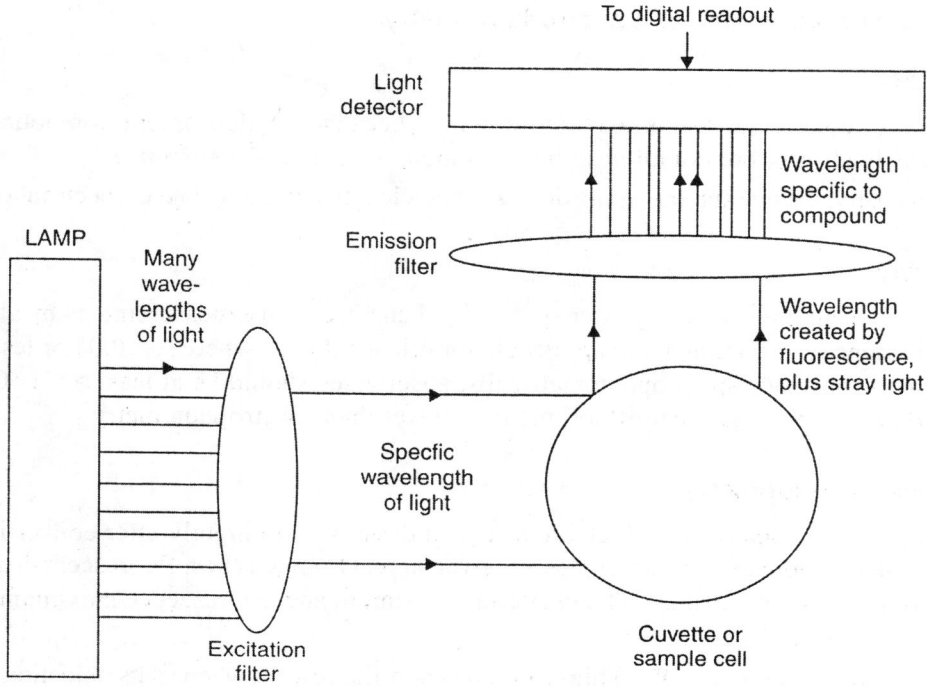

Fig. 7.7. Schematic of the fluorimeter.

In fluorimeter, this function is performed by glass filter. It only transmits the light of narrow band width (50 to 100 nm) and absorb all other radiation. Filters are exchangeable, depending on the requirement of band width, corresponding to the absorption maximum. Quartz prism or grating monochromators are commonly used in spectrofluorimeter. There are more sophisticated and selective in choosing the lines required for excitation of analyte.

Sample cell: The radiation passing through the primary filter, strikes to sample cell. Glass cells are adequate in most of the cases but to work below 320 nm, however, quartz is essential.

Secondary (emission) filter: The fluorescence light is emitted in all the direction by the analyte molecule. The fluorescence intensity is difficult to measure in the direction of propagation due to high intensity background of emitted light. This problem is overcome by observing the fluorescence at a right angle to the beam of excitation light. Some of the light transmitted in this direction is scattered. This undesirable light is removed with the help of secondary filter or monochromator as shown in the chapter of Absorption Spectroscopy. These are selected to provide the most intense fluorescence maximum.

Detector: The fluorescent light goes to detector. Here light signal is converted into electrical signal. The intensity of electrical signal is correspond to intensity of fluorescent light. The most commonly used detector are phototube or photomultiplier as in ultraviolet spectrophotometer or mass spectrometer.

Advantages of Fluorimetry or Spectrofluorometry

A. Selectivity

1. There are fewer compounds that fluorescence, because all fluorescent compounds must necessarily absorb, but not all absorbing compounds emit as fluorescence.
2. In fluorimetry, the measurements are done at 2 wavelengths, it is only one in spectrophotometry.

B. Sensitivity

Fluorescence measurements have greater sensitivity than absorbance measurements by about 100 times. Fluorescence measurement are applicable for dilute solution where A = 0.05 or less, where as to measure a substance spectrophotometrically, absorbance should be at least > 0.1 (0.3–0.9). Therefore, detection limit is spectrofluorometry is lower than spectrophotometry.

Applications of Fluorimetry

There are number of compounds which are analysed directly or indirectly after converting them into fluorescent compounds. Few examples are given here. Quinine is best fluorescent drug and so efficiently assayed by this method. The excitation maximum and fluorescence maximum are 350 mm and 450 mm respectively.

(i) **Determination of vitamin B_1 (Thiamine):** It is non-fluorescent whereas its oxidation product, thiochrome, produces the fluorescence with blue colour. The property is used for the determination of vitamin B_1 in the food samples like meat, cereal etc.

The food sample is hydrolysed to break up the phosphate esters of thiamine present in the sample. The solution on filtration removes phosphates and other insoluble matter. Then, the filtrate is diluted to a known volume. From the filtrate, two equal aliquots are taken, one for analysis and other for a blank. To both aliquots, equal quantities of sodium hydroxide and isobutyl alcohol are added. To the first, oxidizing agent like potassium ferricyanide is added. After shaking, the alcoholic solution is separated from the aqueous solution. Then, the alcoholic solution is examined in the fluorimeter. The excitation maximum is taken at 365 mm and the fluorescence maximum at about 440 mm. The whole procedure, including a blank, is repeated with a standard thiamine solution.

Thiamine hydrochloride   Thiochrome

(ii) **Determination of vitamin B_2 (riboflavin):** The riboflavin can be determined by fluorescence spectrophotometry with excitation wavelength 475.4 nm and emission wavelength 524.7 nm.

Similarly, fluorimetric method of assays are applied to large number of pharmaceuticals (Table 7.1) due to high sensitivity. The fluorescent compounds can be assayed in the range of 10^{-4} to 10^{-9} M.

Table 7.1. Examples of drugs estimated by fluorimetry

S. No.	Drugs	Excitation wavelength (nm)	Emission wavelength (nm)	S. No.	Drugs	Excitation wavelength (nm)	Emission wavelength (nm)
1.	p-Aminosalicylic acid	300	404	10.	Pyridoxal	330	385
2.	Amphotericin B	340	427	11.	Pyridoxamine	335	400
3.	Chlorodiazepoxide	285	510	12.	Pyridoxine	340	400
4.	Cyclizine	305	417	13.	Promazine	320	450
5.	Diphenhydramine	305	412	14.	Ocinine	350	450
6.	Fluphenazine	290	480	15.	Reserpine	390	510
7.	Flurazepam	375	475	16.	Trifluoroperazine	320	470
8.	Oxazepam	365	490	17.	Carbazole	340	370
9.	Pheniramine	275	434				

(iii) **Determination of uranium:** An interesting example is the determination of uranium in salts by Fluorimetry. This is used extensively in the field of nuclear research. The uranium sample is evaporated with nitric acid to bring about oxidation. Then, the sample is fused with sodium fluoride to a melt having fluorides of sodium and uranium. On cooling, this solidifies to a glass which is examined in a specially designed fluorimeter. Hence, by making complex with NaF, one can determine uranium of the order of 5×10^{-9} g in a 1 g of solid sample.

(iv) **Application of fluorimetry in inorganic analysis:** In general, inorganic ions do not exhibit fluorescence. However, some of these inorganic ions form fluorescent chelates with non-fluorescent organic molecules. This has provided the basis for very sensitive analysis of many elements including most of the transition elements.

One interesting example is the determination of aluminium (III) in alloys. Aluminium (III) forms a complex with dye Pontachrome Blue-back RM at pH of 4.8 which fluoresces strongly. One can determine aluminium in the range of 0.2 to 25 μg in a volume of 50 ml with a sensitivity of 1 part in 10^8.

Cadmium can be estimated by precipitating it with 2-(2-hydroxyphenyl)-benzoxazole in the presence of tartrate. The complex on dissolving in glacial acetic acid yields a solution with orange tint and a bright blue colored fluorescence in ultraviolet light. The acetic acid solution thus forms basis for the determination of cadmium.

Similarly, calcium can be estimated by Fluorimetry with calcein solution.

(v) **Fluorescent indicators:** The intensity and color of the fluorescence of many substances depend upon the pH of solution, i.e., their colors depend upon the pH range. These are termed as *fluorescent indicators*. These are mainly used in volumetric titrations. These can be employed in the titration of colored solutions in which the changes in color of indicators get masked. Some examples of fluorescent indicators are given in Table 7.2.

Table 7.2. Examples of some fluorescent indicators

Name of indicator	Approx pH range	Color change
Eosin	3.0–4.0	Colorless to green
Fluorescein	4.0–6.0	Colorless to green
Quinine sulphate	3.0–5.0	Blue to violet
Acridine	5.2–6.6	Green to violet-blue
2-Naphthaquinone	4.4–6.3	Blue to colorless
2-Hydroxycinnamic acid	7.2–9.0	Colorless to green

(vi) **Organic analysis:** Fluorimetry has been used to carry out qualitative as well quantitative analysis for a great many aromatic compounds present in cigarette smoke, air-pollutant, concentrates and automobile exhausts. A specific example is the determination of benzopyrene in the nanogram range in cigarette (approximately 10 nanogram of benzopyrene is present in one cigarette). LSD (lysergic acid diethylamide) can be analysed fluorimetrically especially in a sample of blood or urine. The excitation and fluorescence wavelength used are 335 and 435 nm respectively.

Experiment: Assay of Quinine sulphate solution

Experiment (Procedure)

1. **Preparation of standard quinine sulphate:** Dissolve 0.1 g of Quinine sulphate in 0.1 N H_2SO_4 and dilute to 1 litre with same solvent (100 µg/ml).
2. Dilute 5 ml of this solution to 50 ml with 0.1 N H_2SO_4 (10 µg/ml).
3. Pipette out 1 ml, 2 ml, 3 ml, 4 ml, 5 ml of the above solution into 50 ml volumetric flask and make up the volume with 0.1 N H_2SO_4.
4. Select proper excitation (µ 350 nm) and emission filters (µ 450 nm). Measure fluorescence intensity of each standard solution and prepare calibration curve by plotting a graph of fluorescence intensity versus concentration.
5. Similarly measure the fluorescence intensity of unknown solution and find out the concentration of unknown solution from calibration curve.

CHAPTER 8

Flame Photometry

Flame photometry, also referred to as 'flame atomic emission spectrometry' is a quick, economical and simple way of detecting the metal ions, primarily sodium, potassium, lithium, calcium and barium in a concentrated solution. The process is an extension of the principles used in a flame test, with the main differences having more precision in the results, and the use of more advanced technology.

INTRODUCTION

It is a well known that that several elements like sodium, potassium, calcium and barium when burn in the flame emit out a characteristic flame (Table 8.1). The color is a characteristic of particular element. It means, metal or metallic salts excited in a flame in flame photometry, specific wavelength which is characteristic of element of the visible and ultraviolet radiation emitted out, is observed in qualitative analysis. It means, metal or metallic salts excited in a flame in flame photometry, specific wavelength which is characteristic of element of the visible and ultraviolet radiation emitted out is observed in qualitative analysis.

Table 8.1. Atomic flame emissions of the alkali and alkaline earth metals in terms of the emission wavelength and the color produced

Element	Emission wavelength (nm)	Flame color
Sodium (Na)	589	Yellow
Potassium (K)	766	Violet
Barium (Ba)	554	Lime green
Calcium (Ca)	622*	Orange
Lithium (Li)	670	Red

* Calcium is measured by using the calcium hydroxide band emission at 622 nm as the calcium main atomic emission occurs at 423 nm.

THEORETICAL CONCEPT

Flame photometry (more accurately called flame atomic emission spectrometry) is a branch of atomic spectroscopy (see chapter 6) in which the species examined in the spectrometer are in the form of atoms. In a typical flame photometric experiment, a solution containing the relevant substance to be analysed is aspirated into the burner and dispersed into the flame as a fine spray. This process is called **nebulisation** which serves to increase the surface area of the solution sample, so that the solvent evaporation (desolvation) can proceed more rapidly and the resulting dried solute particles can be volatilised better. In the flame, the solvent evaporates first, leaving finely divided solid particles which move to hottest region of the flame where gaseous atoms and ions are produced. The atoms are excited by absorbing energy available from the flame. As the excited atoms return to a ground state of lower energy, radiation of wavelength, characteristic of the element, is emitted. The intensity of the emitted radiation is then measured, which can be related to the concentration of the element present, which forms the basis of quantitative analysis. The following processes occur in the flame. The various steps occurring in flame photometry can be shown by following sequence of steps:

(i) **Desolvation:** The sample containing metal particles is dehydrated by the heat of the flame and the solvent is evaporated.

(ii) **Vaporisation:** The heat of the flame vaporises the sample constituents. No chemical change takes place at this stage.

(iii) **Atomisation:** At this stage the metal ions that were in the solvent are reduced to metal atoms. For example, Mg^{2+} (aq) + 2e $\longrightarrow$ Mg (g). By heat of the flame and action of the reducing gas (fuel), molecules and ions of the sample species are decomposed and reduced to give atoms.

(iv) **Excitation:** The atoms at this stage absorb energy from the heat of the flame and excited to higher level. The amount of energy absorbed depends on the electrostatic forces of attraction between the negatively charged electrons and the positively charged nucleus.

(v) **Emission of radiation:** The atoms in the excited state are very unstable and move back down to the ground state or a lower energy state quite quickly. As they do so, they emit the energy in the form of radiation of characteristic wavelength, which is measured by a detector. For some metals this radiation corresponds to wavelengths of light in the visible region of the electromagnetic spectrum and is observed as a characteristic color of the flame. As electrons from different energy levels are able to emit light as they relax, the flame color observed will be a mixture of all the different wavelengths emitted by the different electrons in the metal atom under investigation. Fig. 8.1 illustrates various steps representing the processes.

For example, the flame emission spectrum of the element sodium can be obtained by placing a solution of sodium chloride in a suitable flame. At the temperature of the flame (2000°C to 3000°C) the outer electron of the sodium atom is promoted from the ground state $3s$ orbital to excited p orbitals ($3p$, $4p$, $5p$). The relaxation of the excited electron gives rise to the characteristic emission spectrum of the sodium atom. The emission spectrum of the sodium atom is relatively simple and consists of about 40 signals or lines; the most prominent emission signals being in the region of

285 nm, 330 nm and 590 nm. Fig. 8.2 shows a portion of the flame emission spectrum for sodium atom; the excitation being done by an oxyhydrogen flame. There is intense signal at 589 nm in the emission of the sodium atom. This in fact consists of a pair of lines at 589 and 589.6 nm, which could not be resolved due to instrumental limitations. This pair of lines originates from the relaxation of the excited electron in $3p$ to the $3s$ level is responsible for the characteristic yellow glow of the sodium light.

Flame photometry is suitable for qualitative and quantitative determination of several cations, especially for metals that are easily excited to higher energy levels at a relatively low flame temperature (mainly Na, K, Rb, Cs, Ca, Ba, Cu). The metal or metallic salts possessing low excitation energies are most commonly estimated by this method, for example alkali or alkaline earth metals.

Introduction of metallic salt solution
↓
Production of liquid droplet
↓
Evaporation of liquid (formation of solid residue)
↓
Gaseous atoms
↓
Dissociation of free neutral atoms
↓
Excitation of atoms
↓
Emission of radiation from the excited atoms
↓
Measurement of wavelength and intensity of emitted radiation

Fig. 8.1. Various sequences in flame photometry.

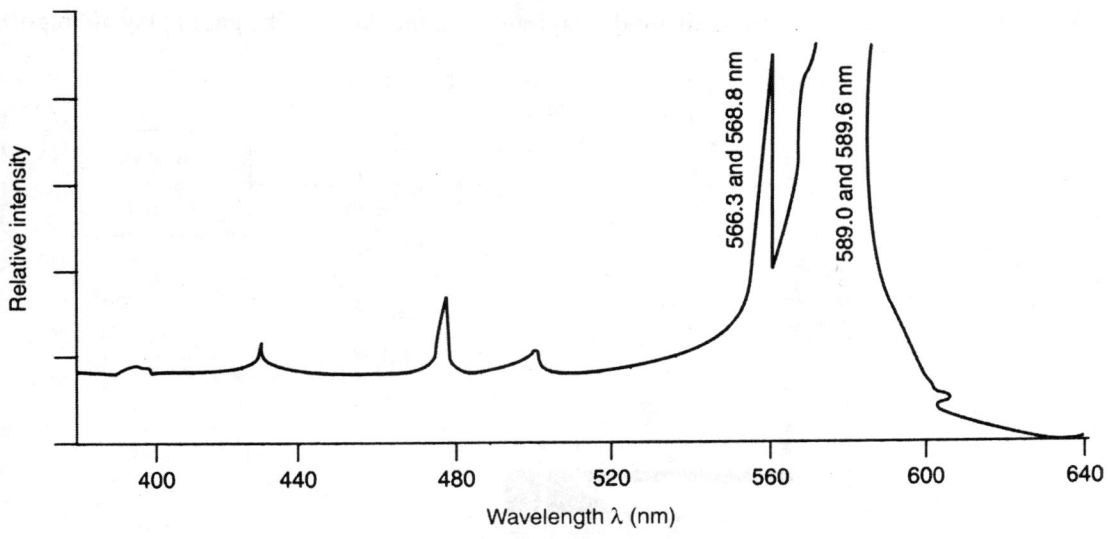

Fig. 8.2. Flame emission spectrum for sodium atom obtained from oxyhydrogen flame.

EMISSION SPECTRA

If the atom loses energy, the electron passes from higher to a lower energy level, energy is released and a spectral line of specific wavelength is emitted. The line constitutes the **emission spectrum**.

The **emission spectra** of two types:
- **Continuous spectra:** When white light from any source such as sun or bulb is analysed by passing through a prism, it splits up into seven different wide bands of color from violet to red (like rainbow). These color are so continuous that each of them merges into the next. Hence the spectrum is called as continuous spectrum.
- **Line spectra:** When an electric discharge is passed through a gas at low pressure light is emitted. If this light is resolved by a spectroscope, it is found that some isolated colored lines are obtained on a photographic plate separated from each other by dark spaces. This spectrum is called line spectrum. Each line in the spectrum corresponds to a particular wavelength. Each element gives its own characteristic spectrum. Line spectra are obtained from atoms of luminous gases or vapours when electric discharge passes through them.

INSTRUMENTATION

The flame photometers are relatively simply instruments (Fig. 8.3) used in this technique. There is no need for source of light, since it is the measured constituent of the sample that emits the light. The energy that is needed for the excitation is provided by the temperature of the flame (2000–3000°C), produced by the burning of acetylene or natural gas (or propane-butane gas) in the presence of air or oxygen. By the heat of the flame and the effect of the reducing gas (fuel), molecules and ions of the sample species are decomposed and reduced to give atoms, e.g.: $Na^+ + e^-$? Na. Atoms in the vapour state give line spectra. (Not band spectra, because there are no covalent bonds). The most sensitive parts of the instrument are the aspirator and the burner. The gases play an important

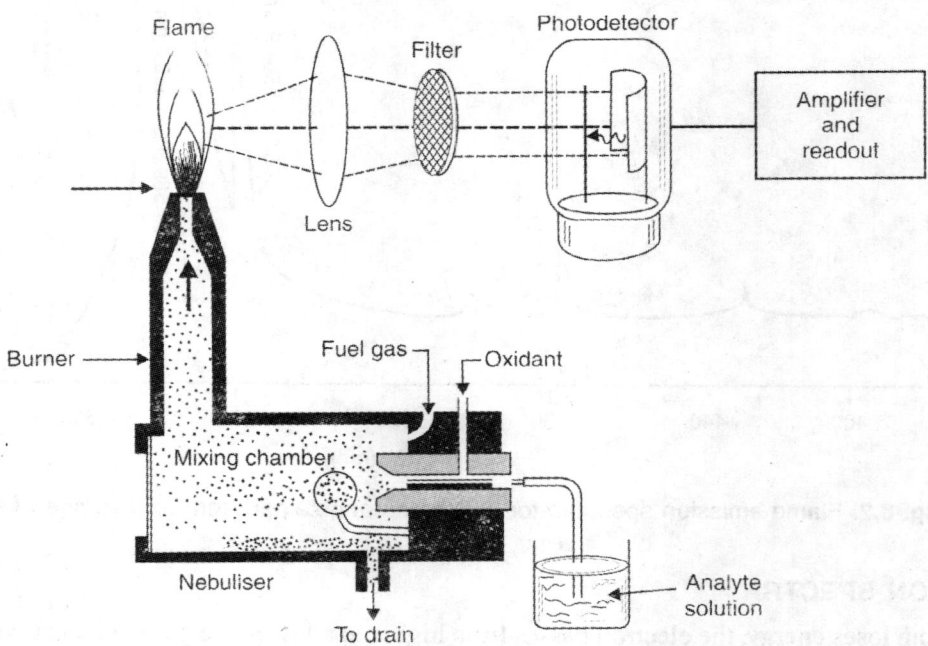

Fig. 8.3. Schematic diagram of flame photometer.

role in the aspiration and while making the aerosol. The air sucks up the sample (according to Bernoulli's principle) and passes it into the aspirator, where the bigger drops condense and could be eliminated.

The monochromator selects the suitable (characteristic) wavelength of the emitted light. The usual optical filters could be used. The emitted light reaches the detector. This is a photomultiplier producing an electric signal proportional to the intensity of emitted light.

A simple flame photometer consists of the following basic components:
(a) **Atomizer and burner:** The burner consists of a flame that can be maintained in a constant form and at a constant temperature. Atomizer is a means of transporting a homogeneous solution into the flame at a steady rate.
(b) **The optical system:** A means of isolating light of the wavelength to be measured from that of extraneous emissions.
(c) **The photosensitive detector:** It is a photo-detector; a means of measuring the intensity of radiation emitted by the flame.
(d) Amplifier and readout device.

(a) Atomizer and burner

In flame-AES, a nebulizer-burner system is used to atomize the minerals in the sample and excite

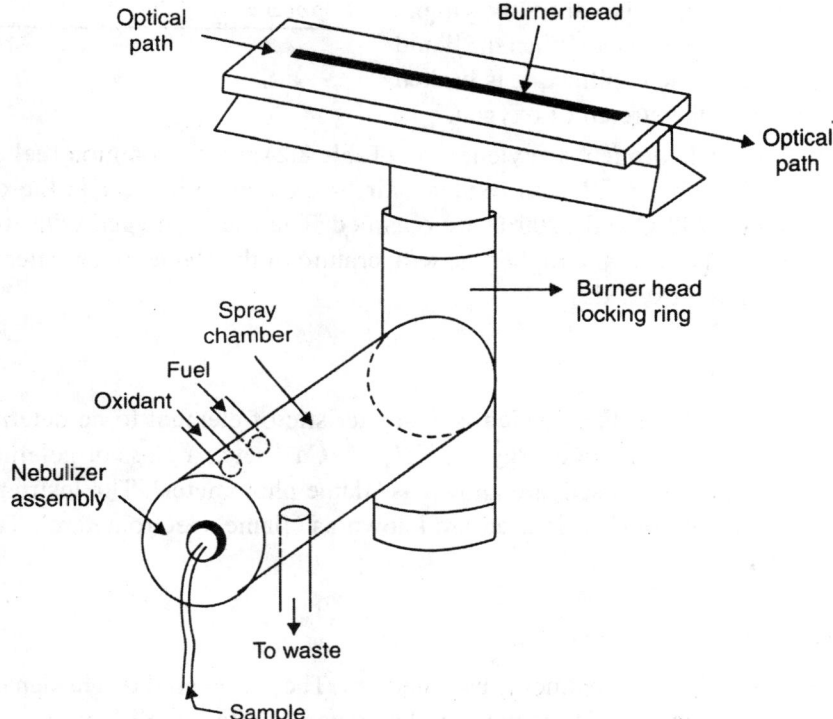

Fig. 8.4. Flame atomization assembly equipped with spray chamber and slot burner.

a large proportion of them to higher energy levels. Atomizer is the most important device of the flame photometer. It produces a fine, uniform spray of analyte solution. The spray is carried to the flame by stream of oxidant (air or oxygen) that supports combustion of the fuel gas used for the flame. Pressure regulators and flow meters regulate the fuel and supporting gases to provide reproducible spray and flame characteristics.

The atomizer may be separate or combined with the burner as single unit. In an atomizer that is separate from the burner (Fig. 8.4), the stream of oxidant atomizes the sample solution in the atomization chamber. The large drops formed, are collected along the walls of the chamber and are drained off. While fine drops are carried as a mist to the burner flame. In the combined atomizer-burner unit (Fig. 8.5) a central capillary tube is immersed in the sample solution. The flow of the oxidant around the capillary tube causes the sample solution to be aspirated up the tube. When the liquid reaches the upper tip of the capillary, it is broken down into fire mist by the stream of oxygen.

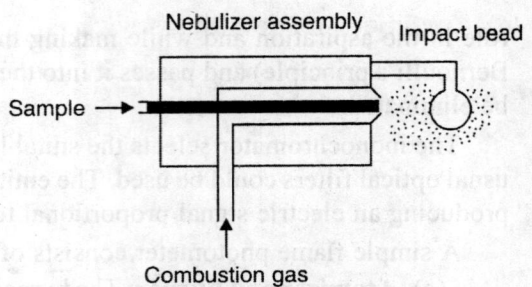

Fig. 8.5. Nebulizer assembly.

Table 8.2. Flame temperature of various fuel/oxidants

Fuel/oxidant	Temperature °C
H_2/Air	2100
H_2/O_2	2750
C_2H_2/Air	2150
C_2H_2/O_2	3100
Propane/Air	1900
Propane/O_2	2800

Natural or coal gas, hydrogen, acetylene, etc. (Table 8.2) are the common fuel gases, used for flame excitation. These are used with oxidant, air or oxygen. When air is the oxidant, flame temperature between 1700°C and 2200°C are obtained. The use of oxygen with fuel gases gives higher temperature. In general, the higher the temperature of the flame, the greater the number of spectral lines that can be excited.

(b) The optical system

It isolate a particular spectral lines which is characteristic of element to be determined. For the element possessing low excitation energy the Na^+, K^+, Ca^{++}, etc., a glass or gelatin filter is used, the instruments where filter is used, are known as 'flame photometer'. The instruments in which prism or grating monochromator is used are known as 'flame spectrometers'. The later one is costly but more efficient.

(c) The detector system

Phototube or photo multiplier is commonly used detector. These convert the light signal into electrical signal (more detail on page), which is measured as much or after amplification.

(d) Amplifier and readout device

The output from the detector is suitably amplified and displayed on a readout device like a meter or a digital display. The sensitivity of the amplifier can be changed so as to be able to analyse samples of varying concentrations. Nowadays the instruments have microprocessor controlled electronics that provides output compatible with the printers and computers thereby minimising the possibility of operator error in transferring data.

QUALITATIVE FLAME PHOTOMETRY

Flame photometric methods are widely used for the determination of alkali and the alkaline earth metals in samples that are easily prepared as aqueous solutions. Some of these elements can be detected visually by the color in the flame, e.g. sodium produces yellow colored flame. However, this method is not very reliable. The best method is to use flame photometer with a filter or monochromator to separate radiation with the wavelengths characteristic of the different metals from other radiations present. If the radiation of the characteristic wavelength is detected, it will indicate the presence of the metal in the sample.

The method to carry out detection of elements by flame photometry is fast, simple and if carried out with care, quite reliable. However, there are some difficulties. It does not provide information about the molecular structure of the compound present in the sample solution. Nonradiating element such as carbon, hydrogen and halides cannot be detected. These can only be determined under special circumstances.

QUANTITATIVE FLAME PHOTOMETRY

This technique uses a flame that evaporates the solvent and also sublimates and atomizes the metal and then excites a valence electron to an upper energy state. Light is emitted at characteristic wavelengths for each metal as electron returns to the ground state that makes qualitative determination possible. Flame photometers use optical filters to monitor for the selected emission wavelength produced by the analyte species. Comparison of emission intensities of unknowns to either that of standard solutions (plotting calibration curve), or to those of an internal standard (standard addition method), allows quantitative analysis of the analyte metal in the sample solution. The intensity of the light emitted could be described by the Scheibe-Lomakin equation:

$$I = k \times c^n$$

where

$c =$ the concentration of the element
$k =$ proportionality constant
$n \sim 1$ (at the linear part of the calibration curve), therefore the intensity of emitted light is directly proportional to the concentration of the sample.

Because of the very narrow and characteristic emission lines from the gas-phase atoms in the flame plasma, the method is relatively free of interferences from other elements. Therefore the flame photometry (as with other atomic spectroscopy methods) is very sensitive; measuring concentration of ppm magnitude (part per million, e.g. mg kg^{-1}) usually does not cause any problem.

The optical concentration range of the solutions for the measured metal ion is 10^{-3}–10^{-4} mol dm^{-3}. Typical precision for analysis of dilute aqueous solutions are about ± 1–5% relative.

The analysis of alkali and alkaline earth metals can be successfully done by flame photometry because their atoms reach the excited state at a temperature lower than that at which most other elements are excited. The analysis of Na, K, Li, Ba and Ca are typically determined at low temperatures, i.e. 1500–2000°C. Table 8.3 lists some of the elements that can be determined by flame photometry and their detection limits.

Table 8.3. Elements, their characteristic emission wavelength and detection limits

Element	Wavelength λ (nm)	Detection limit (mg)	Element	Wavelength λ (nm)	Detection limit (mg)
Al	396	0.5	Cu	326	0.6
	484	0.5			
	253	1.0	Fe	372	2.5
				386	2.7
As	2350	2.2	Pb	406	14
	455	3	Li	671	0.067
	554	1			
Bi	223	6.4	Mg	285	1.0
				383	1.6
Ca	423	0.07	Hg	254	2.5
	554	0.16	Ni	355	1.6
	662	0.6	Pd	363	0.1

APPLICATION OF FLAME PHOTOMETRY

Some of the applications of flame photometric method are given here.
1. Determination of Na$^+$, K$^+$, and Ca^{++} in biological fluid (serum, urine).
   This is commonly used interference free method of measuring Sodium (Na), Potassium (K), and Calcium (Ca) in the biological fluids. Flame photometers have traditionally been used for the measurement of these cations.
2. Determination of hardness of water.
3. Determination of alkalis in cement.
4. Determination of calcium in beer.
5. Estimation of calcium in milk.
6. Determination of potassium in fertilizers.
7. Determination of available potassium in soils.
8. Sodium and potassium in silicates, minerals and ores.

9. The determination of calcium in fruit juice.
10. The determination of potassium/sodium in glass.
11. The determination of calcium in biscuits.
12. The determination of lithium in greases.

INTERFERENCES IN QUANTITATIVE FLAME PHOTOMETRIC DETERMINATIONS

The interferences encountered can be classified as follows:
- Spectral interferences
- Ionisation interferences
- Chemical interferences

Spectral interferences

These refer to the interferences that affect the spectral intensity or resolution. There are several types of spectral interferences which are explained below:
- The **first type** of interference arises when two elements exhibit spectra, which partially overlap, and both emit radiation at same particular wavelength. The detector is unable to distinguish between the sources of radiation and so records the total signal, thus resulting in incorrect answer. Such interferences are more common at high flame temperatures because numerous spectral lines are produced at high temperatures. For example, the Fe line at 324.73 nm overlaps with the Cu line at 324.75 nm. Such interference can be overcome either by taking measurements at an alternative wavelength which has no overlap, if available, or by removing the interfering element by extraction. Alternatively, one may make a calibration curve, which is prepared from a solution having similar quantities of the interfering element.
- The **second type** of spectral interference deals with spectral lines of two or more elements which are close but their spectra do not overlap. This type of interference becomes a problem when a filter is used as the device to isolate spectral lines. A filter may allow spectral lines separated by 5.0–10.0 nm to pass through, thus resulting in an error in the analysis. Such interferences can be reduced by increasing the resolution of the spectral isolation system. However, the interference cannot be eliminated entirely due to the finite width of the spectral isolation system and the finite slit width in such systems.
- A **third type** of spectral interference occurs due to the presence of continuous background which arises due to high concentration of salts in the sample, especially of alkali and alkaline earth metals. Some organic solvents also produce a continuous background. This type of interference can be corrected by using suitable scanning technique.

Ionisation Interferences

In some cases, high temperature flame may cause ionisation of some of the metal atoms, e.g., in case of sodium, it can be given as follows:

$$Na \longrightarrow Na^+ + e^-$$

The Na$^+$ ion possesses an emission spectrum of its own with frequencies, which are different from those of atomic spectrum of the Na atom. This reduces the radiant power of atomic emission. This interference can be eliminated by adding a large quantity of a potassium salt to be standards as well as sample solutions. This addition of potassium salt suppresses the ionisation of sodium, as the potassium atom itself undergoes ionisation due to low ionisation energy. Thus, the sodium atom emission is enhanced. This type of interference is restricted to alkali metals.

Chemical Interferences

The chemical interferences arise out of the reaction between different interferents and the analyte. These are of different types. Some of these are given below.

Cation-anion interference

The presence of certain anions, such as oxalate, phosphate, sulphate and aluminate, in a solution may affect the intensity of radiation emitted by an element, resulting in serious analytical error. For example, calcium in the presence of phosphate ion forms a stable substance, as $Ca_3(PO_4)_2$ which does not decompose easily, resulting in the production of lesser atoms. Thus, the calcium signal is depressed. Another similar example is that of determination of barium in presence of sulphate forming insoluble $BaSO_4$. This type of interference can be removed either by extraction of the anion or by using calibration curves prepared from standard solutions containing same concentrations of the anion as found in the sample.

Cation-cation interference

In many cases, mutual interferences of cations have been observed, resulting in reduced signal intensity of the element being determined. These interferences are neither spectral nor ionic in nature and the mechanism of such interferences is not well understood. Thus, for example, aluminium interferes with calcium and magnesium. Also, sodium and potassium show cation-cation interference on one another.

Interference due to oxide formation

This type of interference arises due to the formation of stable metal oxide if oxygen is present in the flame, resulting in reduced signal intensity. The alkaline earth metals are subject to this type of interference. This type of interference can be eliminated by either using very high flame temperature to dissociate the oxides or by using oxygen-deficient environment to produce excited atoms.

Other factors

A number of other factors affect the intensity of light emission from a given sample solution. For example, the organic solvents in a sample may also influence the intensity of the emission line by changing the viscosity and surface tension of the liquid, which in turn alter the rate at which the sample is aspirated into the flame. They also affect the flame temperature through their contribution to the heat of combustion. An increase in the line intensity is usually observed.

Experiment: Determination of concentration of sodium ions in NaCl solution by flame photometry

Procedure

1. Prepare stock solution of NaCl by dissolving 100 mg in 1 litre of distilled water (100 µg/ml).
2. Dilute 1 ml, 2 ml, 3 ml, 4 ml and 5 ml from stock solution to 50 ml.
3. Insert the sodium optical filter each standard solution (λ 589 nm).
4. Measure the emission intensity by using flame photometer and plot a calibration graph between concentration v/s emission intensity.
5. Similarly, measure the emission intensity of unknown solution and find out the concentration of the unknown solution from the calibration graph.

CHAPTER 9

Turbidimetric and Nephelometric Titrations

The blue color of the sky during the day and the red color of the sun at sunset are due to scattering of light by small dust particles, molecules of water, and other gases in the atmosphere. The efficiency of scattering depends on the wavelength of light. The sky is blue because violet and blue light are scattered to a greater extent than other, longer wavelengths of light. For the same reason, the sun appears to be red when observed at sunset because red light is less efficiently scattered and therefore, transmitted to greater extent than other wavelengths of light. The scattering of radiation has been studied since the late 1800s, with applications beginning soon thereafter. The earliest quantitative applications of scattering, which date from the early 1900s, used the elastic scattering of light to determine the concentration of colloidal particles in a suspension.

ORIGIN OF SCATTERING

When monochromatic light of wavelength λ, is passed through a medium containing particles, whose largest dimensions are less than $3/2\ \lambda$, is scattered in all directions. For example, visible radiation of 500 nm is scattered by particles as large as 750 nm in the longest dimension. With larger particles, radiation also may be reflected or refracted. Two general categories of scattering are recognised:

(i) In elastic scattering, radiation is absorbed by the analyte and re-emitted without a change in the radiation's energy.

(ii) When the radiation is re-emitted with a change in energy, the scattering is said to be inelastic.

Only elastic scattering is considered in this text. Elastic scattering is divided into two types: Rayleigh, or small-particle scattering, and large-particle scattering. Rayleigh scattering occurs when the scattering particles largest dimension is less than 5% of the radiation's wavelength. The intensity of the scattered radiation is symmetrically distributed (Fig. 9.1a) and is proportional to its frequency to the fourth power (n^4), accounting for the greater scattering of blue light compared with red light. For larger particles, the distribution of scattered light increases in the forward direction and decreases in the backward direction as the result of constructive and destructive interferences (Fig. 9.1b).

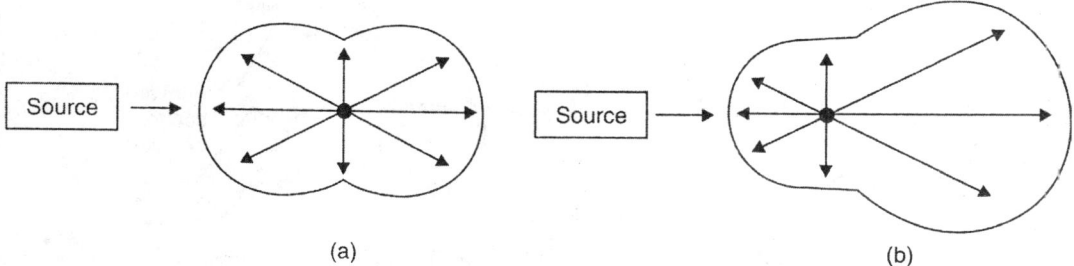

Fig. 9.1. Distribution of radiation for (a) Rayleigh scattering and (b) large-particle scattering.

TURBIDIMETRY AND NEPHELOMETRY

Turbidimetry is the measurement of light-scattering species in solution by means of a decrease in intensity of the incident beam (means intensity of unscattered light) after it has passed through solution while **Nephelometry measure the light scattering species by measuring** the intensity of scattered radiation at an angle of 90° to the source. Infact, this method is based on a comparison of the intensity of light scattered by a standard reference suspension under the same conditions. The higher the intensity of scattered light, the higher the turbidity. Formazin polymer is used as the primary standard reference suspension. The turbidity of a specified concentration of formazin suspension is defined as 4000 Nephelometric Turbidity Unit (NTU). Formazin particles have uniform size and shape. The formazin suspension is prepared by mixing equal volumes of the hydrazine sulphate solution and the hexamethylenetetramine solution.

1. Hexamethylenetetramine + $6H_2O$ + $2H_2SO_4$ (From hydrazine sulphate) $\longrightarrow$ $6\ H_2C=O$ (Formaldehyde) + $2(NH_4)_2SO_4$

2. $n\ H_2C=O$ + $\frac{n}{2}\ H_2N-NH_2$ $\longrightarrow$ [Formazin]$_n$ + nH_2O

Both the techniques are two related techniques in which an incident source of radiation is elastically scattered by a suspension of colloidal particles. In **turbidimetry**, the detector is placed in line with the radiation source, and the decrease in the radiation's transmitted power is measured. In **Nephelometry**, scattered radiation is measured at an angle of 90° to the radiation source. The similarity of the measurement of turbidimetry to absorbance, and of nephelometry to fluorescence, is evident in the block instrumental designs shown in Fig. 9.2. In fact, turbidity can be measured using a UV-Visible spectrophotometer, such as a Spectronic-20, whereas a spectrofluorometer is suitable for nephelometry.

188 Pharmaceutical Analysis

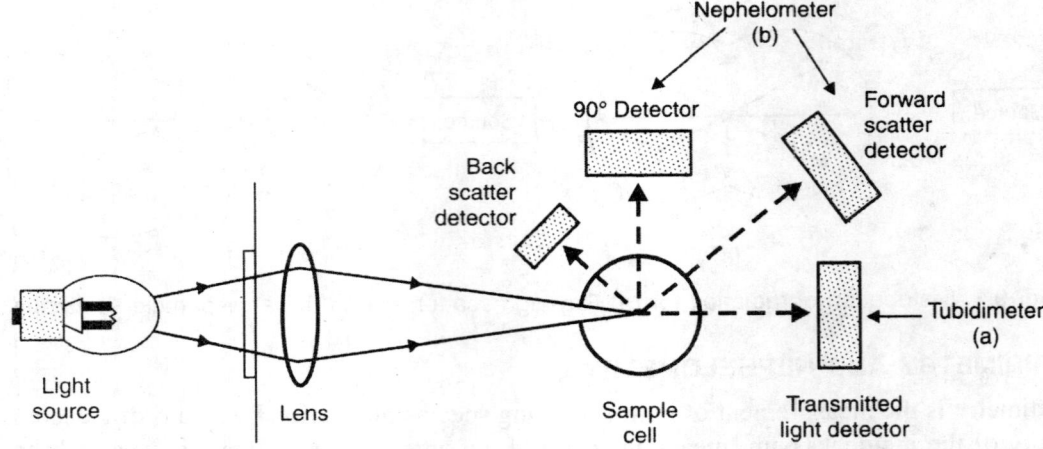

Fig. 9.2. Schematic diagram for (a) a Turbidometer, and (b) a Nephelometer.

Turbidimeters or nephelometers uses a tungsten lamp as light source with spectral sensitivity at about 550 nm operating at a filament temperature of 2700°C or IR LED having an emission maximum at 860 nm with a 60 nm spectral bandwidth. Silicon photodiodes and photomultipliers are commonly used as detectors and record changes in light scattered or transmitted by the sample. The light scattered at 90 ± 2.5° is detected by the primary detector. The instruments used are calibrated against standards of known turbidity and are capable of automatic determination of turbidity. The test results expressed in NTU units, are obtained directly from the instrument and compared to the specifications in the individual monographs.

Turbidimetry versus Nephelometry

The selection between turbidimetry and nephelometry is determined by two principal factors. The most important consideration is the intensity of the transmitted or scattered radiation relative to the intensity of radiation from the source. When the solution contains a small concentration of scattering particles, the intensity of the transmitted radiation, I_T, will be very similar to the intensity of the radiation source, I_U. As we learned earlier in the section on molecular absorption, determining a small difference between two intense signals is subject to a substantial uncertainty. Thus, nephelometry is a more apropriate choice for samples containing few scattering particles. On the other hand, turbidimetry is a better choice for samples containing a high concentration of scattering particles.

The second consideration is choosing between turbidimetry and nephelometry is the size of the scattering particles. For nephelometry, the intensity of scattered radiation at 90° will be greatest if the particles are small enough to produce Rayleigh scattering. For larger particles, as shown in Fig. 9.1, scattering intensity is diminished at 90°. When using an ultraviolet or visible source of radiation, the optimum particle size is 0.1–1 µm. The size of the scattering particles is less important for turbidimetry, in which the signal is the relative decrease in transmitted radiation. In fact, turbidimetric measurements are still feasible even when the size of the scattering particles results in an increase in reflection and refraction (although a linear relationship between the signal and the concentration of scattering particles may no longer hold).

QUANTITATIVE TURBIDIMETRY

In turbidimetry, the measured transmittance T, is the ratio of the transmitted intensity of source radiation, I to the intensity of source radiation transmitted by a blank, I_o:

$$T = \frac{I}{I_o}$$

The relationship between transmittance and concentration of scattering particles is similar to that given by Beer's law:

$$-\log T = kbc \qquad ...(9.1)$$

where
- k is the turbidity constant. Its value depends upon size and shape of particles and wavelength of radiation.
- b is the path length.
- c is the concentration of scattering particles, in mass per unit volume (w/v).

As with Beer's law, equation 9.1 may show appreciable deviation from linearity. The exact relationship is established by a calibration curve prepared using a series of standards of known concentration.

Turbidimetry is similar to colorimetric since both methods measure the amount of transmitted light. Hence, following criteria should be fulfilled to get the linearity:
   (i) The suspension should be dilute.
   (ii) The suspension should be stable and should not allow the particles to settle down.
   (iii) The particles of suspension should be small and fine.
   (iv) The particles should have a uniform shape and size to allow uniform scattering of light.
   (v) For the stability of suspension addition of other salt and protective colloid should be used.
   (vi) Viscosity and temperature should be such as to maintain stable suspension.

QUANTITATIVE NEPHELOMETRY

In nephelometry, the relationship between the intensity of scattered radiation, Is, and the concentration, C (% w/v) of scattering particle is given by:

$$Is = ks\, I_o C \qquad ...(9.2)$$

where ks is an empirical constant for the system, I_o is the intensity of incident source radiation.

The value of ks is determined from a calibration curve prepared using a series of standards of known concentration.

Selection of wavelength for the incident radiation

For turbidimetry, where incident radiation is transmitted through the sample, it is necessary to avoid radiation that is absorbed by the sample. Since absorption is a common problem, the wavelength must be selected with some care, using a filter or monochromator. For nephelometry, the absorption of incident is not a problem unless it induces fluorescent from the sample with a non-fluorescent sample, there is no need for wavelength selection and source of white light may be used for the incident radiation.

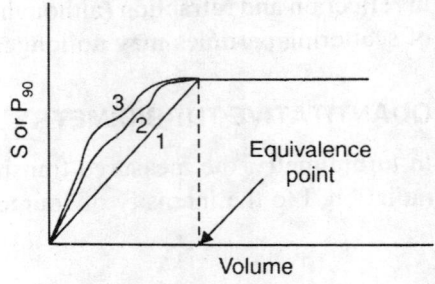

Fig. 9.3. Turbidimetric titration curve: Curve 1 is an ideal curve; curve 2 and 3 might result from precipitates with mixed particle size, poor stirring etc.

Turbidimetric titrations

Turbidimetric titrations may be carried out just as photometric titrations. In these titrations, a graph is obtained by plotting absorbance against the volume of titrant added. An increase in absorbance occurs as more and more of precipitate is formed and the curve declines sharply when the whole of the substance gets precipitated. This is abrupt change in the slope is indicative to end point.

Titrations of the type A + B $\longrightarrow$ C, where C is insoluble precipitates, might be expected to give a curve of either turbidance or scattered intensity which would consist of two intersecting straight lines as the amount of precipitate increase to a maximum and then become constant. This is, however, true only if the number of particles increase linearly to the end point and size of the particles remains the same throughout. This is not possible in practice, because the added reagent will simultaneously form new particles and add to those previously formed. Hence, if the particles become too large, a poorly defined end point or none at all will result.

Sample preparation

Although equations 9.1 and 9.2 relate scattering to the concentration of scattering particles, the intensity of scattered radiation is also influenced strongly by the particle's size and shape. For example, samples containing the same number of scattering particles may show significantly different values for $-\log T$ or Is depending on the average diameter of the particles. For a quantitative analysis, therefore, it is necessary to maintain a uniform distribution of particle sizes throughout the sample and between samples and standards.

Most turbidimetric and nephelometric methods rely on the formation of the scattering particles by precipitation. As we have learned in the discussion of precipitation in gravimetry (see Vol. I), the properties of a precipitate are determined by the conditions used to effect the precipitation. To maintain a reproducible distribution of particle sizes between samples and standards, it is necessary to control parameters such as the concentration of reagents, order of adding reagents, pH, temperature, agitation or stirring rate, ionic strength, and time between the precipitate's initial formation and the measurement of transmittance or scattering. In many cases a surface-active agent, such as glycerol, gelatin, or dextrin, is added to stabilize the precipitate in a colloidal state and to prevent the coagulation of the particles.

APPLICATIONS OF TURBIDIMETRY AND NEPHELOMETRY

(i) At present turbidity is used to verify the quality of water for industrial use and for drinking purpose. It is used as a measure of suspended solids like silt, clay, algae, rust and also bacteria and other microorganisms present in water.

(ii) In food and beverage industries, turbidimetry is used to test the clarity of fruit juices.

(iii) Turbidimetry is used to measure the amount of benzene in alcohol.

(iv) Turbidimetric analysis is used for the analysis of turbidity in sugar products.

(v) Nephelometric measurements are used to determine protein, yeast, glycogen and beta and gamma globulin in blood serum and plasma.

(vi) Both turbidimetry and nephelometry are used for continuous monitoring of air and water pollution.

(vii) Turbidimetric methods are used for determination of end point in precipitation reactions.

(viii) It is employed in soap and detergent industry in determination of cloud point.

Experiment: Turbidimetric determination of sulphate in water

Principle

The sulphate is precipitated as barium sulphate on adding $BaCl_2$ solution to an acidified sample solution. The concentration of SO_4^{2-} may be determined either by turbidimetry or nephelometry using an incident source of radiation of 420 nm. External standards containing known concentrations of SO_4^{2-} are used to standardize the method.

Procedure

A 100 ml sample is transferred to a 250 ml Erlenmeyer flask along with 5.00 ml of a conditioning reagent. The composition of the conditioning reagent is 500 ml glycerol, 30 ml concentrated HCl, 300 ml distilled water, 100 ml 95% ethyl or isopropyl alcohol, and 75 g NaCl. The sample and conditioning reagent are placed on a magnetic stirrer that is operated at the same speed for all samples and standards. A portion of crystalline $BaCl_2$ is added using a measuring spoon whose capacity is 0.2–0.3 ml, precipitating the SO_4^{2-} as $BaSO_4$. Timing begins when the $BaCl_2$ is added to the solution and precipitate are allowed to stir for exactly 1 min. At the end of the stirring period, a portion of the suspension is poured into the turbidimeter or nephelometer cell, and the transmittance or scattering intensity measured at 30-s intervals for 4 min. The minimum transmittance or maximum scattering intensity recorded during this period is the analytical signal. Calibration curves over the range 0–40 ppm SO_4^{2-} are prepared by diluting a 100-ppm SO_4^{2-} standard. The standards and a reagent blank must be treated in exactly the same fashion as samples.

Role of the conditioning reagent

The conditioning reagent is used to stabilize the precipitate of $BaSO_4$. The high ionic strength and acidity, due to NaCl and HCl, prevent the formation of microcrystalline particles of $BaSO_4$, and glycerol and alcohol help in stabilizing the precipitate's suspension.

CHAPTER 10

Potentiometric Titration

Potentiometry is an electroanalytical method which is based on measurement of potential of an electrode system under the conditions of no current flow. Potentiometric measurements enable selective detection of ions in presence of other substances. Before going into main topic, it is necessary to understand some basic fundamentals regarding electrochemistry.

ELECTROCHEMICAL CELL

The electrochemical cell is a device in which a redox reaction takes place indirectly and the decrease in potential energy of the reaction appears largely in the form of electrical energy.

Electric current results from a chemical reaction; in which oxidation (loss of electrons) occurs at one electrode and reduction (gain of electron) at the other electrode. Oxidation and reduction occur simultaneously. Oxidation occur only if reduction place at the same time. This can be illustrated by taking a few examples.

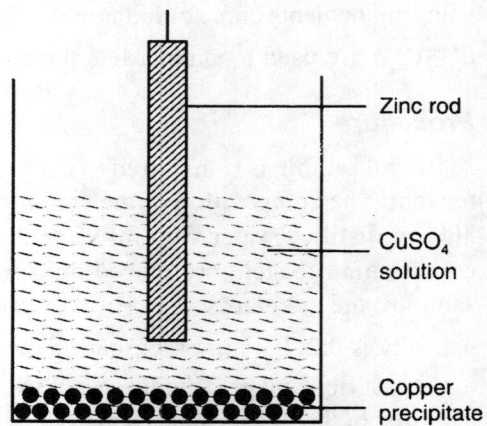

Fig. 10.1. Zn–$CuSO_4$ reaction in a beaker.

1. Zn–$CuSO_4$ reaction in a beaker (oxidation of zinc metal by Cu^{++} ions).

    If a zinc rod is placed in a solution of copper sulphate (Fig. 10.1) the following observation will be made. The zinc strip starts dissolving forming Zn^{2+} ion in a solution (oxidation):

    $$Zn(s) \longrightarrow Zn^{2+}(aq) + e^- \qquad ...(10.1)$$

    At the same time, copper starts precipitating out from the solution is due to reduction of Cu^{2+} present in a solution of copper metal (eq. 10.2):

    $$Cu^{2+}(aq) + 2e^- \longrightarrow Cu(s) \qquad ...(10.2)$$

The reaction (10.1) and (10.2) are called half reaction where the reactions (10.1) and (10.2) are referred as oxidation half reaction and reduction half reaction respectively. The overall redox reaction is obtained by summation of two half reaction (10.1) and (10.2):

$$Zn(s) + Cu^{2+}(aq) \longrightarrow Zn^{2+}(aq) + Cu(s) \qquad ...(10.3)$$

The reaction is exothermic i.e. accompanied by evolution of heat. Hence ΔH is negative. The decrease of potential energy appears as heat.

Possibility of reverse reaction is nil (copper rod in a solution of zinc sulphate); it means, zinc metal can be oxidized by Cu^{2+} ion but Copper metal cannot be oxidized by Zn^{2+} ions.

2. Cu–$AgNO_3$ reaction in a beaker (oxidation of copper metal by Ag^{++} ions).

$$Cu(s) + 2Ag^+(aq) \longrightarrow Cu^{2+}(aq) + 2Ag(s) \qquad ...(10.4)$$

Copper can be oxidized by Ag^+ ion but silver cannot be oxidized by copper.

Redox Reaction in Electrochemical Cells

Due to the redox reaction in electrochemical cells, the decrease of potential energy appear as electrical energy. It can be explained by the following experiment.

Take a dilute (≈ 0.1 ml) solution of copper sulphate in one beaker and a dilute solution of zinc sulphate in an another beaker. Put a copper rod in the copper sulphate solution and zinc rod in the zinc sulphate solution.

Connect one end of metal rod (zinc rod) to one terminal of ammeter and other (copper rod) through variable resistance to the other terminal of the same ammeter as shown in Fig. 10.2. Finally connect the two solution with each other through a glass tube containing a solution of potassium sulphate (salt bridge). If the metal rods are not connected to each other or it salt bridge is taken out, no current flows through the ammeter and no reaction takes place in the cell. But, as soon as the connection is made as shown in Fig. 10.2, the current starts flowing as indicated by the reading.

$$Zn(s) + Cu^{2+}(aq) \longrightarrow Zn^{2+}(aq) + Cu(s)$$

The current continuous to flow as long as chemical reaction continues to take place. If the flow of current is stopped after some time by disconnecting the wire and metal rods are washed, dried and weighed. It will be seen that zinc rod has lost in mass, while copper rod has gained in mass. The gain and loss in mass in copper and zinc rod take place according to Faraday's second law.

Loss in mass of zinc rod/gain in mass of copper rod

Mass of 1 gm equivalent of zinc/mass of 1 gm equivalent of Cu = 32.70/31.70.

The loss in mass of zinc rod is due to passing of zinc metal into solution as Zn^{2+} ions:

$$Zn(s) \longrightarrow Zn^{2+}(aq) + 2e^-$$

This is an oxidation half reaction. The electron thus released accumulate in the zinc rod, move into ammeter and then through the resistance, enter the copper rod there, then taken up the Cu^{2+} ions which are discharged as copper metal(s) on the copper electrode.

$$Cu^{2+}(aq) + 2e^- \longrightarrow Cu(s)$$

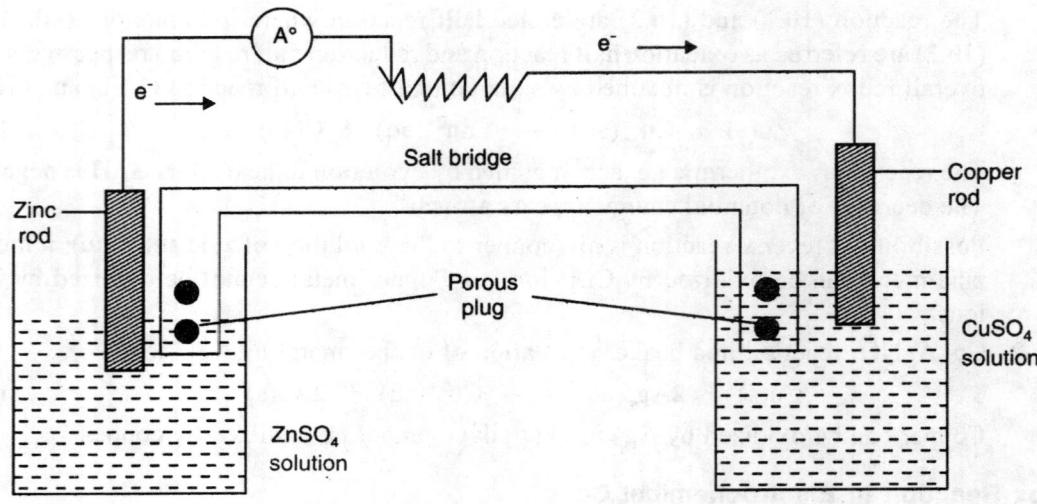

Fig. 10.2. Electrochemical cell.

This is reduction half reaction thus the number of electrons liberated in one half reaction is equal to number of electron consumed in another half reaction.

It is also observed that no heat is evolved in present case, whereas a large amount of heat (about 212 KJ per 'g' of zinc changing into Zn^{2+} ions) is evolved when the same reactions take place in a beaker. The decrease in energy which appears as heat energy (when reaction take place directly by placing zinc rod in $CuSO_4.5H_2O$ solution), appears as an electrical energy when the same reaction take place indirectly in an electrochemical cell.

Direction of flow of electrons

In Fig. 10.2 electrons are flowing from zinc rod to the copper. According to convention, the electrode at which oxidation occurs is called *negative* electrode while the electrode at which reduction occurs is called *positive* electrode. Thus, in the above cell, zinc electrode is called negative electrode while copper electrode is called positive electrode. As mentioned above, the direction of flow of electrons (negative electricity) in the present cell is from zinc electrode to copper electrode. Hence, direction of flow of positive electricity is from copper electrode to zinc electrode.

The Daniel cell

The galvanic cell in which the $Zn–CuSO_4$ reaction takes place is called Daniel cell (Fig. 10.3). It differs from the electrochemical cell.

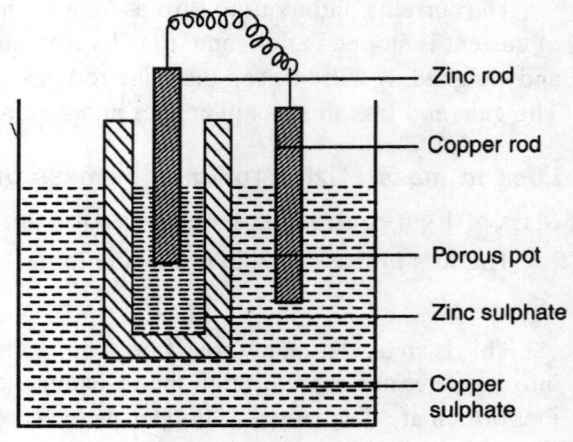

Fig. 10.3. The Daniel cell.

There is no salt bridge in the present case. Zinc sulphate is placed in a porous pot while copper sulphate is placed in a glass vessel. The two solutions can seep through the porous pot with each other automatically.

Relative tendencies of electrodes to liberate electrons

When two electrodes are joined to form a cell, a competition sets in between two electrodes to liberate electrons. In the cell of Zn–Cu electrodes, zinc has greater tendency to liberate electrons than copper. The electrons flows from zinc to copper. Zinc, therefore acts as the negative electrode white copper acts as the positive electrode. In the cell of Cu–Ag electrodes copper electrodes has greater tendency to liberate electron.

In Zn–H_2 cell, zinc has greater tendency to liberate electrons. So it acts as negative electrode while hydrogen (gas) electrode act as a positive electrode. If, however, a Cu–H_2 (g) cell is set up, hydrogen (gas) having greater tendency to liberate electrons than copper act as negative electrode while copper act as the positive electrode. From these observations, various electrodes can be arranged in decreasing order of tendencies to liberate electrons.

$$Zn > H_2 > Cu > Ag$$

According to convention, the electrode at which electrons are released is written to the left while at which electrons are taken up is written on the right while keeping this view, the Zn–Cu cell (Daniel cell) can be written as:

$$Zn/ZnSO_4 \parallel CuSO_4/Cu$$

A single vertical line represents a phase boundary across which a potential difference exists. The double vertical line signifies a boundary between two solutions of different composition across which a potential difference exists.

E.M.F. of cell and its measurement

The flow of electricity from one electrode to other electrode in a galvanic cell indicates that two electrodes have different potential. The difference of potential which causes flow of current from one electrode (at higher potential) to another electrode (at lower potential) is called the electromotive force (E.M.F.).

The (E.M.F.) of cell can be measured by connecting the two electrodes to the two terminals of voltameter. The potential difference is then read directly from the instrument. This method, however, suffers from two defects. Firstly, as some current is drawn from the cell during the process of measurement itself, chemical reaction occurs to some extent. Secondly, with flow of current, a part of the E.M.F. is used up in overcoming the internal resistance of the cell. Hence, the potential difference, as read from the voltameter, will not be correct E.M.F. of the cell.

E.M.F. of a cell can be measured accurately only by a method which involves little or no flow of electricity. Such a method is based on Poggesndorff's compensation principle. In this method, the E.M.F. of another cell or battery until two E.M.F.'s become equal and there is no net flow of current in the circuit. The electrical assembly used is known as *potentiometer*.

A potentiometer in simple form consists of two electrical circuits in combination. The first

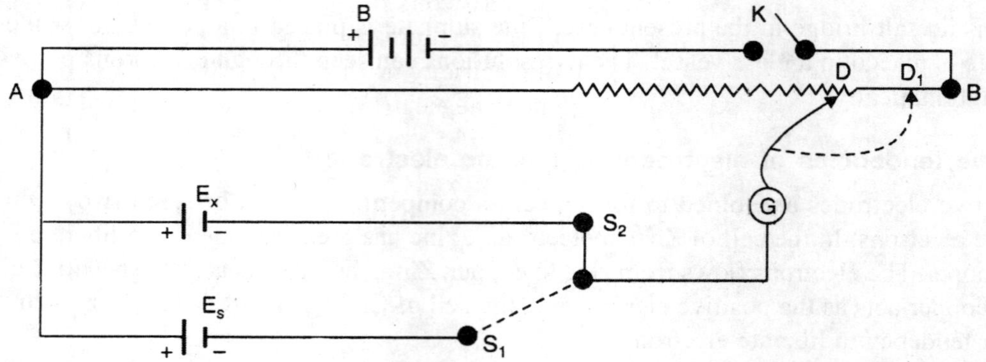

Fig. 10.4. The potentiometer.

circuit consists of uniform wire AB of higher resistance. A storage battery(B) of constant E.M.F. which should be larger than E.M.F. of the cell to be measured, is connected at the ends A and B of the wire (Fig. 10.4). The second circuit is made up of two cell's X and S (one of accurately known potential, the other whose potential is to be determined), a switch, K to include one or other of the cells in the circuit, a galvanometer to show the flow of current, and a sliding contact, D on the length of resistance wire. When switch K is closed, the battery, B sends electricity flowing from the battery B to the end A of the resistance with AB. At point A, the current from battery can divide, part of it flowing through the resistance wire AB and then back to battery B; the remainder tends to flow through the second part of the circuit: the small cell (either X or S), the switches, S_1 and S_2 and via sliding contact D, through the DQ part of the resistance wire AB and then back to the storage battery, B. The tendency for electricity from battery B to flow in the second circuit is opposed by the tendency for electricity to form cells E_x and E_s upto A and through the part AD of the resistance wire and back to X or S through the galvanometer. The galvanometer G then will indicate whether current is flowing in the second part of the circuit and in which direction.

The sliding contact is moved along the wire AB till no current flows through the galvanometer. First of all, the E_x (of unknown E.M.F.) is included through switch, S_1 and the sliding contact is moved till no current flows in galvanometer. Then E.M.F. of the cell, say E_x is proportional to the distance AD.

$$E_x \alpha \ AD$$

The cell, E_x is now replaced by a standard cell, E_s, the E.M.F. of which, say E_s is known.
Then,
$$E_s \ \alpha \ AD^1$$
$$E_x = AD/AD^1 \times E_s \qquad \ldots(10.5)$$

The standard cell, E_s must be capable of giving constant and reproducible E.M.F. and its variation with temperature should be small.

Electrical energy

The electrical energy produced by a cell is given by the product of E.M.F. and the quantity of electricity which is passed.

For example, in daniel cell, the E.M.F. is 1.10 volts the cell reaction involves liberation by taking up of 2 electrons that is deposition of two 'g' equivalents of copper (or dissolution of 2 'g' equivalent of zinc), therefore, the quantity of electricity produced according to Faraday's second law is 2 Faradays (nF) that is 2 × 96,500. Hence, the electrical energy generated in the cell for the complete cell reaction:

$$= 2 \times 96,500 \times 1.1 = 212,300 \text{ joules.}$$

Reversible cell

A cell is said to work in a thermodynamically reversible manner when it is sending out infinitely small current so that cell reaction always remains virtually in a state of equilibrium.

Relation between free energy change and electrical energy

According to Gibbs and Helm Holtz, the electrical energy of reversible cell is measured by the free energy decrease ($-\Delta G$) of the reaction occurring in the cell.

$$-\Delta G = nFE \qquad \ldots(10.6)$$

where
nf = electrical energy produced
E = E.M.F. of cell

Thermodynamics of a reversible cell

Suppose the reaction occurring in reversible cell is represented by the equation:

$$A + B \rightleftharpoons C + D$$

The decrease in free energy $-\Delta G$ is given by the well known thermodynamic equation:

$$-\Delta G = -\Delta G^\circ - RT \ln J \qquad \ldots(10.7)$$

where $-\Delta G^\circ$ is the decrease in free energy accompanying the same process, when all the reactants and products are in their standard states of unit activity and J stands for the reaction quotient of the activity $a_C \times a_D$ of the products and reactants $a_A \times a_B$ at any given stage of the reaction. Substituting the value of J, we have:

$$-\Delta G = -\Delta G^\circ - RT \ln \frac{a_C \times a_D}{a_A \times a_B} \qquad \ldots(10.8)$$

As $\qquad -\Delta G = nFE$ in eq. 10.6

Hence, $\qquad nFE = nFE^\circ - RT \ln \dfrac{a_C \times a_D}{a_A \times a_B} \qquad \ldots(10.9)$

where E° is the EMF of the cell in which the activity or concentration of each reactant and each product of the cell reaction is equal to unity. E° is known as the standard EMF of the cell. Equation

10.9 is known as Nernst equation. Replacing activities by concentrations, the Nernst equation may be written as:

$$E = E^o - \frac{RT}{nF} \ln \frac{C \times D}{A \times B}$$

The Nernst equation enables us to calculate EMF of cell when concentration of reactants and products of the cell reaction are known.

Single electrode potential

The tendency of an electrode to lose or gain electrons when it is in contact with its own ions in solution is called electrode potential. Since the tendency to lose electrons means also tendency to get oxidised, so this tendency is called oxidation potential. Similarly, the tendency to gain electrons means the tendency to get reduced. Hence, this tendency is called reduction potential. It is not possible to determine the potential of single electrode (half two electrodes that we can measure by combining them to give a complete cell). By arbitrarily choosing potential of one electrode as zero, it is possible to assign numerical values to potential of various other electrodes. The standard that has been chosen by convention is:

$$2H^{+1} + 2e^{-1} \longrightarrow H_2 \qquad E^o = 0.00 \text{ volts}$$
$$\text{(aq)} \qquad \text{(gas)}$$

Here, the notation E^o is called the standard electrode potential and is assigned potential of the standard hydrogen electrode when the concentration of H^{+1} is 1.0 M and the pressure of the hydrogen gas is 1.0 atmsphere. The measured cell voltage using the standard hydrogen electrode is therefore potential of other half-reaction.

Accordingly, the potential of reversible hydrogen electrode in which the gas at one atmospheric pressure activity (or unit concentration) has been fixed as zero. The electrode is known as **standard hydrogen electrode**, it is represented as:

$$\text{Pt, } H_2 \text{ (1 atm), } H^+ \text{ (C = 1)}$$

All other single electrode potential are referred to as potential on the hydrogen scale.

Electrometric determination of pH

The relation by which EMF of a suitable pH measuring electrode is related to the hydrogen ion concentration was developed by Nernst:

$$E = E^o - \log [H^+] \qquad \qquad ...(10.10)$$
$$E = E^o - 0.0591 \log [H^+] \qquad \qquad ...(10.11)$$

where E^o is a potential dependent on the electrode system used. R is the gas constant, T is the absolute temperature, F (the Faraday) is 96,485 coulombs/mole and n is the number of electrons involved in the equilibrium for n = 1, the factor RT/nF = 0.0591 (at 25°C). Using the Sorenson expression (pH = $-\log [H^+]$) for pH.

$$E = E^o + 0.0591 \text{ pH} \qquad \qquad ...(10.12)$$

$E°$ is standard electrode potential. It can be determined by using hydrogen electrode, glass electrode and quinhydrone electrode. These electrodes are also called as indicator electrodes.

(a) pH determination by using hydrogen electrode

The potential of hydrogen electrode depend upon the pH value of a solution to which it is in contact. This can be reference electrode. The hydrogen electrode in the unknown solution is usually found to be negative and calomel electrode is generally positive with respect to the hydrogen electrode. The complete cell can be shown by:

Pt, H_2 (1 atm), H^+ (C = unknown || KCl (salt soln), $Hg_2Cl_2(s)$, Hg

$$S_{cell} = S_{cell} \text{ (right)} - S_{cell} \text{ (left)}$$
$$= E(Hg_2Cl_2, Cl^-) - E(H^+, H_2)$$
$$= 0.02422 - (-0.0591 \text{ pH})$$
$$0.0591 \text{ pH} = S_{cell} - 0.2422$$
$$\text{pH} = \frac{E_{cell} - 0.242}{0.0591}$$

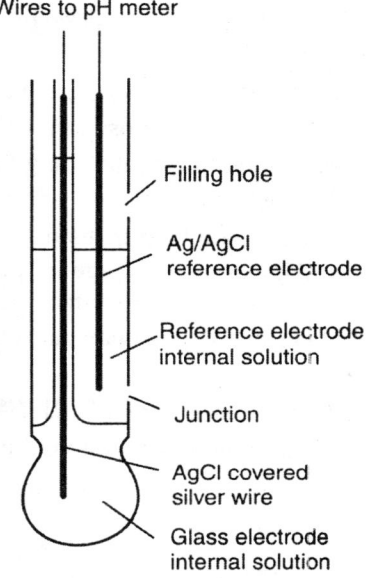

Fig. 10.5. Glass electrode.

(b) pH determination by glass electrode

It is most popular of all electrodes for pH determination. The glass electrode is made of special glass of relatively low melting point and high electrical conductivity. It is blown in the form of bulb which is then sealed to the bottom of a glass tube. A solution of 0.1 M HCl which furnishes a constant hydrogen ion concentration, is placed inside the bulb and a Ag–AgCl electrode or a simply platinum wire is inserted to make the electrical contact as shown in Fig. 10.5, the reference electrode employed is usually the calomel electrode (SCE). The half cell (glass electrode) can be designated Eg, for convenience Ag.AgCl/HCl (01 mol/glass membrane/H^+) (test solution).

Theoretically, this half cell has a standard electrode potential $Eg°$ and because it is sensitive to hydrogen ion, changes in the potential may be shown mathematically as:

$$Eg = Eg° + 0.0591 \log [H^+]$$
$$= Eg° - 0.0591 \text{ pH} \quad \ldots(10.13)$$

The entire cell assembly contain SCE as reference electrode hence:

$$Eg = EHg° - Eg \quad \ldots(10.14)$$
$$= E_{right} - E_{left}$$

Substituting eq (10.13) into (10.14) and rearranging gives:

$$\text{pH} = \frac{Ec - EHg° + Eg°}{0.0591} \quad \ldots(10.15)$$

For any given measurement, $EHg^\circ - Eg^\circ$ remain constant. Therefore, these two values may be combined and designated the glass electrode. Substituting into eq. 10.15 gives:

$$Ec = Eg + 0.0591\, pH$$

$$pH = \frac{Ec - Eg}{0.0591} \qquad \ldots(10.16)$$

To use eq. 10.16 in combination with a glass electrode, it is first necessary to standardize or determine, Eg experimentally since this value is defined on the reference electrode (internal and external). This can be done by using a buffer solution of known pH and determine the potential of the cell, Ec.

The glass electrode can be used for strong oxidising agent which interfere with quinhydrone electrode. It can be used in the presence of metallic ions, poisons. The glass electrode can be used in solution of pH values ranging from 0 to 9. Electrodes of special glass can be used for measuring pH values even upto 12.

The advantage of using glass electrode is its rapid response, unaffected by the presence of oxidizing or reducing agents, dissolved gases and highly coloured liquids. But the main disadvantage of glass electrode is its fragility, small scratches and the presence of dehydrating agents, colloids and surface deposit can cause interference in the measurements.

(c) pH determination by using quinhydrone electrode

The quinone-hydroquinone involves the following equilibrium

$$C_6H_4O_2 + 2H^+ + 2e^- \rightleftharpoons C_4H_6O_2$$
$$\text{Quinone (Q)} \qquad\qquad\qquad \text{Hydroquinone (QH}_2\text{)}$$

For the reduction reaction, the potential developed on platinum electrode:

$$E = E^\circ - \frac{2.303\, RT}{2F} \log \frac{[QH_2]}{[Q][H^+]^2}$$

$$= E^\circ - \frac{2.303\, RT}{2F} \log \frac{[QH_2]}{[Q]} + \frac{2.303\, RT}{2F} \log [H^+]^2$$

Now in aqueous solution of quinhydrone:

$$[QH_2] = [Q]$$

$\therefore \qquad\qquad \log \dfrac{[QH_2]}{[Q]} = \log 1 = 0$

Also $\qquad\qquad \log [H^+]^2 = 2 \log [H^+]$

Hence, $\qquad\qquad E = E^\circ + \dfrac{2.303\, RT}{2F} \times 2 \log [H^+]$

$$= E^o + \frac{2.303 \, RT}{F} \log[H^+]$$

$$= E^o - \frac{2.303 \, RT}{F} pH$$

$$= E^o - 0.0591 \, pH \text{ at } 25°C \qquad \ldots(10.17)$$

Instead of taking quinone and hydroquinone, a small amount of quinhydrone (equimolar compound of quinone (Q) and hydroquinone (QH_2) is taken since hydroquinone QH_2 is a weak acid, its ionisation is very small particularly at pH less than 7. Therefore, concentration of hydroquinone $[QH_2]$ is the same as that of quinone $[Q]$ that is the quantity $[Q]/[QH_2]$ is unity so middle term in eq. (10.17) becomes zero.

$$E^o_{(H^+, Q, QH_2)} = E^o_{(H^+, Q, QH_2)} + 0.0591 \log[H^+]$$

$$= E^o_{(H^+, Q, QH_2)} - 0.0591 \log pH$$

$$= 0.696 - 0.0591 \, pH$$

The standard electrode potential (reduction of the quinhydrone) is +0.6996 V. Thus, potential of quinhydrone electrode depends upon the pH value of a solution with which it is in contact. The potential of quinhydrone electrode is determined by connecting it with calomel (reference) electrode. This cell can be represented as:

$$\text{Hg, } Hg_2Cl_2(s) \text{ KCl (salt solution)} \parallel H^+ \text{ (unknown conc.) Q, } QH_2$$

The EMF of the cell is:

$$E_{cell} = E_{right} - E_{left}$$

$$= E_{(H^+, Q, QH_2)} - E_{(Hg_2, Cl_2, Cl^-)}$$

$$= (0.06996 - 0.0591 \, pH) - 0.2422 \text{ at } 25°C$$

$$0.0591 \, pH = 0.6996 - 0.2422 - E_{cell}$$

$$pH = \frac{0.6996 - 0.2422 - E_{cell}}{0.0591}$$

Limitations

The quinhydrone electrode cannot be used for solutions of pH values more than 8. In more alkaline solutions, hydroquinone ionises appreciably as an acid and also get oxidised partly by atmospheric oxygen. This alters the equilibrium between quinone and hydroquinone which forms the basis of the above equation.

Some reference electrodes used are:

Calomel electrode

The calomel half cell is the most widely used. A calomel half cell is one in which mercury and calomel [Mercury (I)/Chloride] are covered with aqueous KCl solution (Fig. 10.6). The KCl concentration usually used are 0.1 M, 1 M and saturated while the latter being the most convenient to use. The potentials for the calomel electrode against normal hydrogen electrode in saturated, 1.0 M, 0.1 M potassium chloride are + 250, 286, 338 mV at 20°C while at 25°C are +246, 285 and 338 mV respectively.

Silver-silver chloride electrode

It consists of silver wire coated electrolytically by silver chloride, dipping into a solution of potassium chloride of definite strength. The potential of the silver-silver chloride electrode against normal hydrogen electrode in saturated, 1.0 M, 0.1 M potassium chloride is +200, 235.5 and 288 mV respectively at 25°C I (Fig. 10.7).

Salt bridges

A salt bridge of saturated potassium chloride, potassium nitrate or ammonium nitrate is used to prevent the contamination of the reference electrode with the test solutions. When two solutions of electrolyte are brought in contact a potential difference is set up between them due to transference of ions across the boundary. The potential difference is known as junction potential. The salt bridge reduces these potentials almost to zero and they become significant.

Potentiometric titration

EMF measurement is useful in potentiometric titration. It is possible to detect the end point of a titration by measurement of the potential of suitable electrode (indicator electrode).

The solution (10–25 ml) to be titrated is taken in a 100 ml beaker and a suitable indicator and reference electrode are immersed in a solution (if electrodes do not dip properly, some distilled water is added to the solution. The electrodes are connected to a potentiometer (Fig. 10.8). The titrant solution is gradually added from a burette. After each addition, the solution is stirred, preferably by means of an electrical stirrer and potentiometer reading is recorded. Since the potential of reference electrode remains constant throughout the titration, the change in emf shown by potentiometer is actually the change in potential of indicator electrode during the titration.

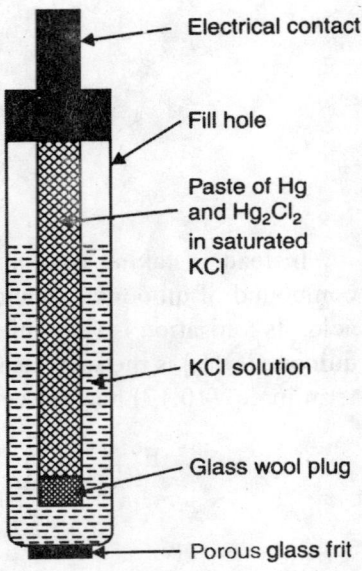

Fig. 10.6. Calomel electrode.

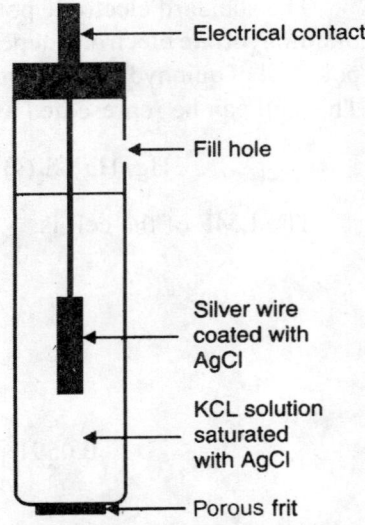

Fig. 10.7. Silver-silver chloride electrode.

Suppose ΔE represents the change in potential when a volume ΔV of titrant is added. If a graph between different values of ΔE against corresponding values of volume of titrant added is plotted, a sharp peak is obtained which gives the end point as shown in Fig. 10.9.

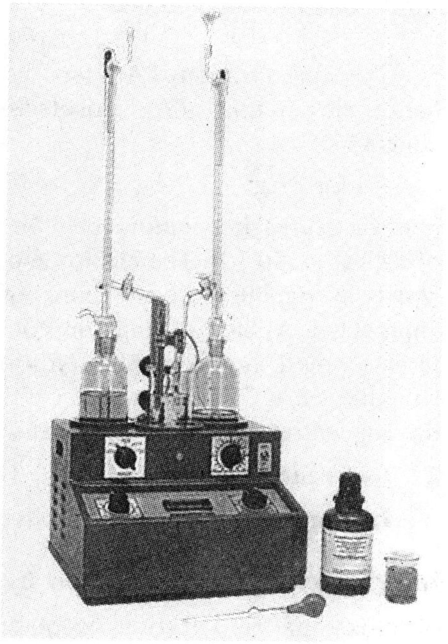

(i) Acid-base titration or Neutralisation titration

Potential of hydrogen electrode varies with concentration of H^+ ions with which it is in contact, according to the equation 10.12.

$$E(H^+, H_2) = E^o(H^+, H_2) + 0.0591 \log[H^+]$$
$$= -0.0591 \log[H^+]$$

Infact, any electrode whose potential depends upon H^+ ion concentration (e.g. quinhydrone or glass electrode), can be used as an indicator electrode.

The potential of the indicator electrode is measured potentiometrically by connecting it with saturated calomel electrode. The concentration of the titrant is usually 5 to 10 times higher than that of the solutions to be titrated to avoid volume change. It is evident that potential of hydrogen electrode shall decrease the 0.0591 volts for every ten fold decrease in concentration of H^+ ions.

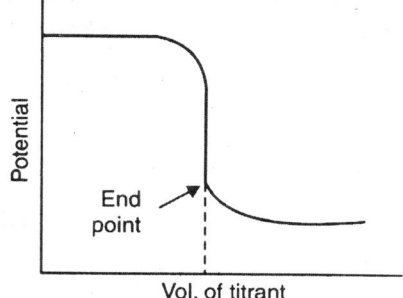

Fig. 10.8. Apparatus for potentiometric titration.

Assuming, for the sake of simplicity of calculation that there is no change in volume during the titration, it is evident that addition of alkali (titrant) to acid will produce little change in potential but more and more rapidly at the end point approaches. After the end point, further addition of NaOH produces very little change in the H^+ ion concentration and there is very little change in electrode potential.

On plotting the electrode potential against the volume of sodium hydroxide, a curve of the type shown in Fig. 10.9 is obtained. The end point corresponding to the point of inflexion (that is the point where slope of curve is maximum). The volume of NaOH solution required for the purpose is read out from graph.

Reference electrode: Saturated calomel electrode.

Indicator electrode: Quinhydrone, glass electrode.

(ii) Precipitation titration

Suppose we want to standardize a solution of silver nitrate. The silver electrode is used as an indicator electrode in this case while the calomel electrode as a reference electrode. The solution is titrated against solution of KCl solution, the strength of which is about 10 times higher. As the reaction proceeds, the Ag^+ ions get gradually precipitated as AgCl:

Fig. 10.9. Titration of acid with NaOH.

$$Ag^+ + NO_3^- + K^+ + Cl^- \longrightarrow AgCl\downarrow + K^+ + NO_3^-$$

The concentration of Ag^+ ions, goes on decreasing and hence, the potential of Ag^+, Ag electrode, given by Nernst equations:

$$E(Ag^+, Ag) = E^o(Ag^+, Ag) + 0.0591 \log [Ag^+]$$

goes on decreasing continuously on progressive addition of KCl (Fig. 10.10). The electrode potential shall change slowly at first but more and more rapidly as the end point approaches. At the end point, the concentration of Ag^+ ion is very small as this is now only on account of slight solubility of AgCl. If the addition of KCl continues further, the concentration of Ag^+ ion remain unaffected.

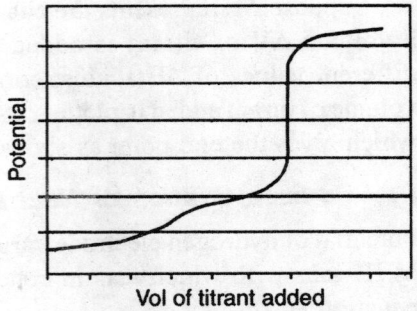

Fig. 10.10. Titration of silver nitrate with standard potassium chloride solution.

Reference electrode: Saturated calomel electrode.

Indicator electrode: Silver-silver chloride electrode.

(iii) Complexometric titration by potentiometry

Complexometric titration by potentiometry has been employed for quantification of ions such as Cu^{2+}. The ethylenediamine tetraacetic acid (EDTA) in the form of its disodium salt is most widely used complexing agent. An indicator, that is sensitive either to pH or to the metal ion is employed for detection of end point (Fig. 10.11).

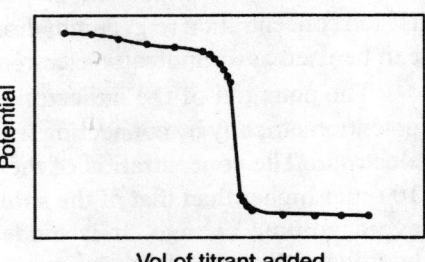

Fig. 10.11. Complexometric titration of copper salt with standard EDTA solution.

Reference electrode: Saturated calomel electrode.

Indicator electrode: Silver electrode or mercury electrode.

(iv) Oxidation reduction titration

The indicator electrode in redox titration usually is a noble metal that ideally, serves merely as a locus of electron transfer from the solution to the internal circuit platinum is used. A reference electrde often the S.C.E. complete the cell. The electrode generate two oxidation states of the reactant or titrant. For example, in titration of iron (ferrous) with cerium.

$$Fe^{2+} \longrightarrow Fe^{3+} + e$$
$$Ce^{4+} \longrightarrow Ce^{3+}$$

$$S_{Fe^{+3}/Fe^{+2}} = E^o_{Fe^{+3}/Fe^{+2}} - \frac{0.0591}{1} \log_{10} \left[\frac{Fe^{+2}}{Fe^{+3}}\right]$$

$$S_{Ce^{+4}/Ce^{+3}} = E^o_{Ce^{+4}/Ce^{+3}} - \frac{0.0591}{1} \log_{10} \left[\frac{Ce^{+3}}{Fe^{+4}}\right]$$

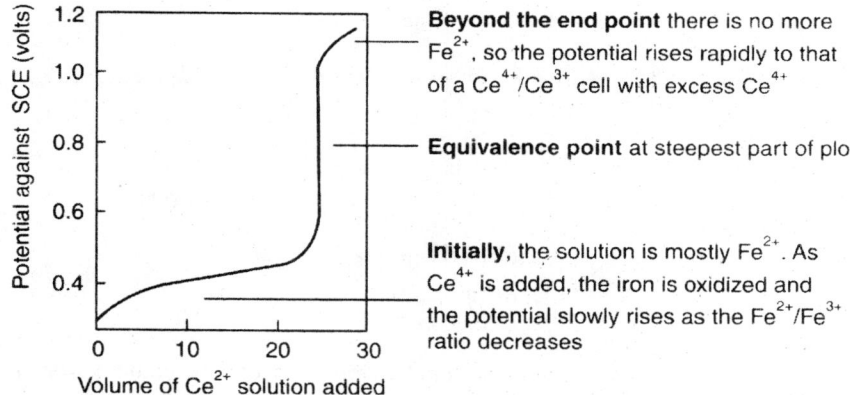

Beyond the end point there is no more Fe^{2+}, so the potential rises rapidly to that of a Ce^{4+}/Ce^{3+} cell with excess Ce^{4+}

Equivalence point at steepest part of plot

Initially, the solution is mostly Fe^{2+}. As Ce^{4+} is added, the iron is oxidized and the potential slowly rises as the Fe^{2+}/Fe^{3+} ratio decreases

Fig. 10.12. Potentiometric titration of ferrous salt.

The electrode potential changes gradually during the major portion of titration (Fig. 10.12). As the equivalence point reaches, the activity ratio changes rapidly.

(v) Diazotisation titrations

Drugs or substances containing aromatic primary amino group can be titrated against sodium nitrite in acidic medium (used as diazotisation titrations). One method of detecting end point is by using starch iodide paper [external indicator method]. The other method, better than the external indicator method is by potentiometric method of determining end point.

Reference electrode: Saturated calomel electrode.

Indicator electrode: Glass electrode.

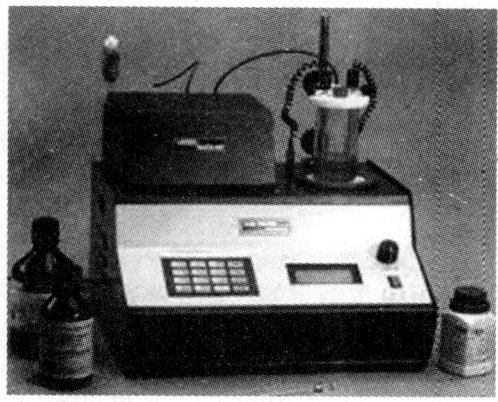

Fig. 10.13. Apparatus for dead stop end point technique.

(vi) Dead stop end point technique

This can be explained by using the following circuit diagram.

Classical example is the determination of water [Moisture content] by **Karl Fischer method** (Fig. 10.13) using dead stop technique.

It contains two platinum electrodes, between which a small emf is applied. No current flows till the solution is free from polarizing substances. Current flows only when both electrodes are depolarized [at the end point]. Normally, the titrant is added through an automatic burette and at the end point the stopper gets automatically closed and titrant stops flowing. This is because there is a sharp transition in the end point between one polarized electrode [beginning of titration] and complete depolarization of both electrodes [at the end point].

The reactions involved in the titration of water using Karl Fischer reagent is given below:

$$3C_5H_5N + SO_2 + I_2 + H_2O \longrightarrow 2C_5H_5NHI + C_2H_5N\overset{O}{\underset{SO_2}{|}}$$

$$C_5H_5N\overset{O}{\underset{SO_2}{|}} + CH_3OH \longrightarrow C_5H_5N\overset{SO_4CH_3}{\underset{H}{\diagup}}$$

Table 10.1. Comparison of potentiometric titrations with conductometric titrations

	Potentiometric titration	*Conductometric titration*
Parameter measured	Potential in mV	Conductivity in mhos
At end point	Rate of change of potential is maximum	Sharp change in conductivity occurs
End point determination	Normal curve, first derivative curve, second derivative curve	End point shown by intersection of two lines
Strength of titrant	Same as that of analyte	5 or 10 times stronger than analyte
Dependency	Temperature dependent	Temperature dependent

Experiment: Find out the normality of given HCl solution with an alkali solution using quinhydrone-calomel electrode system by potentiometric method

Theory

When an acid is titrated with an alkali solution, the H$^+$ ions of acid react with OH$^-$ ions supplied by alkali, so [H$^+$] ion decreases. Suppose an electrode whose potential depends on [H$^+$] (here an indicator electrode). On adding alkali solution from burette, [H$^+$] will change and so potential of indicator electrode changes. If the rate of change of potential is plotted against the volume of alkali, the end point can be from the graph.

In the reference calomel, potential does not depend upon [H$^+$], so its electrode maintains, a constant potential during titration. The change in emf is equivalent to the change in potential of indicator electrode since the potential of reference electrode remains unchanged.

Procedure

1. Prepare 0.1 N oxalic acid solution.
2. Prepare 0.1 N NaOH solution 4 g of NaOH in 1 litre of H$_2$O.
3. Pipette 25 ml of oxalic acid in 100 ml beaker. Dip a quinhydrone electrode (indicator electrode) and a calomel electrode in the beaker. Connect the two electrodes to a potentiometer. Start adding NaOH from burette and measure the potential difference. For example, end point from graph shows volume of NaOH = 25.2.

$$N_1V_1 = N_2V_2$$
$$\text{(NaOH)} \quad \text{(Oxalic acid)}$$
$$N_1 \times 25 = 0.1238 \times 25.2$$

NaOH is standardized potentiometrically:

4. Pipette 25 ml of given HCl solution and titrate potentiometrically with NaOH solution as done in step 3, let us say end point is 25.2.

$$N_1V_1 = N_2V_2$$
$$\text{HCl} \quad \text{(NaOH)}$$

$$\text{Normality of HCl } (N_1) = \frac{0.1238 \times 25.2}{25} = 0.124 \text{ N}$$

CHAPTER 11

Conductometric Titration

Titration is the method of determining the concentration of an unknown solution (the *analyte*) by reacting it completely with a standardized reagent that is a solution of known concentration (the *titrant*). The point at which all of the analyte is consumed is the *equivalent point*. The number of moles of analyte is calculated from the volume of reagent that is required to react with all of the analyte. Previously, a pH electrode was used to measure the pH of the analyte and to determine when the equivalence point was reached. Another method of determining the equivalence point is the conductometric method. It involves the uses of conductometer to measure the conductivity of the analyte. It measures the changes in conductance of solution produced by the ions in the solution. Conductometer works on the principle of Ohm's law.

For example, the titration of barium hydroxide, $Ba(OH)_2$ solution with sulphuric acid solution. Initially the $Ba(OH)_2$ is almost completely dissociated into Ba^{2+} and OH and then with the addition of the H_2SO_4, the following reaction takes place:

$$Ba^{2+} (aq) + 2OH (aq) + 2H^+ (aq) + SO_4^{2-} \longrightarrow BaSO_4 (s) + H_2O$$

The barium sulphate, $BaSO_4$, is fairly insoluble and precipitates out of solution. The hydronium and hydroxide ions combine to form water. Neither of the reaction products contribute very much to the conductivity of the solution, thus as the titration takes place the conductivity will decrease. At the equivalence point, when enough H_2SO_4 has been added to react with the available $Ba(OH)_2$, the conductance of the analyte is at its lowest point. Adding more titrant will cause the conductance of the analyte to increase again. Thus, a plot of conductance vs. volume of H_2SO_4 added will result in a "V" shaped graph (Fig. 11.1). The intercept of the two lines will suggest the exact volume of H_2SO_4 used or the endpoint.

SOME FUNDAMENTAL RELATIONS

The ease of flow of electric current through a body is called its conductance. In metallic conductors, it is caused by the movement of electrons, while in electrolytic solutions it is caused by ions of electrolyte. Electrolytes are substances that produce free ions when they are placed into a solvent

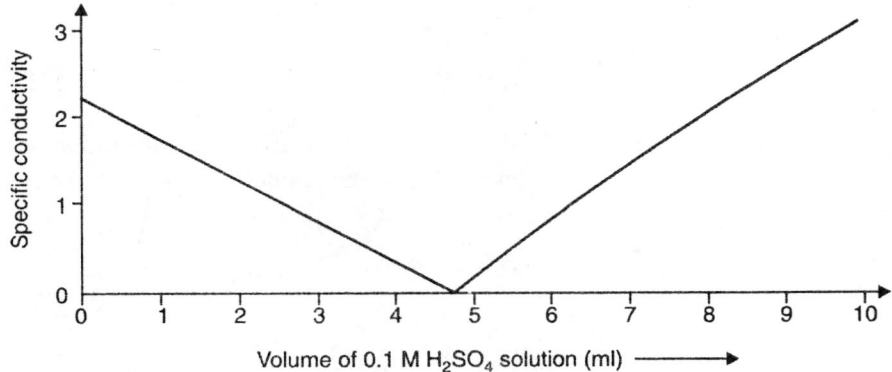

Fig. 11.1. Change in the specific conductivity K in the titration of an approximately 0.1 molar barium hydroxide solution (V = 5 ml) with sulphuric acid.

such as water. Their molecules split up into individual an atomic component, which form ions, in a process, called dissociation. Positively charged ions are cations and those with a negative charge are anions. Due to the presence of free ions, electrolyte solutions behave as an electrically conductive medium. Common electrolytes consist of salts, acids or bases.

Electronic properties of the conductor are described by Ohm's law which states that the current I (amperes) flowing in a conductor is directly proportional to the applied electromotive force U (volts) and inversely proportional to the resistance, R (ohms) of the conductor:

$$I = U/R \qquad \text{...(11.1)}$$

This resistance depends on the intrinsic properties of a conductor and on its shape as:

$$R = \rho \cdot L/S \qquad \text{...(11.2)}$$

where L is a conductor's length and S is a cross-sectional area. Every material is characterized by a specific resistance, ρ, that is given in units of $\Omega.m$ (Ω - ohm, a unit of electric resistance). Electrical properties can be expressed also through quantity, inverse to the resistance, **conductance G**.

$$G = L/R \qquad \text{...(11.3)}$$

Its unit is S (siemens), where $1S = 1/\Omega$.

The **Specific conductance** of any conductor is the reciprocal of specific resistance and is denoted by κ (small kappa).

$$\kappa = L/R.S \qquad \text{...(11.4)}$$

It $l = 1$ cm and $S = 1$ sq cm, then the above equation can be written as:

$$\kappa = 1/R = G \qquad \text{...(11.5)}$$

thus in single words specific conductance can be defined as "the conductivity offered by a solution of length 1 cm and area of 1 sq cm cross section." It is expressed in $ohm^{-1}\,cm^{-1}$ or mhos/cm.

In order to compare quantitatively the conductivities of electrolytes, a quantity called **molar conductivity** is frequently used. The molar conductivity, Λm (capital lambda) is the conductivity per unit molar concentration of a dissolved electrolyte. It is related to conductivity, κ by the relation:

$$\Lambda m = \kappa/c \qquad \ldots(11.6)$$

where c is the concentration in mol m^{-3}. The molar conductivity is usually expressed in Ω^{-1} m^2 mol^{-1} or Ω^{-1} cm^2 mol^{-1}.

The **Equivalent conductance** is defined as the conductance of one gram equivalent of a solute contained between electrodes spaced one cm apart. The equivalent conductivity Λ^* is mainly used in theoretical investigations. Mathematically, it is calculated as:

$$\Lambda^* = \kappa \times V$$

where
k = specific conductivity
V = volume of solution in ml containing 1 'g' equivalent of electrolyte

Relationship between equivalent and specific conductivities in terms of concentration:
Suppose the solution has a concentration of 'c' g equivalent per litre. Then, volume, V containing 1 'g' equivalent to electrolyte will be $\frac{1}{C}$ litre.

$$V = \frac{1}{C} \text{ litre} = \frac{100}{C} \text{ ml}$$

Therefore, equivalent conductance $= \kappa \times \frac{1000}{C} = x \times \frac{1000}{N}$

Relationship between equivalent conductivity and molar conductivity:

$$\Lambda^* = \frac{\text{Molar conductivity}}{\text{No. of charge on an ion}}$$

For example, in KCl, the number of charge on each ion is 1. Therefore,

$$\Lambda^* = \frac{\text{Molar conductivity}}{1}$$

FACTORS AFFECTING CONDUCTANCE

The conductivity of a solution depends on:

(i) **Concentration/Number of ions:** The conductivity of an ionic solution increases with increasing concentration. For strong electrolytes, the increase in conductivity with increase of concentration is sharp. However, for weak electrolytes, the increase in conductivity is more gradual. In both cases, the increase in the conductivity with concentration is due to an increase in the number of ions per unit volume of the solution. For strong electrolytes, which are completely ionised, the increase in conductivity is almost proportional to the concentration. In weak electrolytes, however, the increase in specific conductance is not large due to the low ionisation of the electrolytes, and consequently the conductivity does not go up so rapidly as in the case of strong electrolytes.

(ii) **Ionic mobility in a general way:** The mobility in turn depends on:
   (a) *Type of ion*: The smaller an ion, the more mobile it is and the better it conducts electrical current. Ions of very high conductivity are H_3O^+, OH^-, K^+ and Cl^-. If an ion is surrounded by water molecules (hydratization) and therefore becomes larger, its conductivity decreases.
   (b) *Solvent*: The more polar a solvent, the more completely ionized are the compounds dissolved in it. Water is an ideal solvent for ionic compounds. In alcohols, the ionization decreases with increasing chain length (methanol > ethanol > propanol). In non-polar organic solvents, e.g. chlorinated and non chlorinated hydrocarbons, there is practically no ionization.
   (c) *Temperature*: In contrast to what is found with solids, the conductivity of solutions increases with increasing temperature at a rate that ranges from 1 to 9% per Kelvin, depending on the ion.
   (d) *Viscosity*: The ionic mobility decreases with increasing viscosity, which means that the conductivity also decreases.

How to measure conductance

Principle: Conductance of a solution can be determined by measuring the resistance offered by solution contained within the two electrodes of a conductivity cell. For measuring resistance, the Wheatstone bridge (Fig. 11.2) is employed. It works on the principle of obtaining balance between two arms with the help of a balance indicator (e.g. a galvanometer) at the condition of potential being equal.

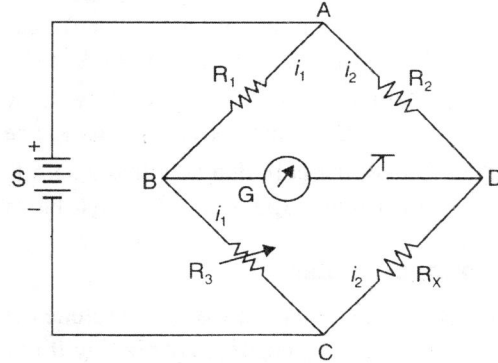

Fig. 11.2. A DC Wheatstone bridge circuit.

Let R_x be an unknown resistor, R_1 and R_2 two standard resistors, R_3 an adjustable resistor and G a galvanometer. The bridge is connected to a source of power S, a battery, and a tapping key K is placed in the path to control the connections. To measure the resistance R_x, the tapping key K is held down momentarily and the bridge is balanced by adjusting R_3 to get no deflection in galvanometer.

In the bridge the total current is divided into two paths: i_1 through R_1 and R_3, and i_2 through R_2 and R_x. Under the balancing conditions, the potential at points B and D must be the same, i.e. the ohmic voltage drop through the resistors R_1 and R_2 must be the same. Hence, the potential at B (EB) must be equal to potential at D (ED).

$$EB = ED \qquad \ldots(11.9)$$
Or
$$i_1 R_1 = i_2 R_2 \qquad \ldots(11.10)$$
Similarly,
$$i_1 R_3 = i_2 R_x \qquad \ldots(11.11)$$

Dividing Eq. (11.10) by Eq. (11.11), we get

$$\frac{R_1}{R_3} = \frac{R_2}{R_x}$$

$$R_x = \frac{R_2 R_3}{R_1} \qquad ...(11.12)$$

Thus,

$$G = \frac{R_1}{R_2 R_3} \qquad 11.13$$

Measurement of conductance of a solution

The Principle of the Wheatstone bridge discussed above can be used to measure the conductance of solutions. However, the following considerations must also be kept in mind:

(i) Since a direct current would polarize the electrodes in the conductivity cell by electrolyzing the solution to avoid polarization an alternating current (ac) source of power must be used in a place of a dc source (battery) usually ac voltages of 3–6 volts with frequency of 50 Hz or 1000 Hz used across points A and C of Fig. 11.2.

(ii) A suitable conductivity cell (with electrodes dipped in the solution) is located between points C and D. Thus, Rx represents the resistance of the conductivity cell.

(iii) Since, the cell also acts like a small capacitor (Cx), and to balance its capacitance resistance a variable capacitor, CB, must be inserted into the bridge.

Conductometer

From above discussion we can conclude that conductance is reciprocal of resistance and the resistance of a cell can be measured by placing it in an arm of a Wheatstone bridge. The inverse of resistance gives the conductance and can be directly read on a conductivity measuring instrument, known as "Conductometer".

A typical conductometer, consists of an ac source, a Wheatstone bridge circuit, a null detector or direct reading display and a conductivity cell.

To avoid the effects of polarization, i.e. the change is composition of the measuring cell, alternating current (ac) is used. The instrument has an arrangement to convert the supply of 50 Hz to higher frequency, say 1000 Hz. For measuring low conductance solution, the lower frequency is preferable and for high conductive solutions higher frequencies are preferably used. Several inexpensive conductometers are

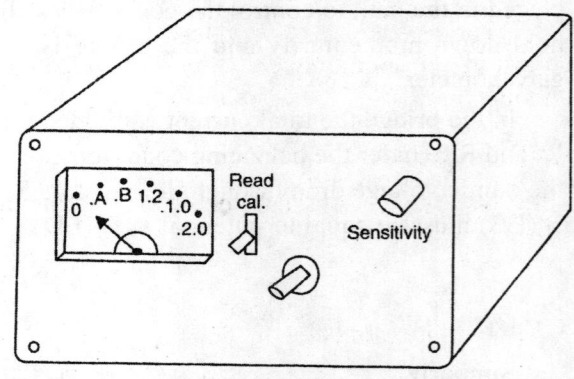

Fig. 11.3. Conductometer.

commercially available. The instruments come as a line-operated unit with and without digital readout. Fig. 11.3 gives the view of a typical conductometer, which can be operated as with given instructions.

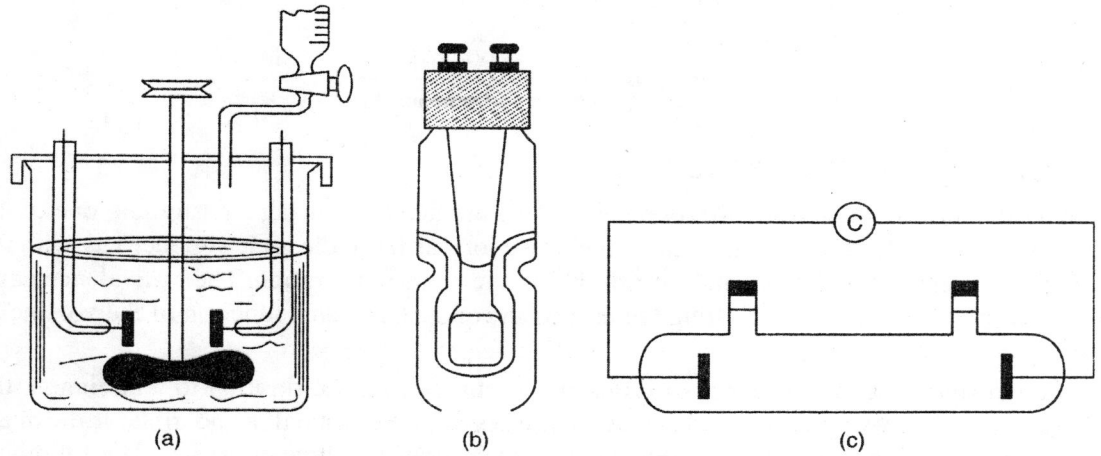

Fig. 11.4. Typical design of conductivity cells.

CELL

Various types of cells have been designed and are in use for the measurement of conductance of a solution (Fig. 11.4). These are made of Pyrex glass fitted with electrodes of platinum or gold. To overcome the imperfections in the current and the other effects at the electrodes, these are coated with a layer of finely divided platinum black. This is achieved by electrolyzing a 3% solution of chloroplatinic acid containing a little of lead acetate. The distance between the electrodes is determined by the conductance of the solution to be measured. For highly conducting solution, solution after each addition from the burette to ensure that the liquid between the electrodes becomes thoroughly mixed. Since absolute conductivity values are not required it is not necessary to know the cell constant.

For spot checking on a process stream or tank, a dip-type of conductivity cell is used.

In some titrations on open beaker with fixed electrodes is sufficient. However, the fairly dilute solutions an open beaker would not be satisfactory because atmospheric CO_2 may alter the conductance.

Cell constant

For a given cell, l and S are constant, and the quantity (l/S) is called the cell constant (κ).

$$K_{cell} = \frac{l}{S} \qquad ...(11.14)$$

Substitute this value in Eq. 11.4

$$\kappa = G\,K_{cell} \qquad ...(11.15)$$

Conductivity = observed conductance × Cell constant

The cell constant is determined by substituting the value of specific conductivity of N/50 KCl solution at 25°C. This value as determined by Kohlrausch was founded to be 0.002765 mhos. The value of conductivity is then oberved with the given cell using N/50 KCl solution. The cell constant is then calculated by using the following relation:

$$\text{Cell constant} = \frac{0.002765}{\text{Observed conductivity}}$$

CONDUCTOMETRIC TITRATIONS

The principle of conductometric titration is based on the fact that during the titration, one of the ions is replaced by the other and invariably these two ions differ in the ionic conductivity with the result that conductivity of the solution varies during the course of titration. The equivalence point may be located graphically by plotting the change in conductance as a function of the volume of titrant added.

In order to reduce the influence of errors in the conductometric titration to a minimum, the angle between the two branches of the titration curve should be as small as possible. If the angle is very obtuse, a small error in the conductance data can cause a large deviation. The following approximate rules will be found useful.

The smaller the conductivity of the ion which replaces the reacting ion, the more accurate will be the result. Thus it is preferable to titrate a silver salt with lithium chloride rather than with HCl. Generally, cations should be titrated with lithium salts and anions with acetates as these ions have low conductivity.

The larger the conductivity of the anion of the reagent which reacts with the cation to be determined, or vice versa, the more acute is the angle of titration curve.

The titration of a slightly ionized salt does not give good results, since the conductivity increases continuously from the commencement.

In the interest of keeping V small, the reagent for the conductometric titration is ordinarily several times more concentrated than the solution being titrated (at least 10–20 times). A micro burette may then be used for the volumetric measurement.

The main advantage to the conductometric titration are its applicability to very dilute, and coloured solutions and to system that involve relative incomplete reactions. For example, neither a potentiometric, nor indicator method can be used for the neutralization titration of phenol ($Ka = 10^{-10}$) a conductometric endpoint can be successfully applied.

Some typical conductometric titration curves are:

1. Strong Acid with a strong base, e.g. HCl with NaOH

Before NaOH is added, the conductance is high due to the presence of highly mobile hydrogen ions. When the base is added, the conductance falls due to the replacement of hydrogen ions by the added cation as H^+ ions react with OH^- ions to form undissociated water. This decrease in the conductance continues till the equivalence point. At the equivalence point, the solution contains only NaCl. After the equivalence point, the conductance increases due to the large conductivity of OH⁻ ions (Fig. 11.5).

2. Weak acid with a strong base, e.g. acetic acid with NaOH

Initially the conductance is low due to the feeble ionization of acetic acid. On the addition of base, there is decrease in conductance not only due to the replacement of H^+ by Na^+ but also suppresses the dissociation of acetic acid due to common ion, acetate. But very soon, the conductance increases on adding NaOH as NaOH neutralizes the undissolved CH_3COOH to CH_3COONa which is the strong electrolyte. This increase in conductance continues raise up to the equivalence point. The graph near the equivalence point is curved due to the hydrolysis of salt CH_3COONa. Beyond the equivalence point, conductance increases more rapidly with the addition of NaOH due to the highly conducting OH⁻ ions (Fig. 11.6).

3. Strong acid with a weak base, e.g. sulphuric acid with dilute ammonia

Initially the conductance is high and then it decreases due to the replacement of H^+. But after the endpoint has been reached the graph becomes almost horizontal, since the excess aqueous ammonia is not appreciably ionised in the presence of ammonium sulphate (Fig. 11.7).

4. Weak acid with a weak base

The nature of curve before the equivalence point is similar to the curve obtained by titrating weak acid against strong base. After the equivalence point, conductance virtually remains same as the weak base which is being added is feebly ionized and, therefore, is not much conducting (Fig. 11.8).

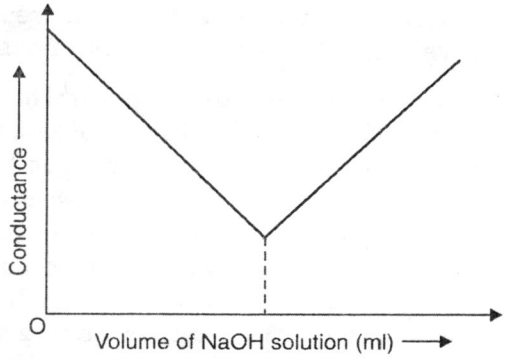

Fig. 11.5. Conductometric titration of a strong acid (HCl) vs strong base (NaOH).

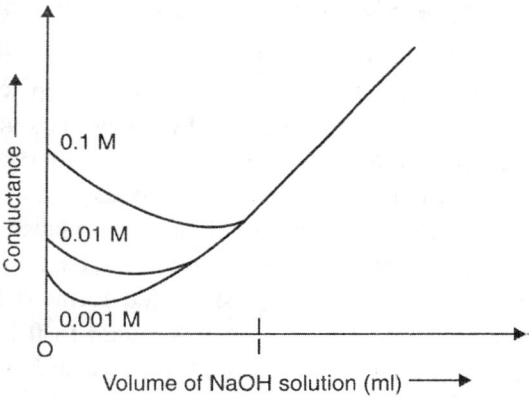

Fig. 11.6. Conductometric titration of a weak acid (acetic acid) vs strong base (NaOH).

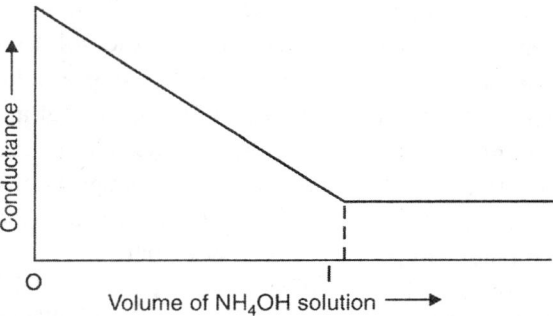

Fig. 11.7. Conductometric titration of a strong acid (H_2SO_4) vs weak base (NH_4OH).

5. Mixture of a strong acid and a weak acid vs a strong base or a weak base

In this curve, there are two break points. The first break point corresponds to the neutralization of strong acid. When the strong acid has been completely neutralized only then the weak acid starts neutralizing. The second break point corresponds to the neutralization of weak acid and after that the conductance increases due to the excess of OH⁻ ions in case of a strong base as the titrant. However, when the titrant is a weak base, it remains almost constant after the end poiont similar to Fig. 11.9.

6. Displacement (or replacement) titrations

When a salt of a weak acid is titrated with a strong acid, the anion of the weak acid is replaced by that of the strong acid and weak acid itself is liberated in the undissociated form. Similarly, in the addition of a strong base to the salt of a weak base, the cation of the weak base is replaced by that of the stronger one and the weak base itself is generated in the undissociated form. If for example, 1M HCl solution is added to 0.1 M solution of sodium acetate, the curve shown in Fig. 11.10 is obtained, the acetate ion is replaced by the chloride ion after the endpoint. The initial increase in conductivity is due to the fact that the conductivity of the chloride ion is slightly greater than that of acetate ion. Until the replacement of nearly complete, the solution contains enough sodium acetate to suppress the ionization of the liberated acetic acid, so resulting a negligible increase in the conductivity of the solution. However, near the equivalent point, the acetic acid is sufficiently ionized to affect the conductivity and a rounded portion of the curve is obtained. Beyond the equivalence point, when excess of HCl is present (ionization of acetic acid is very much suppressed) therefore, the conductivity arises rapidly.

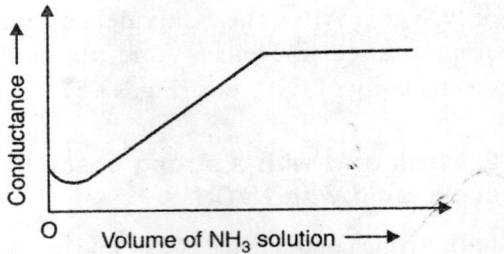

Fig. 11.8. Conductometric titration of a weak acid (acetic acid) vs weak base (NH_4OH).

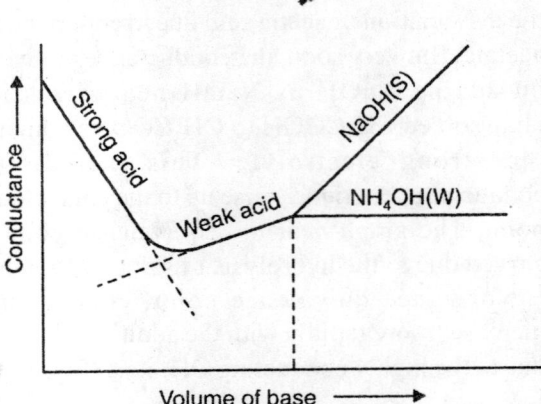

Fig. 11.9. Conductometric titration of a mixture of a strong acid (HCl) and a weak acid (CH_3COOH) vs a strong base (NaOH) or a weak base (NH_4OH).

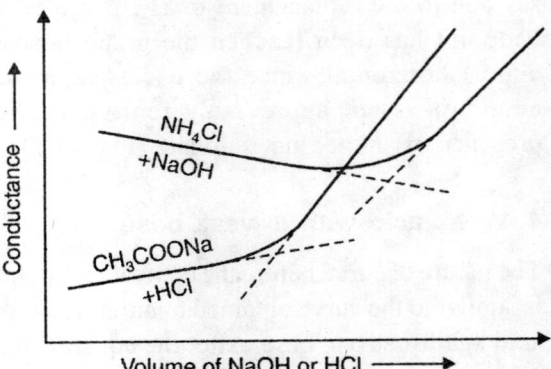

Fig. 11.10. Conductometric titration of a salt of weak acid (sodium acetate) vs. strong acid (HCl); salt of a weak base (NH_4OH) vs. a strong base (NaOH).

7. Precipitation titration and complex formation titration

A reaction may be made the basis of a conductometric precipitation titration provided the reaction product is sparingly soluble or is a stable complex. The solubility of the precipitate (or the dissociation of the complex) should be less than 5%. The addition of ethanol is sometimes recommended to reduce the solubility in the precipitations. An experimental curve is given in Fig. 11.11 (ammonium sulphate in aqueous-ethanol solution with barium acetate). If the solubility of the precipitate were negligibly small, the conductance at the equivalence point should be given by AB and not the observed AC. The addition of excess of the reagent depresses the solubility of the precipitate and, if the solubility is not too large, the position of the point B can be determined by continuing the straight portion of the two arms of the curve until they intersect.

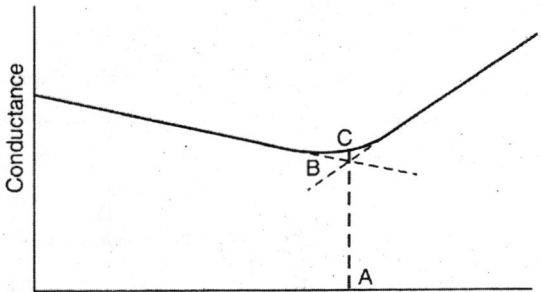

Fig. 11.11. Precipitation titration. Conductometric titration of $(NH_4)_2SO_4$ vs barium acetate.

8. Oxidation-Reduction (Redox) titrations

The conductometric method is not well suited to the study of oxidation-reduction titrations. Almost all such reactions must be carried out in the presence of a large excess of acid or base, which more or less completely masks the change in conductance due to the redox reaction. A typical example is the titration of Fe(II) with potassium permanganate in which, say, a 0.01 M solution of Fe(II) in 0.5 M sulphuric acid is titrated with 0.02 M potassium permanganate. Although the reaction:

$$5Fe^{2+} + MnO_4^- + 8H^+ \longrightarrow 5Fe^{+3} + Mn^{+2} + 4H_2O$$

does consume hydrogen ions, thus decreasing the conductance of the solution up to the equivalence point, the fraction of hydrogen ion thus removed is relatively small. The entire change in conductance is not appreciable and cannot be detected with accuracy by the usual equipment for the conductometric titrations.

APPLICATIONS OF CONDUCTANCE MEASUREMENTS

There are many applications of conductance measurements. The experimental determination of the conducting properties of electrolytic solutions are very important as they can be used to study quantitative behaviour of ions in solution. They can also be used to determine the many physical quantities such as degree of dissociation and dissociation constants of weak acids and bases, ionic product of water, solubility and solubility. Some of these are discussed below:

1. Conductance measurements are employed for the determination of the concentration of solution containing a single strong electrolyte, such as solutions of the common alkalies or acids. An almost linear increase with concentration is observed in conductance for solutions containing as 20 percent weight of solute. Analysis are based on calibration curves. For higher concentration the conductance passes through a maximum because of the hindrance produced

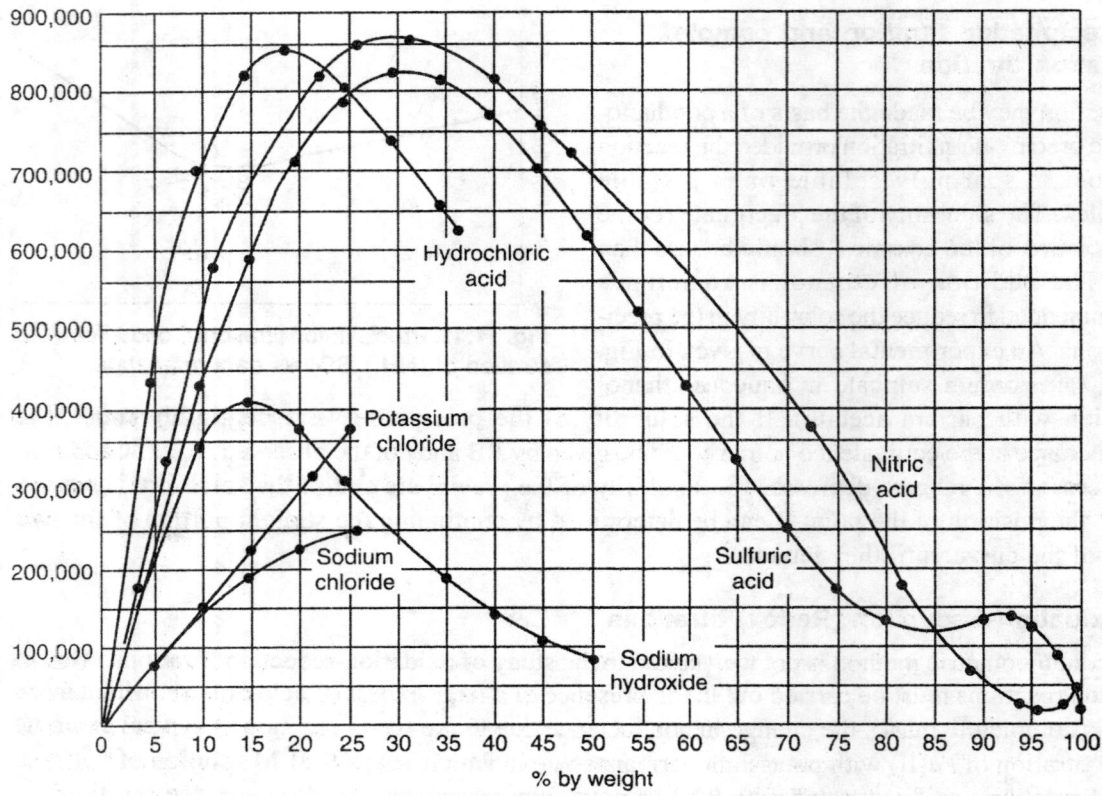

Fig. 11.12. Conductivity (μS/cm) vs chemical concentration.

by interionic attractions for free motion of ions. Some typical curves for some electrolytes are given in Fig. 11.12.

2. Analysis of fuming nitric acid to determine the ratio of NO_2 to H_2O can also done on the basis of calibration curve of the conductance are made: (i) on treated sample and (ii) on a duplicate sample which has been saturated with KNO_3. By this method NO_2 can be determined in the range 0 to 20 percent NO_2 (by weight) and water in the range 0 to 6 percent.

3. Conductance measurements have been useful for the determination of small amounts of ammonia in biological materials. The ammonia is removed from the sample distillation, or swept out with a current of air and absorbed in boric acid solution. The reason for choosing boric acid as absorbent is its small ionization which keeps the specific conductance of the solution a linear function of the concentration of ammonium salt. The specific conductance of the boric acid solution is determined and compared with standards already measured.

4. Conductometric data are also useful for the completion of certain types of elemental analysis, e.g., hydrocarbons can be analysed for their sulphur content by combustion of the sample followed by absorption of the SO_2 and H_2O. The increase in conductance, resulting from the H_2SO_4 that is produced can be related to the concentration of sulphur.

5. Conductance measurements are employed to a considerable extent to measure the salinity of sea water in oceanographic work. These measurements also give information regarding association and dissociation equilibria in aqueous solutions; the condition being that one or more of the reacting species is ionic.
6. Conductometric determination of ash content of cane or beet sugar products has already replaced the tedious gramimetric procedure used earlier.
7. Special electrodes have been designed to determine conductometrically the moisture content of wood before processing it into pulp and paper.
8. The solubility of sparingly soluble salt like $AgCl$, $BaSO_4$, $PbSO_4$ etc. can be determined with the help of conductivity measurements.
9. Determination of vanillin in a vanilla essence.
10. Equilibrium in ionic reaction can be determined, as conductance of solution changes during the progress of reaction.

CHAPTER 12

Polarography

It is an electroanalytical method of analysis where time dependent potential is applied to an electrochemical cell and the current flowing through the cell is measured as a function of total potential. The earliest voltammetric method, polarographic method of analysis was first developed by Jaroslav Heyrovsky in 1922, for that, he received Nobel Prize in 1952 for developing this technique using dropping mercury electrode as the working electrode.

In potentiometry, zero current is maintained. But in polarography, limited current is produced by limited electrolysis. Hence, it is based on the measurement of current resulting from reduction or oxidation of an electro active species, at a given electrode potential under controlled condition. As in potentiometry, there is a reference electrode, saturated calomel electrode (SCE) and an indicator electrode or microelectrode in this technique. The SCE consists of large surface area so that current density (current per unit area) is small at this electrode. Its potential will then essentially constant and unaffected by applied potential (emf). The microelectrode or indicator electrode assumes the potential impressed upon in. The indicator electrodes may be made from quite a large number of materials say for instance mercury, platinum, gold and graphite, having varying shapes and construction. Mostly, DME is used as indicator electrode. The apparatus is designed in such a manner that electrolysis of electroactive species take place at the indicator electrode and the potential of micro electrode is always measured relative to reference electrode.

THEORETICAL CONCEPT

The principle of polarography can be explained with help of simplified polarographic apparatus (Fig. 12.1) which contain a reducible species (RS) such as nitrofurantoin and supporting electrolyte (KCl) in a electrolysis cell. When the movable contact 'm' is placed at the extreme left position (say zero), the potential in the voltameter 'V' will be zero and the current measured in microamp (m amp) on the ammeter 'A' will also register zero. If the contact 'm' is now moved to the light, say to 0.5, a certain voltage will be impressed across the electrode (readable in Voltameter V). Since the microelectrode is negative, ions (impurities in the salt and H_2O) capable of picking up electrons at this low potential and will be reduced and the current flowing through the cell will be registered.

If the movable contact is advanced to 1, a greater voltage will be impressed it across the electrode (more ions will be reduced) and increase in current flowing through the cell will be observed. If we continue moving the contact, we will eventually reach a potential, which will reduce electroactive species.

This effect will be reflected in a relatively large increase in the current flowing through the cell on increasing the voltage shows an increase in the current flowing through the cell because a greater number of reducible species RS (nitrofurantoin) are reduced in the vicinity of electrode. As there is decrease in the concentration of ion in the vicinity of microelectrode, the potential of this electrode will decrease. This is called **concentration polarization**. However, increasing the potential does not bring about an increase in the current. In other words, the current, which is measured in this region, is diffusion controlled and depends on the rates at which the reducible species (nitrofurantoin) move (diffuse) from the bulk of solution to the surface of electrode. The diffusion controlled current (diffusion current or limiting current) is a function of concentration.

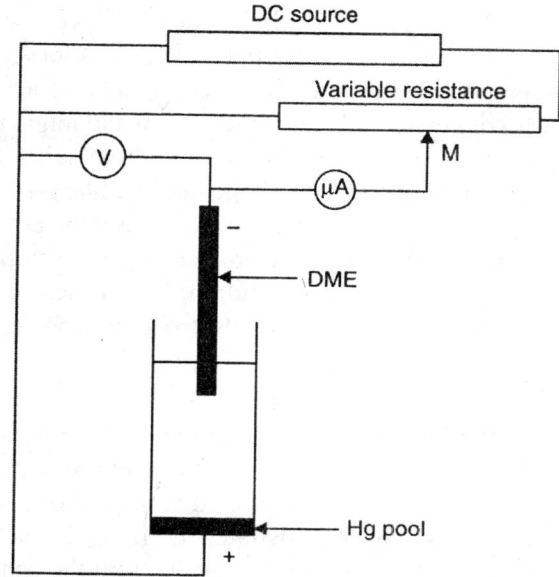

Fig. 12.1. Classical polarographic setup.

Nitrofurantoin + 4H⁺ + 4e → HNOH-... + 4H$_2$O

$$O_2N\text{-furan-}CH-N-N\text{(hydantoin)} + 4H^+ + 4e \xrightarrow{\text{Reduction}} HNOH\text{-furan-}CH-N-N\text{(hydantoin)} + 4H_2O$$

As we want ions should be transferred by diffusion only, we have to avoid the transfer of ion (migration) due to potential gradient. A potential gradient exists between the electrodes with the microelectrode (usually, dropping mercury electrod, DME) negative relative to reference electrode (usually saturated calomel electrode, SCE). Cations will move towards the DME under the influence of this potential and their reduction give rise to the migration current (undesirable). Therefore, to reduce the current carried by the reducible ion, a large concentration of non-reducible electrolyte is added to the solution. This substance, the indifferent electrolyte (or supporting electrolyte) then carries essentially all of the current and **migration current** is eliminated. Commonly used supporting electrolytes are potassium or sodium salts. The potassium ions cannot be discharged at cathode until the impressed voltage becomes large. The large number of potassium ions therefore remains as a crowd around cathode and restrict the potential gradient to a region so very close to the electrode surface. So there is no longer an electrostatic attraction operative to attract other reducible ions from the bulk of the solution. Under these circumstances the limiting current is solely controlled by the diffusion of the electroactive species through the concentration gradient adjacent to the electrode.

Polarogram

The data in polarography are best expressed graphically in which current flow (in amperes) versus potential variation is plotted along the ordinate. This graph is called polarogram. A **polarogram** has the S shape as illustrated in Fig. 12.2. The polarogram is conveniently divided into three regions as A, B and C. Region A results from the charging current of the electrode and reduction of traces of impurities present in the solution. This current is referred to as residual current. Region B results from the reduction of the electro active species in solution. The shape of the curve in this region

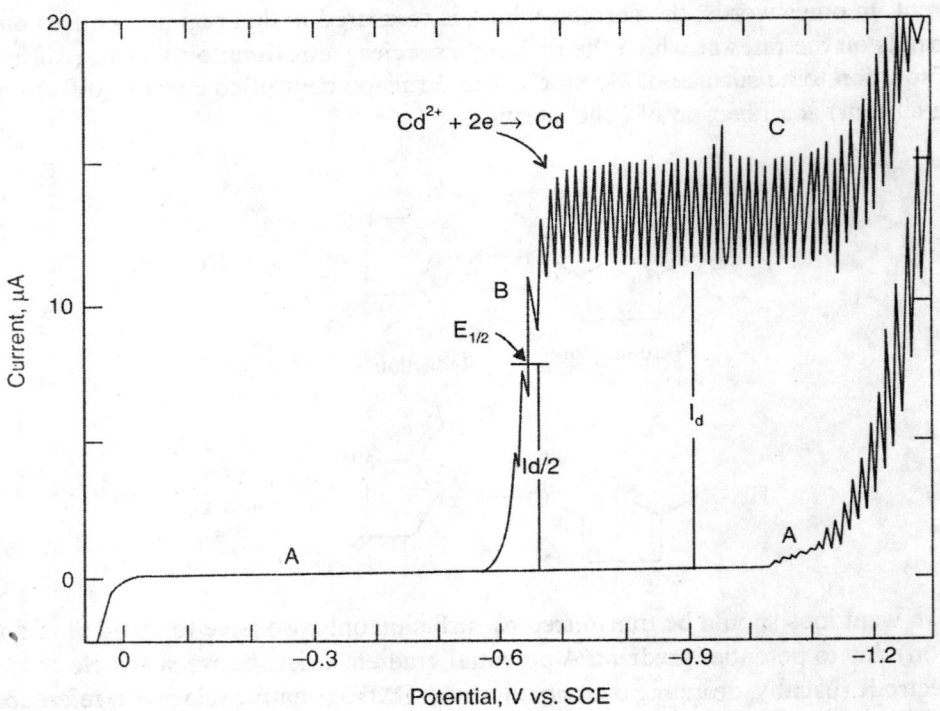

Fig. 12.2. A typical polarogram.

indicates that there are more reducible species in the vicinity of electrode that can be reduced. As the potential of the electrode is increased, more and more of the reducible species are reduced (indicated by the sharp rise in the current) until that point in the curve is reached where an increase in the potential does not give an increase in the current. This indicates that the area in the vicinity of electrode is depleted of reducible species and the reduction is then controlled by the rate at which the species diffuse into this area. The value of the limiting current in region C is called the diffusion current and is directly proportional to the concentration of electro active species.

Half wave potential, $E_{1/2}$

The electro-active material in polarography is characterized by its half-wave potential, $E_{1/2}$. Under any defined set of experimental conditions, each substance has its own characteristic $E_{1/2}$ and this is the basis of qualitative polarographic analysis. The half-wave potential is defined as the potential at which the current due to the reduction or oxidation of the substance responsible for the wave is half as large as on the plateau (Fig. 12.3). The half-wave potential is also independent of the electrode characteristics and concentration of the electroactive substance, therefore serves for the qualitative identification of an unknown substance.

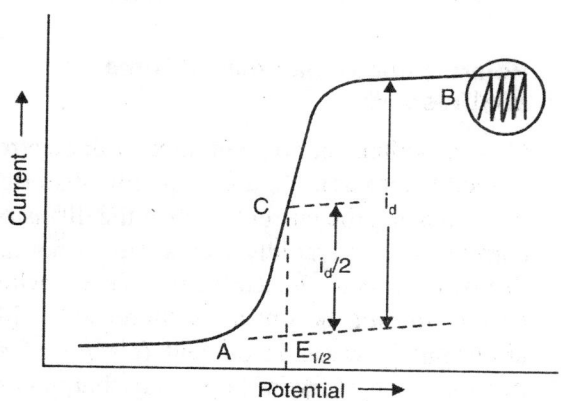

Fig. 12.3. Method for determining half wave potential and diffusion current.

Ilkovic equation

In the presence of excess supporting electrolyte, the electrical force on the reducible/oxidizable ions is nullified and therefore, the limiting current is solely a diffusion current. Ilkovic (1934) examined the various factors which govern the diffusion current and deduced a theoretical equation (12.1) as:

$$i_D = 607\, n\, c D^{1/2}\, m^{2/3}\, t^{1/6} \qquad \ldots(12.1)$$

where

i_d = average diffusion current in microamperes during the life of the drop

n = the number of electrons consumed in the reduction or oxidation of one mole of the electroactive species

D = diffusion coefficient of the reducible or oxidizable substance expressed as cm²/second

c = concentration of electroactive species in millimoles per dm³

m = the rate of flow of mercury from the dropping mercury electrode expressed in mg/second

t = drop time of mercury in seconds

The constant 607 is a combination of natural constants, including the Faraday. This is an important equation because it accounts for the linear dependence of i_d upon c keeping all other factors constant. It is useful in quantitative polarographic analysis. In practice, the limiting current is not exactly the diffusion current. The supporting electrolyte which is 50 to 100 times that of electroactive substance contains impurities which may contribute a small current in addition to non-faradaic condenser current. This is known as 'Residual Current'.

Polarographic maxima: Maxima suppressors

Current-voltage curves obtained with electro-reducible ions at DME are frequently distorted by increasing the current beyond the diffusion current value and rapidly decrease to the normal diffusion plateau after a critical value is reached as the applied potential is increased. This abnormal increase in current is referred as maxima which vary in shape from sharp peaks to rounded humps (Fig. 12.4). To measure the true diffusion currents, the maximum must be eliminated. This can be done by adding small amount of surface-active agents such as gelatin, dye stuff, Triton X-100 etc. which are likely to form an adsorbed layer on the mercury-solution interface to prevent streaming movement of the diffusion layer at the interface. Gelatin is widely used in the concentration range of 0.002 to 0.01%. Higher concentration will suppress the diffusion currents also. Others frequently used are, Triton X-100 (a non-ionic detergent) in the range of 0.002 to 0.004% and methyl cellulose (0.005%).

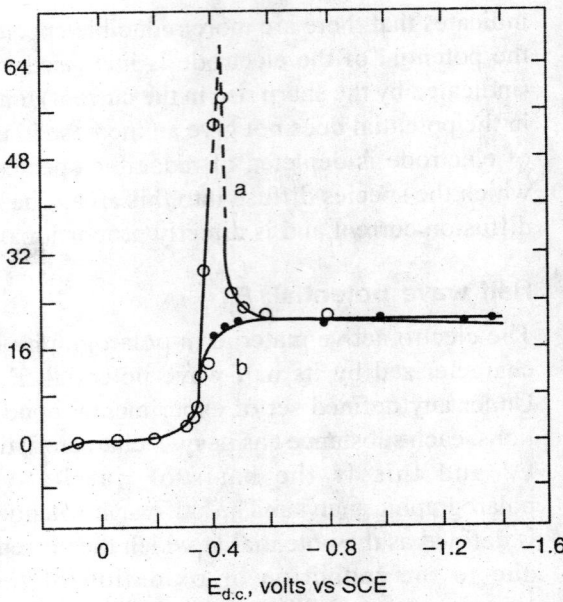

Fig. 12.4. Polarogram of 2.3 mM lead (II) in 0.1 M potassium chloride. (a) In absence of a maximum suppressor. (b) After addition of 0.0002% sodium methyl red.

Dissolved oxygen

Dissolved oxygen present in solution give rise to two reduction waves (Fig. 12.5), as shown by the following equations:

Acid solution:

$$O_2 + 2H^+ + 2e \longrightarrow H_2O_2 \quad \text{first wave} \qquad ...(12.2)$$

$$H_2O_2 + 2H^+ + 2e \longrightarrow 2H_2O \quad \text{second wave} \qquad ...(12.3)$$

Alkaline solution:

$$O_2 + 2H_2O + 2e \longrightarrow H_2O_2 + 2OH^- \quad \text{first wave} \qquad ...(12.4)$$

$$H_2O_2 + 2e \longrightarrow 2OH^- \quad \text{second wave} \qquad ...(12.5)$$

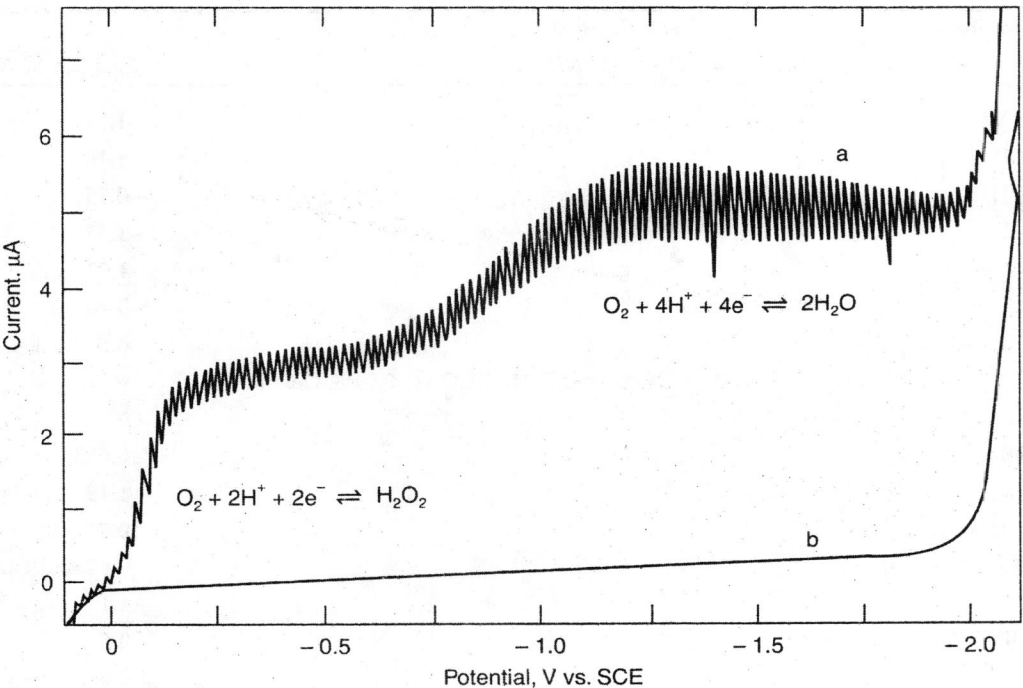

Fig. 12.5. Polarogram of 0.1 M KCl. (a) Saturated with air, (b) after deoxygenation by nitrogen bubbling.

Since these waves occur at the potential, which normally interfere with other wave, it is necessary to remove oxygen by bubbling nitrogen gas through the solution for 10 to 15 min before analyzing the sample.

QUALITATIVE AND QUANTITATIVE POLAROGRAPHIC ANALYSIS

The qualitative analysis of a sample is carried out by matching its $E_{1/2}$ with the tabulated values of the ions (given in the Table 12.1) in the supporting electrolytes used. It is also advisable to use the log-plot for knowing the correct $E_{1/2}$.

Table 12.1. The half-wave potentials of some of the common ions

Metal ion	Supp. electrolytes (i) M NH_3 + 1M NH_4Cl	$E_{1/2}$ V vs. SCE
Cd(II)		−0.81
Co(II)		−1.29
Cu(II)		−0.24
Fe(II)		−0.34 and −1.49
Mn(II)		−1.66

(Contd.)

226 Pharmaceutical Analysis

Metal ion	Supp. electrolytes (i) M NH_3 + 1M NH_4Cl	$E_{1/2}$, V vs. SCE
Mo(VI)		–1.71
Ni(II)		–1.10
Pb(II)		–0.75
Se(II)		–1.53
Te(IV)		–1.21
Tl(I)		–0.48
U(VI)		–0.8 and 1.4
	(ii) 2 M HOAc and 2 M NH_4OAc, 0.01% Gelatin	
(ii)		
Cd(II)		–0.653
Co(II)		–1.19
Cu(II)		–0.07
Mo(VI)		–0.61 and 1.2
Ni(II)		–1.1
Pb(II)		–0.5
Pd(II)		–0.6
Se(II)		–1.11
Te(IV)		–1.18
Tl(I)		–0.47
U(VI)		–0.12
Zn(II)		–1.1
	0.1 M KCl, LiCl, 0.2 $(CH_3)_4NCl$ or NH_4Cl	
(iii)		
Cd(II)		–0.60
Co(II)		–1.20
Cu(II)		>0
Fe(II)		–1.3
Ni(II)		–1.1
Pb(II)		–0.4
Te(IV)		–1.1 and 1.45
Tl(I)		–0.46
U(VI)		–0.185
Zn(II)		–0.995
$E_{1/2}$ of some anions		

(Contd.)

Metal ion	Supp. electrolytes (i) $M\ NH_3 + 1M\ NH_4Cl$	$E_{1/2}$, V vs. SCE
(iv) Anion	Supporting electrolyte	E1/2, V vs. SCE
Br^-	0.1 M KNO_3	0.12
Cl^-	0.1 M KNO_3	0.25
I^-	0.1 M KNO_3	−0.03
CN^-	0.1 M NaOH	−0.36
IO_3^-	0.1 M phosphate buffer, pH 6.4	−0.79
NO_2	−2M citrate, pH 2.5	−1.06
S^-	0.1 M NaOH	−0.43
SCN^-	0.5 M KNO_3	0.10
$S_2O_3^{3-}$	0.2 M NaOAc, pH 5	−0.40

QUANTITATIVE POLAROGRAPHIC ANALYSIS

Polarographic analysis can be used between 10^{-3} to 10^{-5} M concentrations of electroactive substances. If solutions have more than one electroactive substance and if their half-wave potentials in a particular supporting electrolyte differ by about 0.4 V for single charged ions and 0.2 V for doubly charged ions, they can be determined. If the half-wave potential of two ions are close, then various experimental devices can be employed. These include:

(i) Precipitation of one (e.g. lead and zinc mixture – lead may be removed as lead sulphate precipitate for allowing the determination of zinc).

(ii) Complexation: By adding complexing agent, $E_{1/2}$ of one of the ions may be shifted to more negative potential thereby Δ-$E_{1/2}$ of ions become more (e.g. Cu(II) ion can be complexed by potassium cyanide and thereby $E_{1/2}$ is shifted to more negative potential than lead or cadmium).

There are three methods which have been widely used in practice for quantitative analysis. In all these methods, oxygen is removed before taking polarograms of solutions.

1. Wave height – Concentration plots (calibration/working plots)

Standard solutions of different concentrations of ions under investigation are prepared using the same supporting electrolyte and 0.005% maximum suppresser (say gelatin) and polarograms are drawn with the known concentrations of ions. Wave heights of all known concentrations are noted down and after making correction for residual current a plot is drawn as function of concentration (calibration curve). Keeping the supporting electrolyte and gelatin as above, polarogram of unknown is also recorded keeping temperature

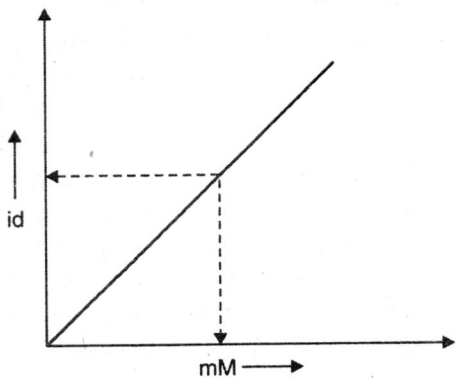

Fig. 12.6. Calibration plot.

constant at 25°C. The wave height of this unknown is referred to the working curve and its concentrations is noted.

2. Internal standard (pilot ion) method

Polarogram of the unknown solution in a supporting electrolyte and gelatin is recorded and to the same solution a standard or pilot ion is added in known amount and current-voltage curve is recorded. The only condition is that $\Delta E_{1/2}$ of pilot ion and unknown should be differed by 0.4 V. The ratio of these two waves is compared with the ratios of known amounts of the two ions previously determined.

3. Method of standard addition

The polarogram of the unknown is first recorded and then a known amount of standard solution of the same ion is added and a second polarogram is taken. The calculations are made as below. If i_{d1} is the wave height the first polarogram of unknown solution of volume V and of concentration, C_u and i_{d2} is the wave height of second polarogram after adding v cm³ of standard solution of concentration C_s, then according to Ilkovic equation:

$$i_{di} = kC_u$$

and

$$i_{d2} = \frac{k(VC_u + vC_2)}{(V + v)}$$

thus

$$k = \frac{i_{d2}(V + v)}{(VC_u + vC_s)}$$

therefore

$$C_u = \frac{i_{d1} vC_s}{(i_{d2} - i_{d1})(V + v) i_{d1} v}$$

Cencentration of unknown, C_u is therefore calculated. This procedure is sometimes reported as spiking used in environmental analysis.

Polarographic apparatus

The basic apparatus for polarographic analysis is given in Fig. 12.7. The commonly used polarographic cell has an external reference electrode and is the H-cell. It consists of two compartments, one containing the solution to be studied and the other containing reference electrode. These compartments are separated by a cross-member filled with 4% agar-saturated potassium chloride gel, which held in place by a medium-porosity sintered disc. The second compartment is the solution compartment into which DME is inserted and this has N_2 inlet and outlet provision. This simple recording polarogram unit has a potentiometer, 'P' by which any emf upto 3 Volts may be gradually applied to the cell. 'R' is a pen recorder and 'V' is voltmeter. In the DME, a very pure mercury, obtained through distillation under vacuum (99.99% pure) is used. Each drop represents a fresh electrode with a new exposed surface. The reproducibility of geometry of each drop with the laps of time is another advantage of the DME over other electrodes. The large **activation overpotential** for hydrogen gas evolution makes this electrode valuable for the study of cathodic processes. One of the most important drawbacks of the Hg as electrode is its **ease of oxidation**. Thus, Hg undergoes **anodic dissolution at +0.25 V vs. SCE** and is oxidized to insoluble Hg_2Cl_2 in presence of chloride ions at zero V vs. SCE so it cannot be used for anodic oxidation above +0.25 V vs. SCE. Also it is important to mention that **Mercury vapors are very poisonous** besides Hg itself is considered to be one of the major pollutants of the environment.

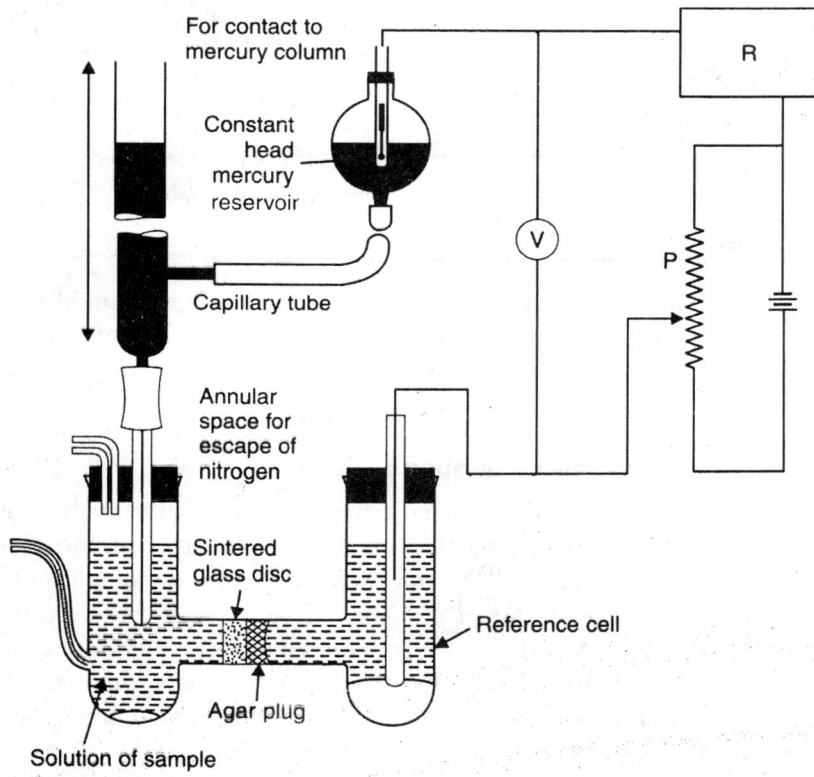

Fig. 12.7. Apparatus for polarographic analysis.

APPLICATIONS OF POLAROGRAPHY

Most metal ions are reducible at DME, and multicomponent mixtures can often be analysed by selecting an appropriate supporting electrolyte so that the half-wave potentials of two ions are differed by about -0.2 V vs SCE or by using complexing agents by taking the advantage of complexing ability of the metal ions.

Based on this, polarography is used predominantly for trace metal analysis of alloys, ultra-pure metals, minerals/metallurgy, environmental analysis (air, water, soil and sea water contaminants), foodstuffs, beverages and body-fluids, toxicology and clinical analysis. Reducible anions such as $-3BrO_3^-$, IO_3^-, $Cr_2O_7^{2-}$ and NO_2^- can also be determined using well buffered solutions (Table 12.2).

Table 12.2. Different samples and element or compound determined

Element or compound determined	Types of sample
Cu, Pb, Sn, Zn	Foodstuffs
Ga, Zn, Cd, Ni	High purity aluminium
Cu, Pb, Ni, Co	Steels
Sn, Pb	Beer and soft drinks
Transition metals	High-purity salts
Free sulphur	Petroleum fractions
Antioxidants	Fuels
Riboflavin	Milk, pharmaceuticals
Vitamin C	Fruit and vegetables
Oxygen	Sea water, gases

It is also useful in the analysis of vitamins, alkaloids, hormones, terpenoid substances and natural colouring substance, analysis of drugs and pharmaceutical preparations, determination of pesticide or herbicide residues in foods, in the structure determination of many organic compounds etc.

Polarographic analysis of organic compounds

This technique is used in organic chemistry for qualitative and quantitative analysis and structure determinations. Most of the organic compounds are insoluble in pure aqueous medium and also in mercury to form amalgam. Therefore, the solvent in which the organic compound and its electrode product is soluble is added to the supporting electrolyte. These solvents include various alcohols or ketones, dimethyl formamide, acetonitrile, ethylene diamine and others. The commonly used supporting electrolytes which are easily mixed with organic solvents are various quaternary ammonium salts such as tetrabutyl ammonium iodide. Some of the organic functional groups that are reducible at DME are given in Table 12.3.

Table 12.3. Reducible organic functional groups

$>C=O$	Ketone	$-C=N$	Nitrile	$-NO_2$	Nitro
$-CHO$	Aldehyde	$-N=N-$	Azo	$-NO$	Nitroso
$>C=C<$	Alkene	$-NO=N-$	Azoxy	$-NHOH$	Hydroxylamine
$-C\equiv C-$	Aryl alkyne	$-O-O-$	Peroxy	$-ONO-$	Nitrite
$>C=C-$	Azomethine	$-S-S-$	Disulfide	$-ONO_2$	Nitrate

In addition, dibromides, aryl halides, α-halogenated ketone or aryl methane, and ketones, polynuclear aromatic ring systems, and heterocyclic double bond reduce at DME. The $-S-S-$, $-SH$ (mercaptanes get oxidized at DME and give anodic currents). Non-polarographic active groups can be converted into active polarographic groups to determine them (Table 12.4).

Table 12.4. Organic functional group analysis of non-polarographic active groups

Functional group	Reagent	Active polarographic group
Carbonyl	Girard T and D	Azomethine
	Semicarbazide	Carbazide
	Hydroxylamine	Hydroxylamine
Primary amine	Peperonal	Azomethine
	CS_2	Dithiocarbonate (anodic)
	$Cu_3(PO_4)_2$ suspension	Copper (II) amine
Secondary amine	HNO_2	Nitrosoamine
Alcohols	Chromic acid	Aldehyde
1,2-Diols	Periodic acid	Aldehyde
Carboxyl	(Transform to thiouranium salts)	–SH (anodic)
Phenyl	Nitration	$-NO_2$

Experiment: Polarographic determination of ascorbic acid in fruit juice

Principle: Ascorbic acid gives a well defined polarographic oxidation wave.

Ascorbic acid $\xrightarrow{-2e^-}$ Dehydroascorbic acid $+ 2H^+$

Use freshly prepared diluted juice.

Calibration curve method

Prepare a fresh stock solution of 0.2% ascorbic acid solution. Prepare 5 standard solutions of ascorbic acid in volumetric flasks of 25 ml. To each one, add 0.5 ml of 0.5 M acetate buffer and different volumes of 0.2% ascorbic acid, 0, 200, 400, 600 and 800 ml. Dilute to the mark with distilled water. For each solution record polarograms over the potential range –150 to +200 mV vs Ag/AgCl/1M KCl reference electrode. Plot id vs 'C' of ascorbic acid (calibration curve).

Standard addition method

Squeeze an orange, grape fruit or lemon until about 10 ml of juice is obtained. Filter the juice through a porous funnel (pore size about 1 mm). Prepare four 25 ml volumetric flasks. Add to each 0.5 ml of 0.5 M acetate buffer, 2.0 ml of the juice and standard addition of 0, 200, 400, and 600 ml of 0.2% ascorbic acid. Dilute to mark with distilled water. Record polarograms under the same conditions as in the calibration step. Draw the standard additions plot and determine the concentration of ascorbic acid. Report the concentration of ascorbic acid (Vitamin C) in the original sample (juice) in mol/l and also ppm.

CHAPTER 13

Amperometric Titrations

In a simple polarographic experiment, the diffusion current between an indicator electrode and reference electrode is recorded (Fig. 13.1). The diffusion current is consequence of polarisation at a microelectrode. So, if some of the electroactive material in the solution is removed by interaction with some other reagent (e.g. EDTA reagent for Zn^{2+} determination), the diffusion current will decrease proportionally.

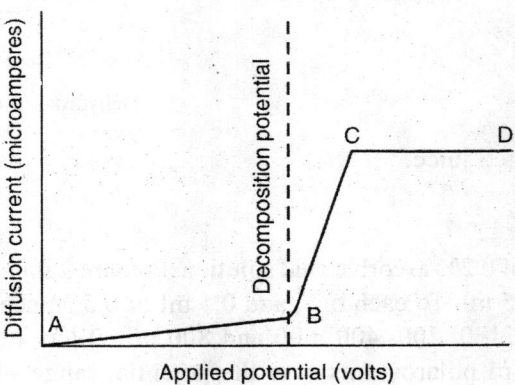

Fig. 13.1. A typical polarogram.

The Fig. 13.2 (at potentials –0.8 V) shows the set of polarogram provided titrant is not reducible. This shows reduction of diffusion current from I_0 to I_1, I_2, I_3 and finally I, at which point all the reducible ions have been exhausted. When this condition is reached, the current value remains constant as the residual value characteristic of the supporting electrolyte. This is the fundamental principal of amperometric titrations or polarographic titrations. The diffusion current at an appropriate applied voltage is measured as a function of the volume of the titrating solution. The end point is the intersection of two lines giving the change of current before and after the equivalence point.

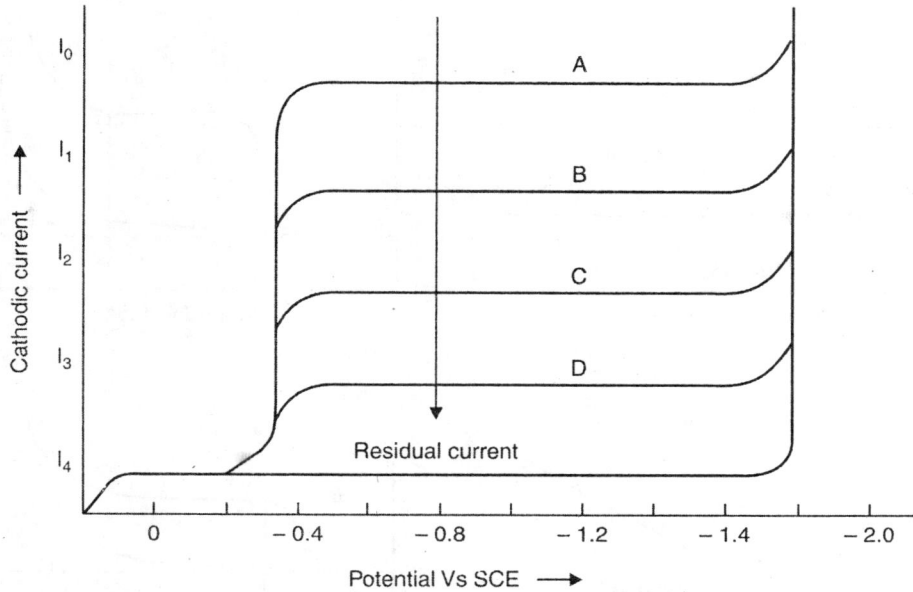

Fig. 13.2. Concept of amperometric titrations.

The voltage applied at the beginning of the titration must be selected so that the diffusion current of the substance to be titrated or of the reagent or of the both, is obtained. Depending on the selection of the applied voltage between indicator electrode (DME) and reference electrode various types of titration curves are obtained as shown in Fig. 13.3.

For each titration the applied voltage is selected to the value between X and Y as shown in figures A to D (S is the substance to be determined and R the reagent).

Fig. 13.3(A). Electroactive material is being removed from the solution by precipitation or complex formation with an inactive titrant at that potential applied, e.g. Pb^{+2} vs Oxalate or Zn^{2+} vs EDTA.

The 13.3(B). Substance to be determined does not give diffusion current but the titrant (reagent) gives current at the applied potential (e.g. SO_4^{2-} ions titrated with Pb^{2+} ions). As long as the substance is available to the titrant, that titrant reacts with substance and current remains zero. After the substance is completely removed by reagent the excess reagent gives its diffusion current in proportional to the excess volume added. So, the reverse L shaped curve obtained.

Fig. 13.3(C). Both, substance to be determined and the titrating reagent give diffusion currents at the potential selected (e.g. Pb^{2+} titrated with $Cr_2O_7^-$).

Fig. 13.3(D). At the applied potential, substance gives anodic current and titrant cathodic current (e.g. I^- ion with $Hg(NO_3)_2$). It is type of compensation titration. In this the 'reagent' and "the substance being titrated" give currents of opposite sign at some potential but ideally donot react with each other at all. The endpoint of such a titration is the point where cathodic current due to the reduction of one of them is just equal to the anodic current due to oxidation of the other. In such

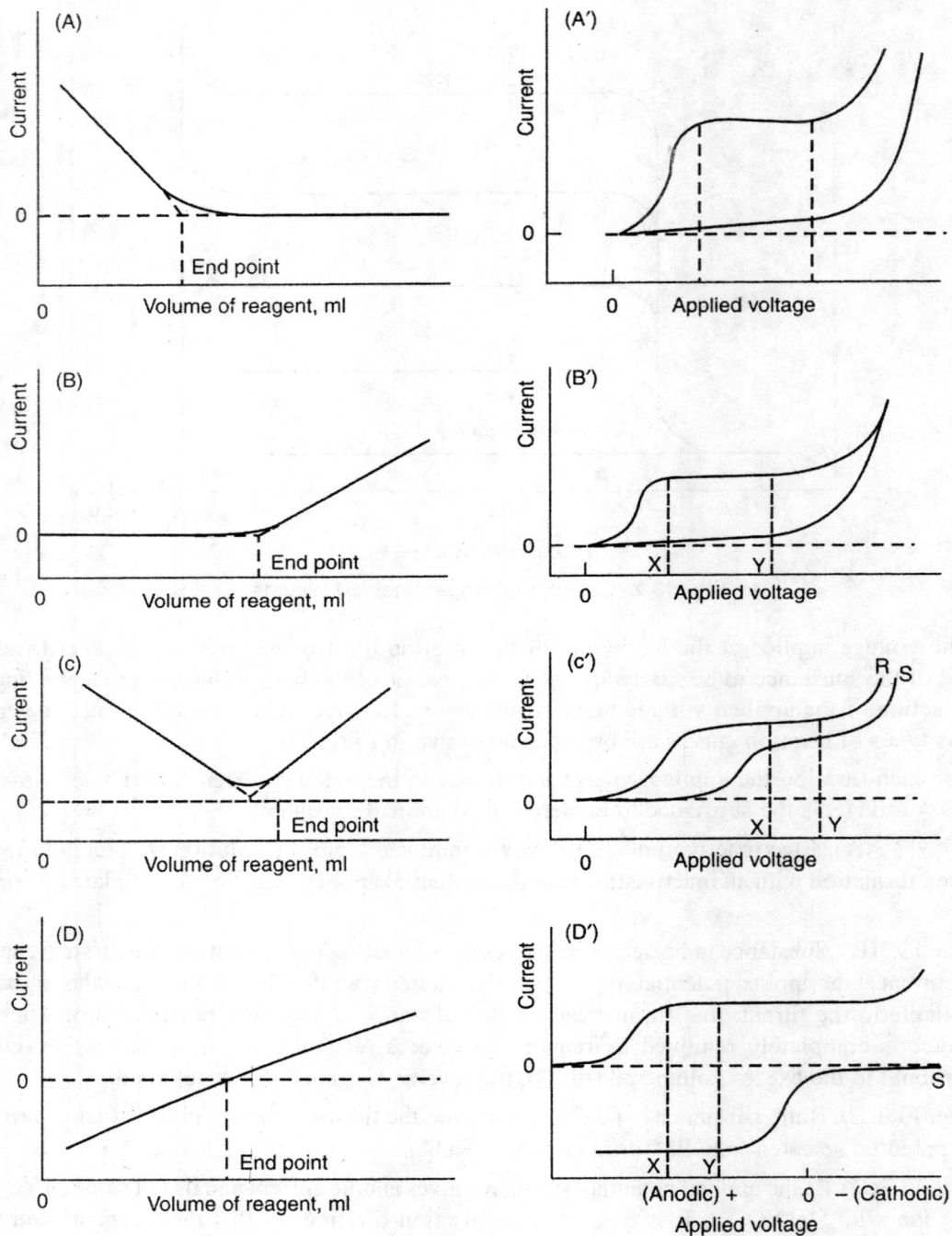

Fig. 13.3. A–D. Common types of curves of amperometric titrations A–D polarograms of individual substances (substance 'S' and reagent 'R').

case, the measured current is just equal to the residual current. This occurs when the electrode itself is oxidized in the anodic half reaction. This is quite possible if the electrode is made of mercury, Al, Ag or some base metal.

Apparatus and Titration Procedure

The titration cell is of Pyrex glass, that is a three necked, flat-bottomed flask. There is a micro burette, dropping mercury electrode, gas outlet tube for N_2 with an additional inlet N_2 provision (Fig. 13.4) in it. The cell is connected to a reference electrode in the form of an attachment with a sintered glass disc separating the titration cell and the RE.

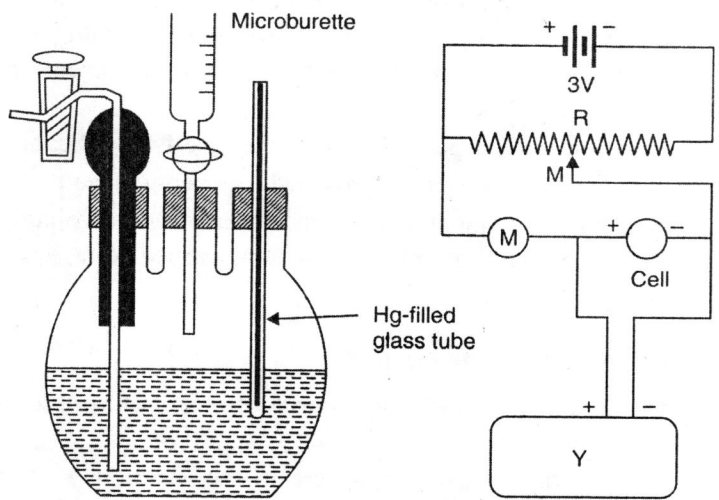

Fig. 13.4. (a) Titration cell, (b) Simple polarograph unit.

The general procedure is as follows:

A known volume of the solution for estimation is placed in the titration cell, required amount of supporting electrolyte is added and the cell is connected to the terminals of the instrument. Dissolved oxygen is expelled by passing pure nitrogen gas for 10–15 minutes and initial current is noted. The known volume of the reagent is added from a microburette, N_2 is passed for 2 minutes and then stopped. The current and burette readings are both noted. This procedure is repeated until sufficient readings are obtained and the graph obtained gives end point at the intersection.

Advantages of Amperometry

1. The titration can usually be carried out rapidly, since the end point is found graphically; a few current measurements at constant applied voltage before and after the end point are sufficient. The chief advantage over other types of titration is the selectivity offered by the electrode potential, as well as by the choice of titrant. For instance, lead ion is reduced at a potential of –0.60 V (relative to the saturated calomel electrode), while zinc ions are not; this allows the determination of lead in the presence of zinc.

2. Titrations can be carried out in cases in which the solubility relations are such that potentiometric or visual indicator methods are unsatisfactory. For example, when the reaction product is markedly soluble (precipitation titration) or appreciably hydrolysed (acid-base titration). This is because the readings near the equivalence point have no special significance in amperometric titrations.

   Readings are recorded in regions where there is excess of titrant, or of reagent, at which points the solubility or hydrolysis is suppressed by the Mass Action effect; the point of intersection of these lines gives the equivalence point.
3. A number of amperometric titrations can be carried out at dilutions (e.g. 10^{-4} M) at which many visual or potentiometric titrations no longer yield accurate results.
4. 'Foreign' salts may frequently be present without interference and are, indeed, usually added as the supporting electrolyte in order to eliminate the migration current which is not possible in case of conductometric titration.
5. The results of the titration are independent of the characteristics of capillary.
6. The temperature used need not be known provided it is kept constant during the titration.
7. Although a polarograph is convenient as a means of applying the voltage to the cell, its use is not essential in amperometric titrations. The constant applied voltage may be obtained with a simple potentiometric device.

Disadvantages of Amperometric Titrations

1. These titrations are subject to the ordinary source of errors of volumetric determinations, such as coprecipitation effects.
2. The foreign substances which do not interfere in the titration, must not be present in concentration many times larger than substances to be titrated. In their presence, the relative changes of the current during the titration become smaller.

Applications of Amperometric Titrations

Some examples of amperometric titrations are illustrated in Table 13.1.

Examples of Amperometric Titration

1. **Determination of Zinc with EDTA solution**
   Reagents required:
   (i) 0.005 M zinc ion solution
   (ii) 0.01 M EDTA solution
   (iii) Cyclohydroxylamine
   The titrant should be lean 10 times strong than the ion taken in the cell.
   Procedure: Place 5.00 ml of zinc ion solution in the titration cell, add 1.0 ml of cyclohexylamine and 19.0 ml of distilled water, set the applied potential at -1.4 V vs SCE corresponding to Zn^{2+}. Deaerate the solution and titrate with standard EDTA solution. Pass

Table 13.1. Examples of amperometric titrations

Titrant	Electrode	Species determined
Complexation reactions		
EDTA	DME	Many metallic ions
Precipitation reactions		
Dimethylglyoxime	DME	Ni_{2+}
Lead nitrate	DME	SO_4^{2-}, MoO_4^{2-}, F^-
Mercury (II) nitrate	DME	I^-
Silver nitrate	Rotating Pt	Cl^-, Br^-, I^-, CN^-, Thiols
Thorium (IV) nitrate	DME	F
Potassium dichromate	DME	Pb, Ba
Oxidation reactions		
Iodine	Rotating Pt	As(III), $Na_2S_2O_3$
Potassium bromate/KBr	Rotating Pt	As(III), Sb(III), N_2H_4
Additions	Rotating Pt	Alkenes
Substitutions	Rotating Pt	Some phenols, aromatic amines

N_2 for 1 minute than take readings of both burette and the galvanometer. Large initial current will be decreased as the titration proceeds to a very small value at the equivalence point and remains constant beyond the equivalence point. Use volume correction and plot the readings. The graph is as shown in the titration curve (Fig. 13.3A).

Factor: Each ml of 0.01 M EDTA solution = 0.0006537 g of Zn.

2. **Determination of SO_4^{2-} with $Pb(NO_3)_2$ solution**

At the potential applied –1.2 V vs SCE only Pb^{2+} is reduced to give diffusion current and is used as a titrant.

Reagents required: 0.01 M K_2SO_4 and 0.1 M lead nitrate solution, ethyl alcohol, conc. HNO_3 and thymol blue indicator solution.

Procedure: Take 25 ml of potassium sulphate into the titration cell, add 2 to 3 drops of thymol blue indicator and few drops of conc. HNO_3 until a red colour is obtained (pH is 1.2). To this, add 25 ml of ethyl alcohol which will reduce the solubility of $PbSO_4$ precipitate formed. The reaction is:

$$K_2SO_4 + Pb(NO_3)_2 \longrightarrow PbSO_4 + 2KNO_3$$

Pass N_2 gas for 15 minutes to remove dissolved O_2 and connect the DME and reference electrode to the respective terminals of the polarograph. Titrate with lead nitrate solution adding in small volumes and pure N_2 for 1 minute after each addition.

Note down readings of burette and galvanometer after stopping the passage of N_2. Draw the graph between volume of lead nitrate added and the current recorded from the galvanometer after making volume correction. A reverse L shaped curve will be obtained (Fig. 13.3 B type) from which the end point is detected. Calculate the amount of SO_4^{2-} present in the given solution.

Factor: Each ml of 0.1 M $Pb(NO_3)_2$ solution = 0.009609 g SO_4^{2-}.

3. **Determination of lead with standard dichromate solution**

   The potential selected is –1.0 V vs SCE at which both lead ion and dichromate ions give diffusion current. So, the graph obtained will be V-shaped (Fig. 13.3C).

   Reagents required: 0.001 M $Pb(NO_3)_2$ AR, 0.005 M potassium dichromate and 0.01 M potassium nitrate.

   Procedure: To 25.0 ml of 0.001 M $Pb(NO_3)_2$ solution in the cell, add 25 ml of 0.01 M potassium nitrate solution as supporting electrolyte and pass N_2 for 15 minutes. Apply –1.0 V vs SCE and make necessary connections on the polarograph. Add 0.005 M dichromate solution from the microburette in 0.5 ml portion and pass N_2 each time for 1 minute. Note down the readings of the burette and the galvanometer. Initially the current due to Pb^{2+} decrease as dichromate added and increases after the end point with excess dichromate. After making volume corrections draw the graph and note down the end point reading. Repeat this with unknown $Pb(NO_3)_2$ given.

Biamperometry or Dead-Stop End Point Method

In amperometry, there is one polarized electrode which may be DME or solid electrode or metallic electrode like platinum and the other reference electrode (non-polarized). Mostly SCE electrode is used as reference electrode. In this, the potential corresponding to the limiting current plateau is fixed and diffusion current is measured as function of reagent volume.

In the biamperometry, a pair of identical metallic or solid microelectrodes/polarized electrodes are used. The instrumental setup (Fig. 13.5) is the same as used in amperometry and only SCE is replaced with platinum electrode in the electrolysis cell and a magnetic stirrer is used. A fixed potential difference of 10–20 mV is applied between the two electrodes through the adjustment of resistance variable potentiometer, R (1000 ohms). In such potential difference, one electrode will function as an anode and the other cathode. The shape of the titration curves depend on the reversibilities of the oxidation-reduction couples at the electrodes of both sample and titrant used.

For example, in titration of iodine with sodium thiosulphate solution, iodide-iodine couple is reversible and titrant thiosulphate-tetrathionate couple is irreversible.

$$I_2 + 2e^- \rightleftharpoons 2I^-$$
$$2S_2O_3^{2-} \longrightarrow S_4O_6^{2-} + 2e^-$$

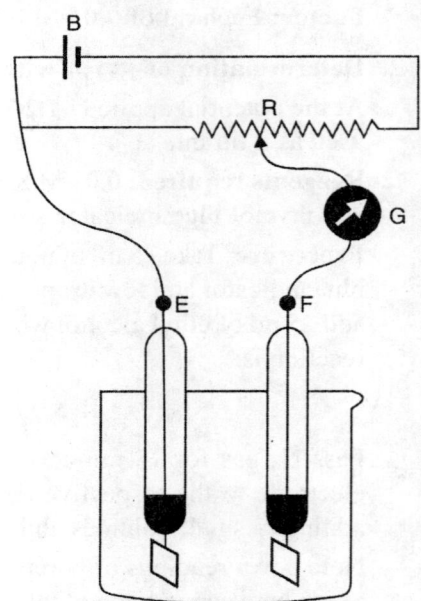

Fig. 13.5. Biamperometry instrument.

Initially, a small amount of electrolysis takes place and an appreciable current flow through the cell. The amount of reduced form oxidized at the anode is equal to that formed by reduction of the oxidized form at cathode. At this stage, both the electrodes are equally depolarized. When iodine in a solution is consumed by thiosulphate, the only one electrode remains depolarized.

Thus after the endpoint, only one electrode is depolarized. Thus **current** will flow until the endpoint has been reached, after **the endpoint, current** will be zero or nearly zero. Due to this **reason, it is called** dead stop endpoint. The titration curve of Fig. 13.6 is obtained where there is decrease in current until dead stop endpoint.

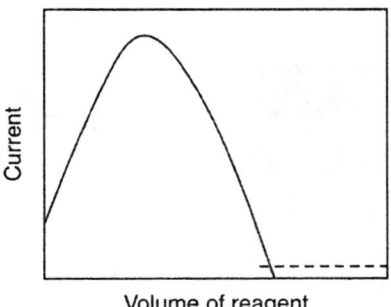

Fig. 13.6. Titration curve of iodine vs sodium thiosulphate.

Another example is titration of ferrous ion with cerric ion where both couples (sample and titrant) involved in titration are reversible.

$$Fe^{2+} \rightleftharpoons Fe^{3+} + 1e^-$$

and Ce(IV) reduced to Ce (III) as:

$$Ce^{4+} + 2e \rightleftharpoons Ce^{3+}$$

In this, at the equivalence point corresponding to complete consumption of ferrous ion before excess ions are added, the current flow is zero or nearly zero. After the endpoint, further addition of cerric ion, current flow is increase to give the V-shaped curve (Fig. 13.7).

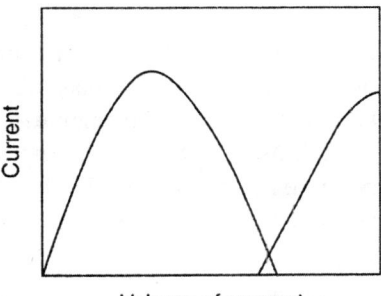

Fig. 13.7. Titration curve of ferrous ions.

CHAPTER 14

Polarimetry

In a ray of natural light, the vibrations are transverse means vibrations take place in plane at a right angles to the direction of propagation but the vibrational directions is constantly changing. In a ray of plane-polarized light (polarized light), the vibrations are also transverse but they take place in only one direction (Fig. 14.1).

Many organic substances e.g. volatile oil, alkaloids and sugars possess the power of rotating the plane of polarized light when it is passed through solution containing them. It can be shown by the following simple experiment. The polarized light is produced by Nicol prism, called *polarizer*. Now if second Nicol prism (analyzer) is placed in the path of emergent light

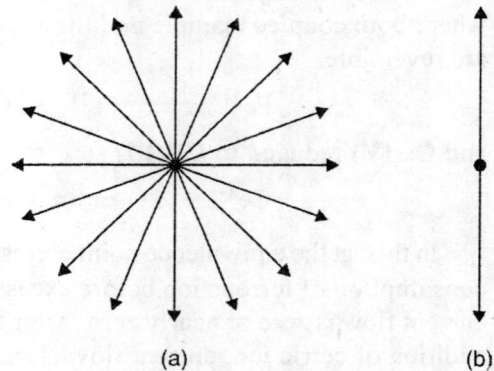

Fig. 14.1. End view of (a) unpolarized light; (b) plane polarized light.

with its axis parallel to that of polarizer, the light remains visible. But if this axis of second prism is at the right angles to that of the first, no light will get through and field will be dark. Now if turpentine oil or cane sugar solution is placed in the path of these two prisms, the fields get lighted and the second prism has to be rotated through a certain angle for extinction of light. These substances that possess a power of rotation are called *optically active* and are designated as dextrorotatory when direction of rotation toward right and as levorotatory when it is toward the left. This phenomenon is due to lack of symmetry in the molecular structure. The measurement of the degree of rotation of the plane of linearly polarized light is called *polarimetry*.

The optical activity of many substances is a function of their chemical constitution as well as of their concentration. Consequently, a determination of the rotatory power or lack of rotatory power of a substance may serve as a tool for identification and determination of purity. In some cases, the measurement of optically activity of a substance may also give some indication of its therapeutic value e.g. the levorotatory alkaloid hyocyamine is much more active as mydriatic than its optically inactive isomer atropine.

The angle of rotation of the polarized light on passage through a optically active substance depend on:

1. Nature of substance: Some substances rotate the light to the right (or clockwise) as viewed looking towards the light source, we sign this rotation, α as + and some of the left (or anticlockwise), signing, α as.
2. Length of the column of substance through which the light passes.
3. In a homogeneous mixtures or solutions, the angle of rotation depends on the concentration of optically active substance.
4. When more than one optically active substance is present in a solution, the resultant rotation will be the same as the sum of the several rotation of each separate constituent in the same volume of solution provided these do not react each other.
5. The angle of rotation also varies with the wavelength of the employed (the shorter the λ, the greater the angle of rotation). The influence of the wavelength of a light source for sugar solutions is seen in the Table 14.1.

Table 14.1. Effect of wavelength on specific rotation

Light source	Wavelength (nm)	Specific rotation $[\alpha]_D^{20}$
Mercury, green	546.23	+ 78.4178
He Ne Laser	632.99	+ 57.2144
Near infrared (NIR)	882.60	+ 28.5462

6. Temperature of sample solution. Temperature dependence of specific rotation is for sugar solutions can be calculated as follows:

$$\alpha(t) = \alpha(20.0°C) [1.0 - 0.000471 (t - 20.0)]$$

The calculation of specific rotation of sucrose solution at different temperatures at same concentration is shown below.

Temperature °C	Rotation of a sucrose solution α [0 angle deg]
20	40.000
21	39.981
25	39.906

There is small decrease of the rotation of sucrose solution with rising temperature.

All above these parameters are combined in the Biot's law which calculates the results in terms of specific rotation. The specific rotation may be defined as angle of rotation of plane of polarized light produced by a liquid, which in a volume of one ml, contain 1 'g' of the active substance when the length of column through which light passes is one decimeter (100 mm). It is calculated by the following general formula.

For liquid substances,

$$[\alpha]_D^{20} = \frac{\alpha}{l \times d}$$

For solutions,

$$[\alpha]_D^t = \frac{100}{lpd} \text{ (or) } [\alpha]_D^t = 100\frac{\alpha}{lc}$$

where
- α = observed rotation in degrees of the liquid at temperature 't' using sodium light, indicated by 'D'.
- l = length of tube in decimeter.
- d = the specific gravity of the liquid or solution at the temperature of observation.
- p = concentration of solution (number of g of active substance in 100 g of a solution.
- c = concentration of solution in g in 100 ml of solutions.

POLARIMETER

The instrument (Fig. 14.2) used to measure the angle of rotation is called 'Polarimeter'. There are following basic components:
(i) Light source
(ii) Polarizer
(iii) Analyzer attached to a disc graduated in degrees
(iv) Sample tube

It may also contain half-shadow device.

Sodium vapour and mercury vapour lamps are the most common sources of monochromatic light for polarimeter. The D-line of the sodium lamp at the visible wavelength of 589 nm is most often employed. Specific rotation determined at the D-line is expressed by the symbol D in the biots law. Use of lower wavelengths, such as those available with the mercury lamp lines isolated by means of filters of maximum transmittance at approximately 578, 546, 436, 405 and 365 nm in a photoelectric polarimeter, have been found to provide advantages in sensitivity with a consequent reduction in the concentration of the test compound. In general, the observed optical rotation at 436 nm is about double and at 365 nm about three times than at 589 nm.

The Polarizer and the analyzer is the Nicol prism. Monochromatic light is plane polarized by Polarizer (stationary). The analyzer can be rotated about the axis of the instrument. A tube containing an optically active liquid is placed in the path of light between two Nicol prisms. A beam of monochromatic light is passed through the sample container in an instrument containing the liquid. The light gets polarised by first Nicol and then falls on second, which is rotated gradually so as to cut out light completely, polarize the lights. This reading corresponds to zero reading. Now, tube containing the optically active liquid is inserted. On looking through Polarimeter, the field will appear bright since polarized light has been rotated. Then analyzer is turned left or right to make the light out. The difference between two reading is the angle of rotation.

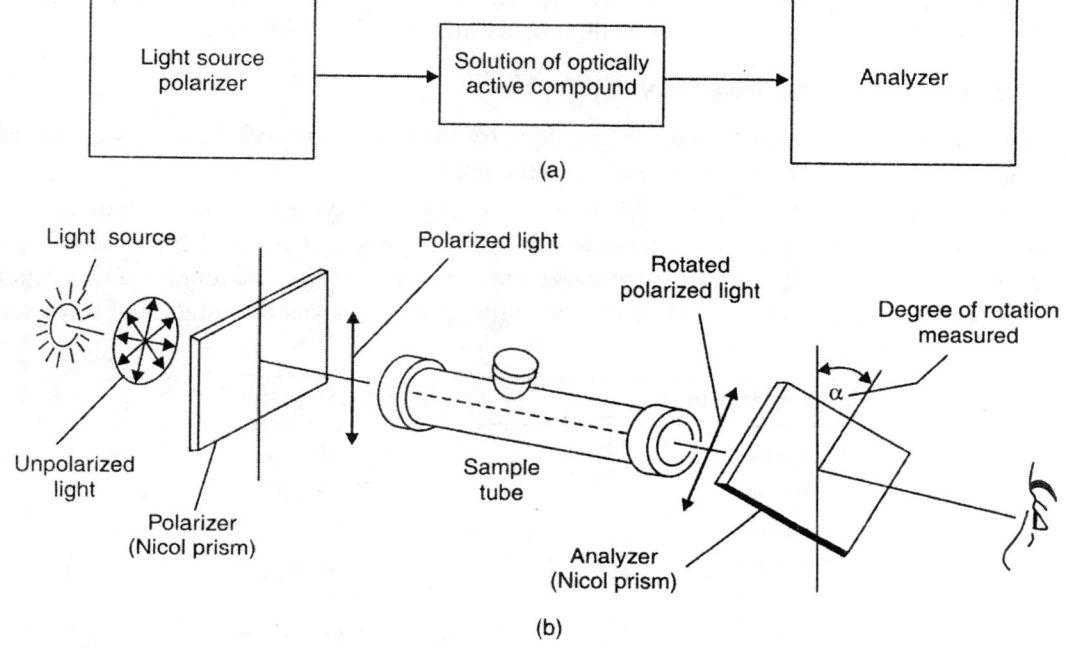

Fig. 14.2. (a) Principle of a polarimeter set up; (b) components of a polarimeter.

Because, it is easier for the human eye to match two adjacent areas to the same degree of brightness in comparison to determine a point of maximum darkness or maximum brightness, so, a third prism (half-shadow prism) is placed behind the Polarizer and rotated through a small angle to divide the field into two halves of unequal brightness. An eyepiece focusses on the field and by rotating the analyzer the two halves may be brought to equal brightness. This field of equal brightness is taken as zero point (Fig. 14.3). When an optically active substance is placed between polarizer and analyzer, one half of the field will appear dark while other will appear light. Rotation of analyzer either in left direction (levorotatory) or right direction (dextrorotatory) returns the two halves to an equal intensity of illumination. The number of degrees through which analyzer is rotated measure the angle of rotation.

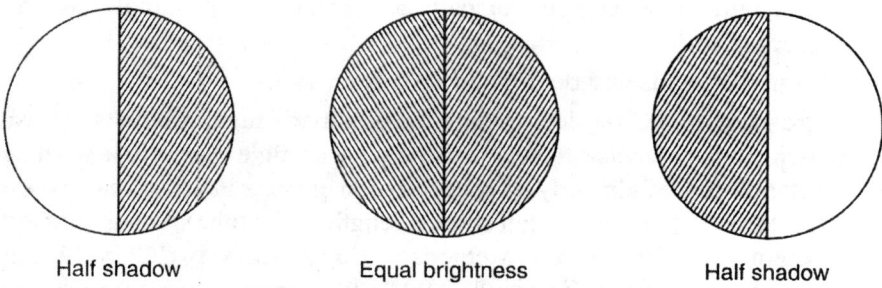

Fig. 14.3. Half shadow prism.

In one complete rotation of the analyzer through 360°, there are two positions on the analyzer 180° apart at which there is maximum of light or darkness in the field view.

APPLICATIONS OF POLARIMETRY

Polarimetry is a sensitive, nondestructive technique for measuring the optical activity exhibited by inorganic and organic compounds. It has following uses:

1. Like melting or boiling point, specific rotation is a physical property of the compound. Hence, it is useful for the qualitative analysis of various drugs. It is used for evaluating and characterizing optically active compounds by measuring their specific rotation and comparing this value with the theoretical values found in literature. This specific rotation of some sugars are given below:

Substance in H_2O	Specific rotation $[\alpha]_D^{20}$
Sucrose	+ 66.54
Glucose	+ 52.74
Fructose	− 93.78
Maltose	+ 137.5
Lactose	+ 55.3
Dextrose	+ 194.9

2. It is useful for determination of purity of various drugs.

Example

The observed specific rotation of a compound is +7.00°. The specific rotation for the pure enantiomer is +28.00°. Calculate the optical purity.

Solution

Optical purity = observed specific rotation/specific rotation of pure enantiomer
= (+ 7.00°/+28.00°) × 100% = 25%

This means that the sample consisted of 75% of the racemic form (= equimolar mixture of the enantiomers, $\alpha = 0°$) and an excess of 25% of the enantiomer in question.

3. Optical activity is helpful in selecting biologically active isomer. For example, only one isomer of chloramphenicol is active.
4. It is also helpful in distinguishing dextro and levo isomers.
5. Polarimetry is frequently used for determining the quality of sugar products. Measurements are made by polarimeters or saccharimeters with the scale in angle degree (0) and sugar degrees (0Z). Angle of rotation depends linearly on concentration of sugar in the solution while keeping some other parameters (temperature, light source, length of the tube). Sugar industry with its International Commission for Uniform Methods of Sugar Analysis (ICUMSA) introduced International Sugar Scale (ISS) in 0Z units. 100.00 0Z units (sugar degrees) belong to Normal

Sucrose Solution prepared from exactly 26 g of sucrose dissolved in pure water to 100 ml. At 20°C andD sodium lamp rotation for this solution in a tube of 200 mm will be a = +34.626°. The ISS is linearly divided, i.e. a rotation of +17.313° (13 g/100 cm^3) equals to a reading of 50.00 0Z. The 0 0Z point in ISS is fixed by the indication given by the saccharimeter for pure water. Normal Sucrose Solution was used to calibrate and standardize polarimetric methods and instruments. Sugar solutions are not very stable and have to be renewed regularly.

Experiment: Quantitative analysis of dextrose solution by polarimetric method

1. Dissolve accurately weighed amount (about 1, 2, 3, 4, 5 and 6 g) of dextrose in water into six 100 ml volumetric flask.
2. Add 0.2 ml of 10% ammonia solution, dilute to 100 ml with water, and allow to stand at room temperature for 30 minutes.
3. Measure the optical rotation of each solution with the help of polarimeter.
4. Make a graph of optical rotation against dextrose concentration.
5. Measure the optical rotation of unknown solution in a similar way.
6. Read the concentration of dextrose from standard curve.

CHAPTER 15

X-ray Absorption, Diffraction and Fluorescence Spectroscopy
(Crystal Tonography)

INTRODUCTION

A variety of X-ray methods are in use. But all methods are mainly classified into three main categories. These are X-ray absorption, X-ray fluorescence and X-ray diffraction methods. We shall discuss these one by one as follows:

(a) X-ray Absorption Methods

These are analogous to absorption methods in the other regions of electromagnetic spectrum. In these methods, a beam of X-rays is allowed to pass through the sample and the attenuation or fraction of X-ray photons absorbed is considered to be a measure of the concentration of the absorbing substance.

X-ray absorption methods are only helpful in certain cases like elemental analysis and thickness measurements. As compared with other X-ray methods, these are undoubtedly the least used.

(b) X-ray Diffraction Methods

These methods are based on the scattering phenomenon of X-rays by crystals. By these methods, one can identify the crystal structures of various solid compounds. These methods are extremely important as compared with X-ray absorption and X-ray fluorescence methods.

(c) X-ray Fluorescence Methods

In these methods, X-rays are generated within the sample and by measuring the wavelength and intensity of the generated X-rays, one can perform qualitative and quantitative analysis. X-ray fluorescence method is non-destructive and frequently requires very little sample preparation before the analysis can be carried out.

Each of the above methods depends upon a different property of the radiation and each has specific applications in analytical chemistry. For example, X-ray absorption is used to detect an imperfection in the internal structure of physical body through which it passes; X-ray diffraction is used to determine crystalline structure. X-ray fluorescence is used for quantitative and qualitative elemental analysis. All three techniques are non-destructive. In many cases the application of X-ray analysis yields information which is unattainable from other instrumental procedures.

GENERALISED THEORETICAL CONCEPTS

1. Origin of X-rays

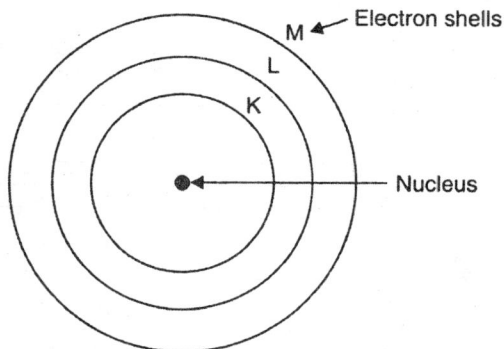

Fig. 15.1. Schematic diagram of the electronic structure of an atom.

The X-ray region lies in the region of about 0.1 to 100Å in electromagnetic spectrum. For analytical purposes, the range of 0.7 to 2.0Å is the most useful region.

The process of production of X-rays may be visualised in terms of Bohr's theory of atomic structure. An atom is composed of nucleus and numerous electrons. The electrons are arranged in layers or shells with the valence electrons in the outer shell. The different shells, are layers of electrons, are called the K shell, L shell, M shell, and so on. For example, a structure of sodium atom contains filled K and L shells and one electron in the M shell. An atom is shown schematically in Fig. 15.1.

Whenever a fast moving electron impinges on an atom, it may knock out an electron completely from one of the inner shells of that atom. Following the loss of inner shell electron one of the outer electrons occupies the vacated orbital, with the simultaneous emission of an X-ray photon. The energy of the emitted X-ray photon is equal to the difference in energy between the two levels involved. For instance, if a K-shell loses its one electron, and it is replaced by the electron from the L-sheli, the resulting X-ray is termed as 'K' X-ray and its energy E_K' is given as follows:

$$E_k' = E_L - E_K$$

where E_L and E_K are the energies of L- and K-shell electrons respectively. These K lines have been further divided in to K_α and K_β depending on whether the electron falling in to the K shell comes from the closest shell or the next nearest shell, i.e., L or M shell.

Similar to above, the L series of X-rays is obtained when an electron in the L shell is ejected and replaced by the electron from the outer shell. Again, L-lines have been further divided into L_α and L_β depending upon whether electron falling into the L orbit comes from the closest shell or the next nearest shell, i.e., M or N shell.

The customary notations used to identify the emitted X-rays are illustrated in Fig. 15.2.

If an electron is dislodged from K shell, it may be replaced by an electron from an L or M shell. The electrons descended from the shell would emit X-rays with a frequency, C.

$$C = \frac{E_L - E_K}{h} \qquad \ldots (15.1)$$

where h is the plank constant.

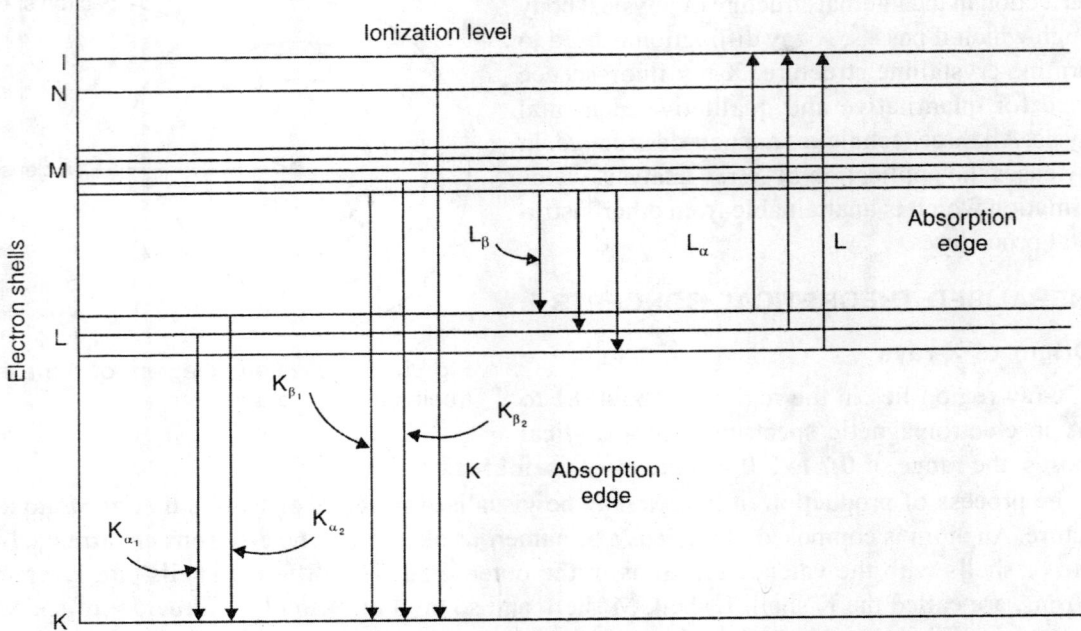

Fig. 15.2. Energy level diagram for a hypothetical atom.

Lines originating from transitions between L and K shells are termed as K lines. The slight difference in the energy levels of the different electrons in the L shell results in the emission lines at slightly different frequencies. These lines are termed as $k_{\alpha 1}$ and $k_{\alpha 2}$. Similarly, electrons descending from the M shell to the L shell would emit X-rays with the frequency, C. This type of transitions causes the emission of L lines x-ray.

$$C = \frac{E_M - E_L}{h} \quad \ldots (15.2)$$

Continuous and Characteristic X-ray Spectra

Generally, the spectrum of X-rays emitted from a given target element may have either a series of sharp and characteristic lines, as discussed above or may have complicated spectrum of X-rays with fairly sharp spectral lines superimposed on the continuum. The difference depends on whether we are using primary X-rays (in the former case) or high-energy electrons (in the latter case) to bombard the target element and eject an inner electron.

In Fig. 15.3, a typical spectrum emitted by a copper target when bombarded by electrons accelerating at 8.9 kV is shown. If instead of electrons, the primary X-rays are used to excite the target material, the spectrum does not contain continuous but will have only the sharp characteristic lines.

The X-ray spectrum of a copper target consists of few sharp and intense lines superimposed on a polychromatic background called "white radiation". The sharp spectral lines comprise the

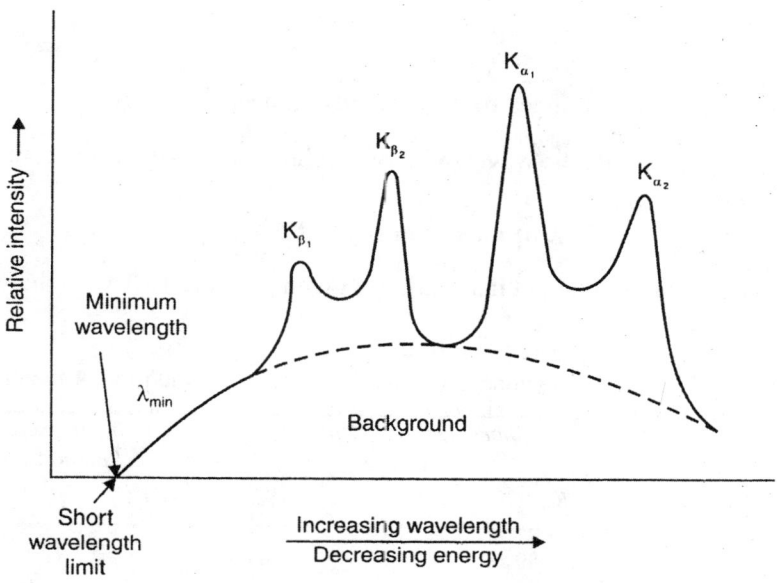

Fig. 15.3. X-ray spectrum of a copper tangent. The intensity of K_β line is about 10 per cent of the K_α doublet.

characteristic radiation of the target material. These lines are produced due to electron transitions which are resulted due to the complete ejection of electrons of the target atom by the incident electron beam. For example, the ejection of a $1s$ electron followed by the transitions $2p \rightarrow 1s$ and $3p \rightarrow 1s$ results in the production of K_α and K_β radiation.

In Fig. 15.3, λ_{min} is called the minimum wavelength. This corresponds to maximum energy of the electrons. λ_{min} is also called cutoff wavelength and is inversely proportional :

$$\lambda_{min} = \frac{hc}{Ve} \qquad \ldots (15.3)$$

to applied voltage (Fig. 15.4); as given by where h is a plank's constant, c is the speed of light in vacuum, e is the charge on electron and V is accelerating voltage applied to the X-ray tube. On substituting the values of h and c in equation (15.3). The cut off wavelength depends upon the accelerating potential but independent of the target material. Thus λ_{min} for the spectrum produced with a molybdenum target at 35 kV is identical to λ_{min} for a tungston target at the same voltage.

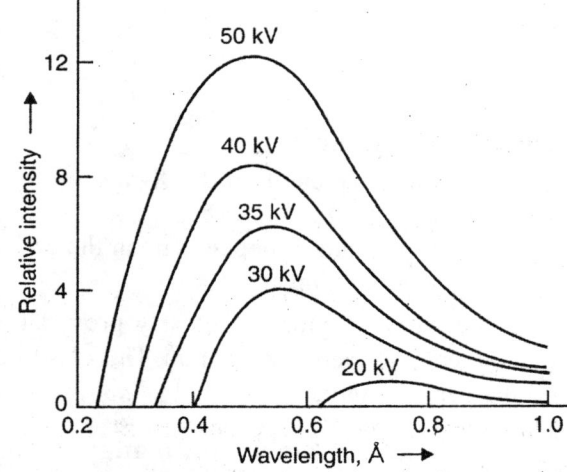

Fig. 15.4. Distribution of continuous radiation from an X-ray tube with tungston target.

$$\lambda_{min} = \frac{12400}{V}$$

where λ_{min} and V have units of angestroms and volts respectively.

With this, one can calculate the wavelength of maximum intensity of the continum by applying the following relation :

$$\lambda \text{ of max intensity} = 1.5 \times \lambda_{min} \qquad \ldots (15.4)$$

Some of the more common target materials are given in Table 15.1 with the wavelength of the characteristic radiation.

Table 15.1. The characteristic radiations of some common target materials

Target material	Characteristic radiation (Angstrom)			Minimum excitation (Potential (kV)
	K_{α_1}	K_{α_2}	K_{β_2}	
Co	1.7889	1.7928	1.6208	7.7
Cr	2.2896	2.2935	2.0848	6.0
Cu	1.5405	1.5443	1.3921	8.9
Fe	1.9360	1.9399	1.7565	7.1
Mo	0.7093	0.7135	0.6325	20.0
Ni	1.6578	1.6618	1.5001	8.3

During the First World War, Henry Moseley, a young scientist working at Cambridge, England, recorded the spectra of the numerous elements. From his work, he enunciated an empirical relation between the atomic number of the element and wavelength of the emitted X-ray lines. This relation is as follows:

$$\frac{C}{\lambda} = a(Z - \sigma)^2$$

where
- C = speed of light,
- λ = the wavelength of the X-ray,
- a = a constant,
- σ = a constant; it depends upon the series of lines (e.g., K_α or K_β or L_α lines)
- z = atomic number

The work of Moseley clearly proved that atomic number, and not atomic weight, is the fundamental property of the atom. This clarified disputes concerning the position of all the elements in the periodic table.

2. Interaction of X-ray with matter

The X-rays can interact with matter in three ways: absorption, scattering, diffraction and fluorescence. We shall now discuss these one by one.

(a) Absorption

If a beam of X-rays is allowed to pass through matter, it loses energy partly by scattering (generally very small part of the total loss) and partly by true absorption. The absorption of X-rays means that the electrons of the atoms constituting the matter absorb energy from these rays and get excited. Then, these excited electrons emit secondary (secondary fluorescent) radiation characteristic of those atoms.

The absorption of X-rays follows the Beer's law which may be written as:

$$I = I_0 \, e^{-\mu l \rho} \qquad (15.5)$$

where
- I_0 = incident intensity of X-rays,
- I = intensity after passing through the absorbing sample,
- l = thickness of material, cm,
- μ = mass absorption coeffecient, cm²/g and
- ρ = the density of the absorbing material, g/c²

The mass absorption coefficient of elements is nearly independent of the physical state of the absorber. However, it decreases rapidly with decreasing wavelength of the X-rays, according to the following relationship of formula:

$$\mu = \frac{CN}{A} Z^4 \lambda^3 \qquad \ldots\, (15.6)$$

where
- C = Proportionality constant,
- N = Avogadro's number,
- A = Atomic weight of absorbing element, and
- λ = wavelength of X-ray radiation.
- Z = atomic number

The equation (15.6) becomes more accurate as Z and λ increases because scattering then becomes less important. However, if mass absorption coefficient plotted against wavelength of X-rays, the curves obtained are not smooth but show a series of discontinuities known as absorption edges, which occur at definite wavelengths for each element. At these wavelength the energy of X-ray beam is sufficient to cause ejection of electrons from the lower atomic orbital (i.e., 1s → transitions) and the mass absorption coefficient therefore rises sharply.

A typical curve of wavelength versus μ is shown in Fig. 15.5. This curve shows the variation of the mass absorption coefficient with wavelength.

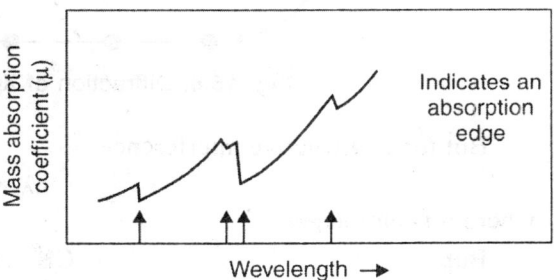

Fig. 15.5. The variation of the mass absorption coefficient with wavelength.

252 Pharmaceutical Analysis

It is important to emphasise that the extent of absorption by a given element depends upon the number of atoms of that element in the path of X-rays but is independent of the physical or chemical state of that element. For example, the amount of absorption by a given number of iodine atoms will remain same whether we take iodine in the form of diatomic gas, a liquid, or a solid or in a compound (NaI, RI or iodobenzene).

(b) Scattering and diffraction

As the phenomenon of scattering forms the basis of diffraction, we will consider them together.

When a beam of X-radiation is incident upon a substance, the electrons constituting the atoms of the substance become as small oscillators. These, start oscillating at the same frequency as that of incident X-radiation, emit electromagnetic radiations in all directions at the same frequency as the incident X-radiation. These scattered waves are coming from electrons which are arranged in a regular manner in a crystal lattice and then travelling in certain directions. If these waves undergo constructive interference, they are said to be diffracted by the crystal plane. Every crystalline substance scatters the X-rays in its own unique diffraction pattern producing a fingerprint of its atomic and molecular structure. The conditions for diffraction are governed by **Bragg's law** and the diffracted beams are often referred to as reflections Constructive interference of the reflected beam emerging from two different planes will take place if the difference in the path length of two rays is equal to whole number of wavelengths. This can be understood from Fig. 15.6. If one X-ray is striking the top crystal plane at A and the other X-ray is striking the second crystal plane at B, the path difference between two parallel X-rays is equal to CB + BD.

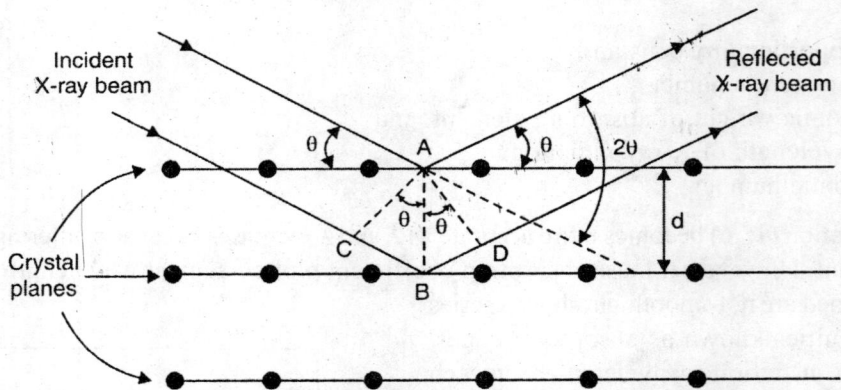

Fig. 15.6. Diffraction of X-ray from a set of crystal planes

But for constructive interference,

$$n\lambda = CB + BD$$

where n is an integer.

But
$$CB = BD = d \sin \theta$$
$$n\lambda = 1 + 1 = 2d \sin \theta \qquad \qquad ...15.7$$

where d is the lattice spacing.

Equation (15.7) is the familiar Bragg's law and is of fundamental importance. The X-rays appear to be reflected only if angle of incidence satisfies the condition that

$$\sin\theta = \frac{n\lambda}{2d}$$

At all the other angles, destructive interference occurs. For Miller's indices, equations (15.7) becomes as X-ray Absorption, Diffraction, and Fluorescence Spectroscopy.

Where θ is the glancing angle of incidence, d_{hkl} is the spacing between the set of crystal planes of Miller's indices $_{hkl}$ and n is an integer.

On putting the integer n equal to 1, 2, 3, etc., a series of angle is obtained at which reflections will occur for a given set of planes off spacing d_{hkl}. These reflections are referred to as first order, second order, third order, etc. respectively.

Bragg's equation (15.7) is obeyed so well that it is possible to use this equation for highly precise determination of the lattice spacing d_{khl}.

Through X-ray diffraction we can identify the crystal structures of various solid compounds and identify a compound from its structure. We can also determine the arrangement of molecules in a crystal. This has enabled us to obtain invaluable information on the structure of such diverse materials as chemical crystals, metals, and living tissue.

(c) Fluorescence

If a sample is irradiated with an X-ray beam, the sample sometimes emits other X-rays beam; this process is called X-ray fluorescence. The wavelength of the X-ray fluorescence enables us to determine what elements are present in a sample. The intensity of the X-rays that are emitted enables us to determine how much is present. It provides us with a method of elemental analysis that is independent of the molecular structure in which the element finds itself. The method is also nondestructive and frequently requires very little sample preparation before the analysis can be carried out.

COMPONENTS OF INSTRUMENTS

Absorption, emission, fluorescence and diffraction of X-rays all find applications in analytical chemistry. Instruments for these applications contain components that are analogous in function to the five components of instruments for optical spectroscopic measurement; these components include a source, a device for restricting the wavelength range of incident radiation, a sample holder, a radiation detector or transducer, and a signal processor and readout. These components differ considerably from their optical counterparts. Their functions, however, are the same.

Like optical instruments, both X-ray photometers and spectrophotometers are encountered, the first using filters and the second using monochromators to restrict radiation from the source. In addition, however, a third method is available for obtaining information about isolated portions of an X-ray spectrum. Here, isolation is achieved electronically with devices that have the power to discriminate between various parts of a spectrum based on the energy rather than the wavelength of the radiation. Thus, X-ray instruments are often described as wavelength dispersive instruments or energy dispersive instruments, depending upon the method by which they resolve spectra.

(i) Sources

Three types of sources are encountered in X-ray instruments: tubes, radioisotopes, and secondary fluorescent sources.

The X-ray tube

The most common source of X-rays for analytical work is the X-ray tube (sometimes called a Coolidge tube), which can take a variety of shapes and forms; one design is shown (Fig. 15.7) schematically. An X-ray source is a highly evacuated tube in which a tungsten filament is mounted as cathode. The anode generally consists of a heavy block of copper with a target metal plated on or imbedded in the surface of the copper. Target materials include such metals as tungsten, chromium, copper, molybdenum, rhodium, scandium, silver, iron, and cobalt. Separate circuits are used to heat the filament and to accelerate the electrons to the target. Electrical current is run through the tungsten filament, causing

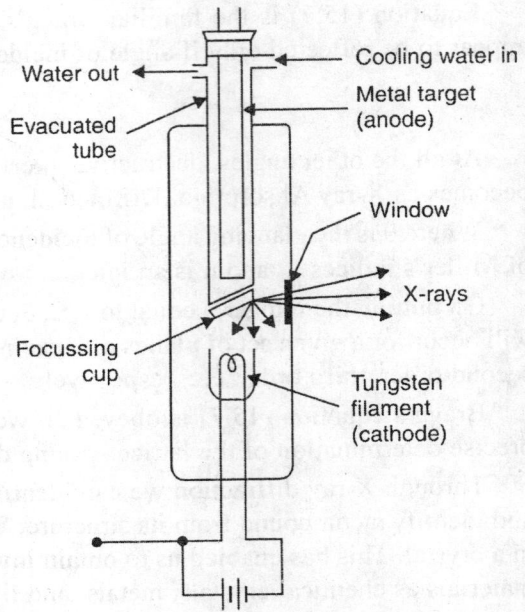

Fig. 15.7. Schematic diagram of an X-ray tube.

it to glow and emit electrons. A large voltage difference is placed in between the cathode and the anode causing the electrons to move at high velocity from the filament to the anode target. Upon striking the atoms in the target, the electron dislodge inner shell electrons resulting in outer shell electrons having jump to lower energy shell to replace the dislodged electrons. These electrons transitions result in the generation of X-rays. The X-ray then move through a window in X-ray tube and used. The heater circuit provides the means for controlling the intensity of the emitted X-rays while the accelerating potential determines their energy, or wavelength. For quantitative work, both circuits must be operated with stabilized power supplies that control the current or the potential to 0.1% relative.

The production of X-rays by electron bombardment is a highly inefficient process. Less than one percent of the electrical power is converted to radiant power, the remainder being dissipated as heat. As a consequence, until relatively recently, water cooling of the anodes of X-ray tubes is required. With modern equipment, however, cooling is often unnecessary because tubes can be operated at significantly lower power than formerly. This reduction in power is made possible by the greater sensitivity of modern X-ray transducers.

Radioisotopes

A variety of radioactive substances have been used as sources in X-ray fluorescence and absorption methods (Table 15.2). Generally, the radioisotope is encapsulated to prevent contamination of the laboratory and shielded to absorb radiation in all but certain directions.

X-ray Absorption, Diffraction and Fluorescence Spectroscopy

Table 15.2. Isotopes useful as source of X-ray

Isotope	Half life	Radiations
^{55}Fe	2.60 years	EC: MnK$_\alpha$, 210.2 pm
^{57}Co	270 days	EC: FeK$_\alpha$, 193.7 pm, FeK$_{\beta 1}$ 175.7 pm
^{66}Co	5.26 years	Gamma: 86.1, 10 M pm
^{141}Am	458 years	EC: NpL$_\alpha$, 88.9 pm, NpL$_\beta$, 69.8 pm, NpL$_\gamma$, 59.7 pm
		Gamma: 20.8, 47.0 pm

The activity of the radioisotopic source decrease with time. After a time equal to half life, the intensity of source is reduced to 50% of its initiatial value. The most common radioactive sources are ^{55}Fe, ^{109}Cd, ^{57}Co, ^{125}I, ^{250}Pb, ^{241}Am. The ^{109}Cd is suited to determine the elements from calcium to zirconium.

Many of the best radioactive sources provide simple line spectra; others produce a continuum. Because of the shape of X-ray absorption curves, a given radioisotope will be suitable for excitation of fluorescence or for absorption studies for a range of elements. For example, a source producing a line in the region between 0.3 and 0.47 Å is suitable for fluorescence or absorption studies involving the K absorption edge for silver. Sensitivity improves and the wavelength of the source line approaches the absorption edge. Iodine-125 with a line at 0.46 Å is ideal for determining silver from this standpoint.

Secondary Fluorescent Sources

In some applications, the fluorescence spectrum of an element that has been excited by radiation from a X-ray tube serves as a source for absorption or fluorescence studies. This arrangement has the advantage of eliminating the continuum emitted by a primary source. For example, an X-ray tube with a tungsten target could be used to excite the K$_\alpha$ and K$_\beta$ lines of molybdenum. The resulting fluorescence spectrum would then be similar to the spectrum a except that the continuum would be absent (Fig. 15.8).

Synchroton

A specialised sources of X-rays which is becoming widely used in research is synchroton radiation which is generated by particle acceleration. Its unique features are brightness many orders of magnitude greater than X-ray tubes wide spectrum, high collimation and linear polarization.

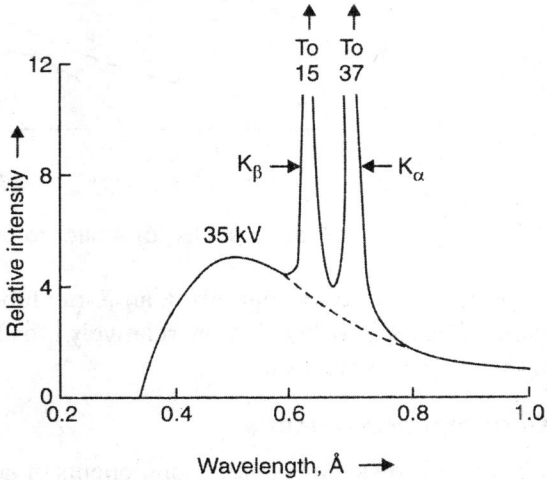

Fig. 15.8. Line spectrum for a tube with a molybdenum target.

(ii) Filters for X-rays

In many applications, it is desirable to employ an X-ray beam that is restricted in its wavelength range. As in the visible region, both filters and monochromators is used for this purpose.

Fig. 15.9 illustrates a common technique for producing a relatively monochromatic beam by use of a filter. Here, the K_β line and most of the continuum emitted from a molybdenum target is removed by a zirconium filter having a thickness of about 0.01 cm. The pure K_α line is then available for analytical purposes. Several other target–filter combinations of this type have been developed, each of which serves to isolate one of the intense lines of a target element. Monochromatic radiation produced in this way is widely used in X-ray diffraction studies. The choice of wavelengths available by this technique is limited by the relatively small number of target-filter combinations that are available.

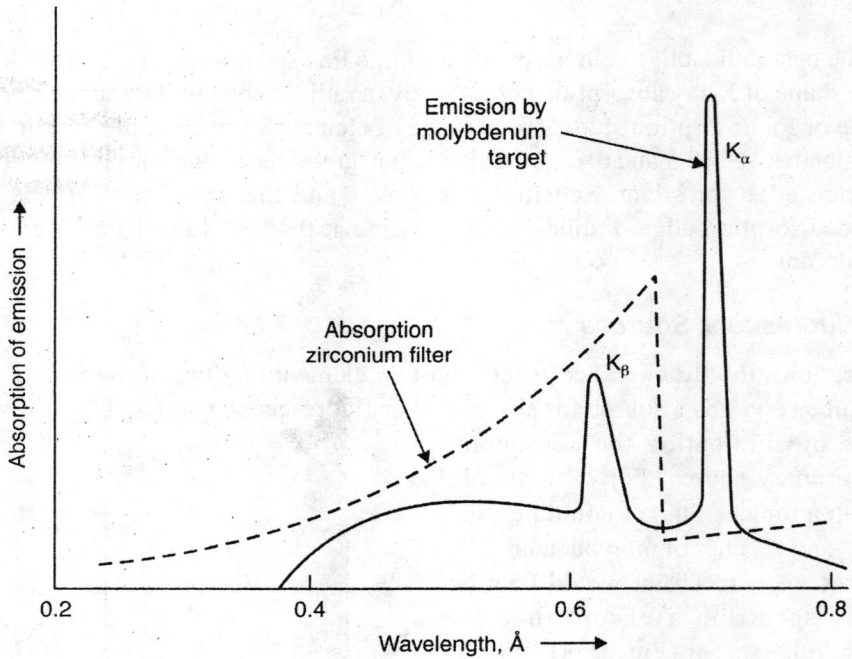

Fig. 15.9. Use of a filter to produce monochromatic radiation.

Filtering the continuum from an X-ray tube is also feasible with thin strips of metal. As with glass filters for visible radiation, relatively broad bands are transmitted with a significant attenuation of the desired wavelengths.

X-ray monochromators

Fig. 15.10 shows the essential components of an X-ray spectrometer. The monochromator consists of a pair of beam collimators, which serves the same purpose as the slits in an optical instrument, and a dispersing element. The later is a single crystal mounted on a goniometer or rotatable table

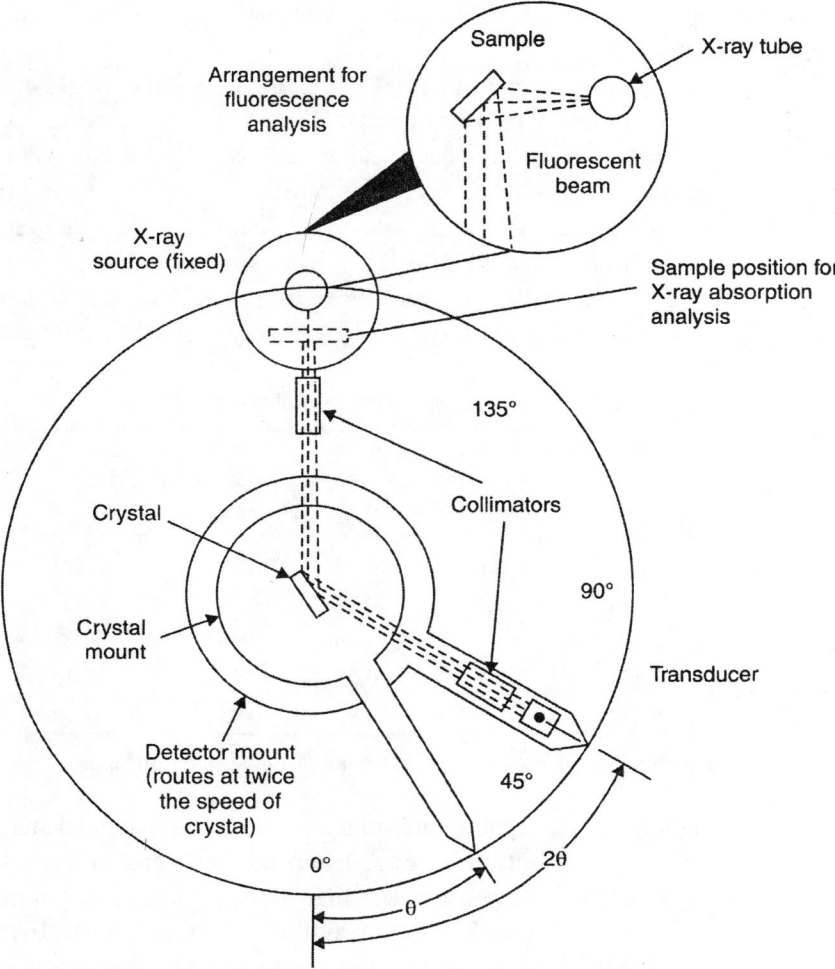

Fig. 15.10. An X-ray monochromator and detector.

that permits variation and precise determination of the angle between the crystal face and the collimated incident beam. From equation 15.7, it is evident that for any given angular setting of the goniometer, only a few wavelengths are diffracted (λ, $\lambda/2$, $\lambda/3$, ..., λ/n where $\lambda = 2d \sin \theta$).

In order to produce a spectrum, it is necessary that the exit beam collimator and the detector be mounted on a second table that rotates at twice the rate of the first; that is, as the crystal rotates through an angle θ, the detector must simultaneously move through an angle 2θ. Clearly, the inter planar spacing d for the crystal must be known precisely (Equation 15.7).

The collimators for X-ray monochromators ordinarily consist of a series of closely spaced metal plates or tubes that absorb all but the parallel beams of radiation.

X-Radiation longer than about 2 Å is absorbed by constituents of the atmosphere. Therefore, provision is usually made for conti-nuous flow of helium through the sample compartment and monochromator when longer wavelengths are required. Alternatively, provisions may be made to evacuate these areas by pumping.

The loss of intensity is high in a monochromator equipped with a flat crystal because as much as 99% of the radiation is sufficiently divergent to be absorbed in the collimators. Increased intensities, by as much as a factor of ten, have been realized by using a curved crystal surface that acts not only to diffract but also to focus the divergent beam from the source on the exit collimator.

As mentioned in Table 15.1, most analytically important X-ray line lie in the region between about 0.1 and 10 Å. A consideration of data in Table 15.3, however, leads to the conclusion that no single crystal satisfactorily disperses radiation over this entire range. As a consequence, an X-ray monochromator must be provided with at least two (and preferably more) interchangeable crystals.

Table 15.3. Properties of typical diffracting crystals

Crystal	Lattice spacing d, Å	Wavelength range^a Å		Dispersion $d\theta/d\lambda$, deg/Å	
		λ_{max}	λ_{min}	at λ_{max}	at λ_{min}
Topaz	1.356	2.67	0.24	2.12	0.32
LiF	2.014	3.97	0.35	1.43	0.25
NaCl	2.820	5.55	0.49	1.02	0.18
EDDT^b	4.404	8.67	0.77	0.65	0.11
ADP^c	5.325	10.50	0.93	0.54	0.09

b = Ethylenediamine-d-tantrate;   c = Ammonium dihydrogen phosphate

The useful wavelength range for a crystal is determined by its lattice spacing d and the problems associated with detection of the radiation when 2θ approaches zero or 180 deg. When a monochromator is set at angles of 2θ that are much less than 10 deg., the amount of polychromatic radiation scattered from the crystal surface becomes prohibitively high. Generally, values of 2θ greater than about 160 deg cannot be measured because the location of the source unit prohibits positioning of the detector at such an angle. The minimum and maximum values for λ_{max} in Table 15.2 were determined from these limitations.

It will be seen from Table 15.3 that a crystal with large lattice spacing, such as ammonium dihydrogen phosphate, has a much greater wavelength range than a crystal in which this variable is small. The advantage of large values of d is offset, however, by the consequent lower dispersion. This effect can be seen by differentiation of Equation 6 of which lead to:

$$\frac{d\theta}{d\lambda} = \frac{n}{2d \cos\theta}$$

Here, $d\theta/d\lambda$ a measure of dispersion, is seen to be inversely proportional to d. Table 15.3 provides dispersion data for the various crystals at their maximum and minimum wavelengths. The low dispersion of ammonium dihydrogen phosphate prohibits its use in the region of short wavelengths; here, a crystal such as topaz or lithium fluoride must be substituted.

(iii) X-ray Transducers and Signal Processors

Early X-ray equipment employed photographic emulsions for detection and measurement of radiation. For reasons of convenience, speed, and accuracy, however, modern instruments are generally equipped with transducers that covert radiant energy into an electrical signal. Three types of transducers encountered are (a) gas-filled transducers, (b) scintillation counters, and (c) semiconductor transducers. Before considering how each of these devices functions, it is worthwhile to discuss photon counting, a signal-processing method that is often used with X-ray transducers as well as detectors of radiation from radioactive sources. As it was mentioned earlier, photon counting is also used in ultraviolet and visible spectroscopy.

Photon Counting

In contrast to the various photoelectric detectors, we have thus far considered, X-ray detectors are usually operated as photon counters. In this mode of operation, individual pulses of charge are produced as quanta of radiation are absorbed by the transducer and are counted; the power of the beam is then recorded digitally as the number of counts per unit of time. Photon counting requires rapid response times for the transducer and signal processor with respect to the rate at which quanta are absorbed by the transducer. In addition, the technique is applicable only in beams of relatively low intensity. As the beam intensity increases, photon pulses begin to overlap and only a steady-state current, which represents an average number of pulses per second, can be measured. If the response time of the transducer is long, pulse overlaps occurs at relatively low photon intensities. As its response time becomes shorter, the transducer is more capable of detecting individual photons without pulse overlap.

For weak sources of radiation, photon counting generally provides more accurate intensity data than are containable by measuring average currents. The improvement can be traced to the fact that signal pulses are generally substantially larger than the pulses arising from background noise in the source, transducer, and associated electronics; separation of the signal from can then be achieved with a pulse-height discriminator, an electronic device that will be further discussed in a later section.

Photon counting is used in X-ray work because the power of available sources is often low. In addition, photon counting permits spectra to be obtained without the noise of a monochromator.

(a) Gas Filled Transducers

When X–radiation passes through an inert gas such as argon, xenon, or krypton, interactions occur that produce a large number of positive gaseous ions and electrons (ion pairs) for each X-ray quantum. Three types of X-ray transducers, namely, ionization chambers, proportional counters, and Geiger tubes, are based upon the enhanced conductivity resulting from this phenomenon.

A typical gas-filled transducer is shown schematically in Fig. 15.11. Radiation enters the chamber through a transparent window of mica, beryllium, aluminum, or Mylar. Each photon of X-radiation may interact with an atom of inert argon gas, causing it to lose one of its outer electrons. This photoelectron has a large kinetic energy, which is equal to the difference between the X-ray photon

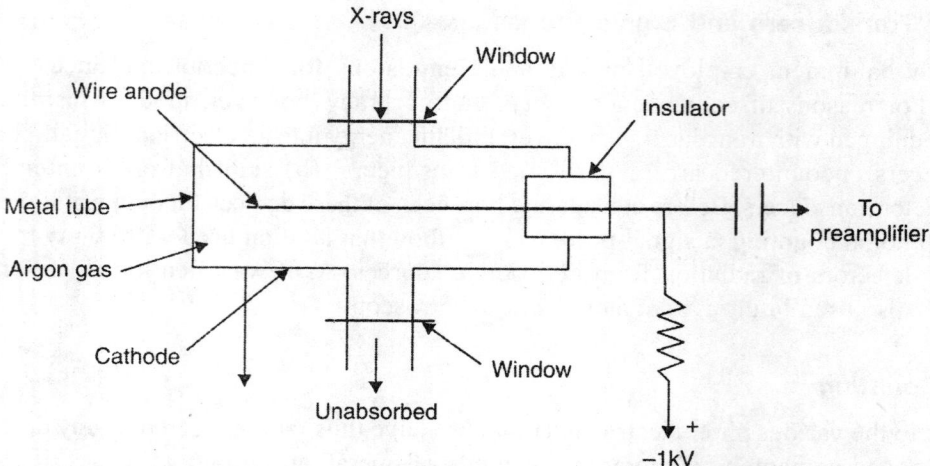

Fig. 15.11. Cross-section of a gas filled detector.

energy and the binding energy of the electron in the argon atom. The photoelectron then loses this excess kinetic energy by ionizing several hundred additional atoms of the gas. Under the influence of an applied potential, the mobile electrons migrate toward the central wire anode while the slower moving cations are attracted toward the cylindrical metal cathode.

Fig. 15.12 shows the effect of applied potential on the number of electrons that reach the anode of a gas-filled transducer for each entering X-ray photon. Three characteristic voltage regions are indicated. At potentials less than V_1, the accelerating force on the ion pairs is low, and the rate at which the positive and negative species separate is insufficient to prevent partial recombination. As a consequence, the number of electrons reaching the anode is smaller than the number produced initially by the incoming radiation.

In the ionization chamber region between V_1 and V_2, the number of electrons reaching the anode is reasonably constant and represents the total number formed by a single photon.

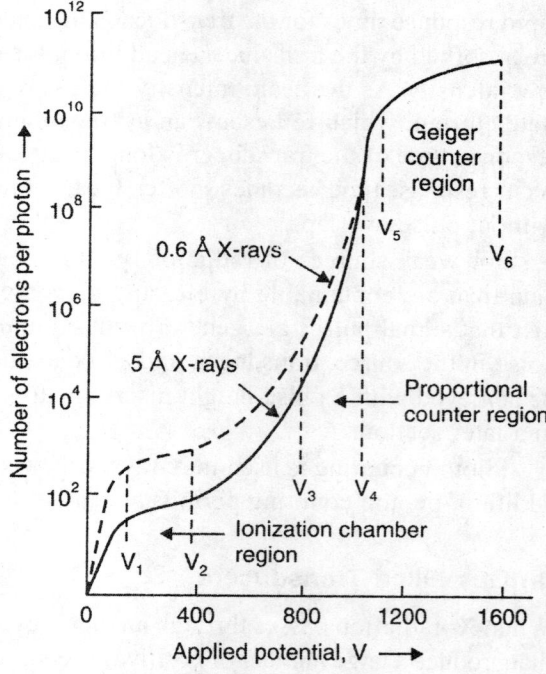

Fig. 15.12. Gas amplification for various types of gas-filled detectors.

In the proportional counter region between V_3 and V_4, the number of electrons increases rapidly with applied potential. This increase is the result of secondary ion-pair production caused by collisions between the accelerated electrons and gas molecules; amplification (gas amplification) of the ion current results.

In the Geiger range V_5 to V_6, amplification of the electrical pulse is enormous but is limited by the positive space charge created as the faster moving electrons migrate away from the slower positive ions. Because of this effect, the number of electron reaching the anode is independent of the type and energy of incoming radiation and is governed instead by the geometry and gas pressure of the tube.

Fig. 15.12 also illustrates that a large number of electrons is produced by the more energetic 0.6 Å radiation than the longer wavelength 5 Å X-rays. Thus, the size of the pulse (the pulse height) is greater for high-frequency X-rays than for low-frequency X-rays.

The Geiger Tube

The Geiger tube is a gas-filled transducer operated in the voltage region between V_5 and V_6 in Fig. 15.12; here, gas amplification is greater than 10^9. Each photon produces an avalanche of electrons and cation; the resulting currents are thus large and relatively easy to detect and measure.

The conduction of electricity through a chamber operated in Geiger region, and in the proportional region as well, is not continuous because the space charge mentioned earlier terminates the flow of electrons to the anode. The net effect is a momentary pulse of current followed by an interval during which the tube does not conduct. Before conduction can again occur, this space charge must be dissipated by migration of the cations to the walls of the chamber. During the dead time, when the tube is nonconducting, response to radiation is impossible; the dead time thus represents a lower limit in the response time of the tube. Typically, the dead time of Geiger tube is in the range from 50 to 200 µs.

Geiger tubes are usually filled with argon; a low concentration of an organic quenching gas often alcohol or methane, is also present to minimize the production of secondary electrons when the cations strike the chamber wall. The lifetime of a tube is limited to some 10^8 to 10^9 counts, by which time the quencher has been depleted with the Geiger tube, radiation is determined by counting the pulses of current. The device is applicable to all types of nuclear and X-radiation. However, it lacks the large counting range of other detectors because of its relatively long dead time; its use in X-ray spectrometers is limited by this factor. Although quantitative applications of Geiger tube transducers have decreased, transducers of this type are still frequently encountered whenever portability is important.

Proportional Counters

The proportional counter is a gas-filled transducer that is operated in the V_3 to V_4 voltage region in Fig. 15.12. Here, the pulse produced by a photon is amplified by ions produced in small enough so that the dead time is only about 1 µs. In general, the pulses from a proportional counter tube must be amplified before being counted.

The number of electrons per pulse, which is proportional to the pulse height, produced in the proportional region depends directly upon the energy, and thus the frequency, of the incoming radiation. A proportional counter can be made sensitive to restricted range of X-ray frequencies with a pulse-height analyzer, which counts a pulse only if its amplitude falls within certain limits.

A pulse-height analyzer in effect permits electronic sorting of radiation; its function is analogous to that of a monochromator.

Proportional counters have been widely used as detectors in X-ray spectrometers.

Ionization Chambers

Ionization chambers are operated in the voltage range from V_1 to V_2 in Fig. 15.12. Here, the currents are small (10^{-13} to 10^{-16} Å typically) and relatively independent of applied voltage. Ionization chambers are not employed in X-ray spectrometry because of their lack of sensitivity. They do, however, find application in radiochemical measurements.

(b) Scintillation Counters

The luminescence produced when radiation strikes a phosphor represents one of the oldest methods of defecting radioactivity and X-rays, and one of the newest as well. In its earliest application, the technique involved the manual counting of flashes that resulted when individual photons or radiochemical particles struck a zinc sulfide screen. The tedium of counting individual flashes by eye led Geiger to develop gas-filled transducers, which were not only more convenient and reliable but more responsive to radiation. The advent of the photomultiplier tube and better phosphors, however, has reversed this trend, and scintillation counting has again become one of the important methods for radiation detection.

The most widely used modern scintillation detector consists of two parts, the phosphor (scintillator) and the photomultiplier (Fig. 15.13). The phosphor is typically a transparent crystal of **sodium iodide that has been activated by the introduction of 0.2% thallium iodide.** Often, the crystal is shaped as a cylinder that is 3 to 4 inch in each dimension; one of the plane surfaces faces the cathode of a photomultiplier tube. As the incoming radiation traverses the crystal, its energy is first lost to the scintillator; this energy is subsequently released in the form of photons of fluorescence radiation. Several thousand photons with a wavelength of about 400 nm are produced

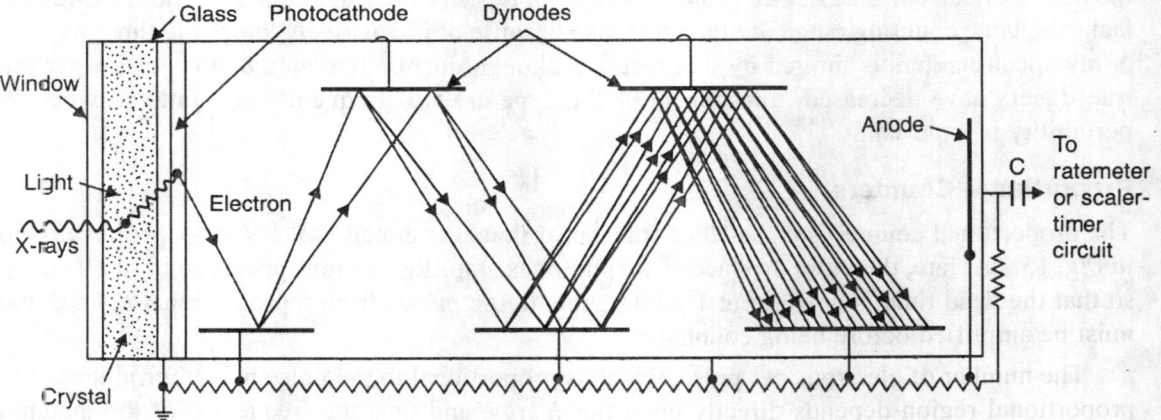

Fig. 15.13. Schematics of a scintillator detector.

by each primary particle of photon over a period of about 0.25 µs which is the dead time. The dead time of a scintillation counter is thus significantly smaller than the dead time of a gas-filled detector.

The flashes of light produced in the scintillator crystal are transmitted to the photocathode of a photomultiplier tube and are in turn converted to electrical pulses that can be amplified and counted. An important characteristic of scintillators is that the number of photons produced in each flash is proportional to the energy pulse-height analyzer to monitor the output of a scintillation counter forms the basis of energy dispersive photometers, to be discussed later.

In addition to sodium iodide crystals, a number of organic scintillators such as **stilbene, anthracene,** and **terphenyl** have been used. In crystalline form, these compounds have decay times of 0.01 and 0.1 µs. Organic liquid scintillators have also been developed and are used to advantage because they exhibit less self-absorption of radiation than do solids. An example of a liquid scintillator is a solution of p-terphenyl in toluene.

(c) Semiconductor Transducers

Semiconductor transducers have assumed major importance as detectors of X-radiations. These devices are sometimes called lithium-drifted silicon detectors, Si(Li), or lithium-drifted germanium detectors, Ge(Li).

Fig. 15.14 illustrates one form of a lithium drifted detector, which is fashioned from a wafer of crystalline silicon. Three layers exist in the crystal, a p-type semi conducting layer that faces the X-ray source, a central intrinsic zone, and an n-type layer. The outer surface of the p-type layer is coated with a thin layer of gold for electrical contact, often; it is also covered with a thin beryllium window that is transparent to X-rays. The signal output is taken from an aluminum layer that coats the n-type silicon; this output is fed into a preamplifier with an amplification factor of about 10. The preamplifier is frequently a field-effect transistor that is made an integral part of the detector.

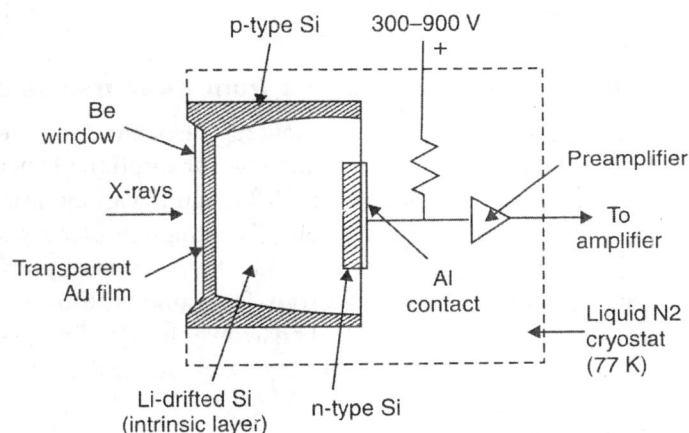

Fig. 15.14. Vertical cross section of a lithium-drifted silicon detector for X-rays and radiation from radioactive sources.

A lithium-drifted detector is formed by vapor-depositing lithium on the surface of a p-doped silicon crystal. Upon heating to 4000 to 5000°C, the lithium diffuses into the crystal; because this element easily loses electrons, its presence converts the p-type region to an n-type region. While still at an elevated temperature, a *dc* potential is applied across the crystal to cause withdrawal of the electrons from the lithium ions replace the holes lost by conduction. Upon cooling, this central layer has a high resistance relative to the other layers because the lithium ions in this medium are less mobile than the hole they displaced.

The intrinsic layer of a silicon detector functions in a way that is analogous to argon in the gas-filled transducer. Initially, absorption of a photon results in formation of a highly energetic photoelectron, which then loses its kinetic energy by elevating several thousand electrons in the silicon to the conduction band; a marked **increase in conductivity** results. When a potential is applied across the crystal, a current pulse accompanies the absorption of each photon. In common with a proportional detector, the size of the pulse is directly proportional to the energy of the absorbed photons. In contrast to the proportional detector, however, secondary amplification of the pulse does not occur.

As shown in Fig. 15.14 the detector and preamplifier of a lithium-drifted detector must be thermo stated at the temperature of liquid nitrogen (77 K) to decrease electronic noise to a tolerable level. The original Si(Li) detectors had to be cooled at all times because at room temperature the lithium atoms would diffuse throughout the silicon thereby degrading the performance of the detector. Modern Si(Li) detectors need to be cooled only during use.

Germanium is used in place of silicon to give lithium-drifted detectors that are particularly useful for detection of radiation that is shorter in wavelength this 0.3 A. These detectors must be cooled at all times. Germanium detectors that do not require lithium drifting have been produced from very pure germanium. These detectors, which are called intrinsic germanium detectors, need to be cooled only during use.

Distribution of Pulse-Heights from X-ray transducers

To understand the properties of energy dispersive spectrometers, it is important to appreciate that the size of current pulses resulting from absorption of successive X-ray photons of identical energy by the transducer will not be exactly the same. Variations arise because the ejection of photoelectrons and their subsequent generation of conduction electrons are random processes governed by the laws of probability. Thus, a Gaussian distribution of pulse heights around a mean is observed. The breadth of this distribution varies from one type of transducer to another, with semiconductor detectors providing significantly narrower bands of pulses. It is this property that has made lithium-drifted detectors so important for energy dispersive X-ray spectroscopy.

Signal Processors

The signal from the preamplifier of an X-ray spectrometer is fed into a liner fast response amplifier whose gain can be varied by a factor up to 10,000. The result is voltage pulses as large as 10 V.

Pulse-Height Selectors

All modern X-ray spectrometer (wavelength dispersive as well as energy dispersive) are equipped with discriminators that reject pulses of about 0.5 V or less (after amplification). In this way, transducer and amplifier noise is reduced significantly. In lieu of a discriminator, many instruments are equipped with pulse-height selectors, which are electronic circuits that reject not only pulses with heights below some predetermined minimum level but also those above a preset maximum level; that is, they remove all pulses except those that lie within a limited channel or window of

X-ray Absorption, Diffraction and Fluorescence Spectroscopy

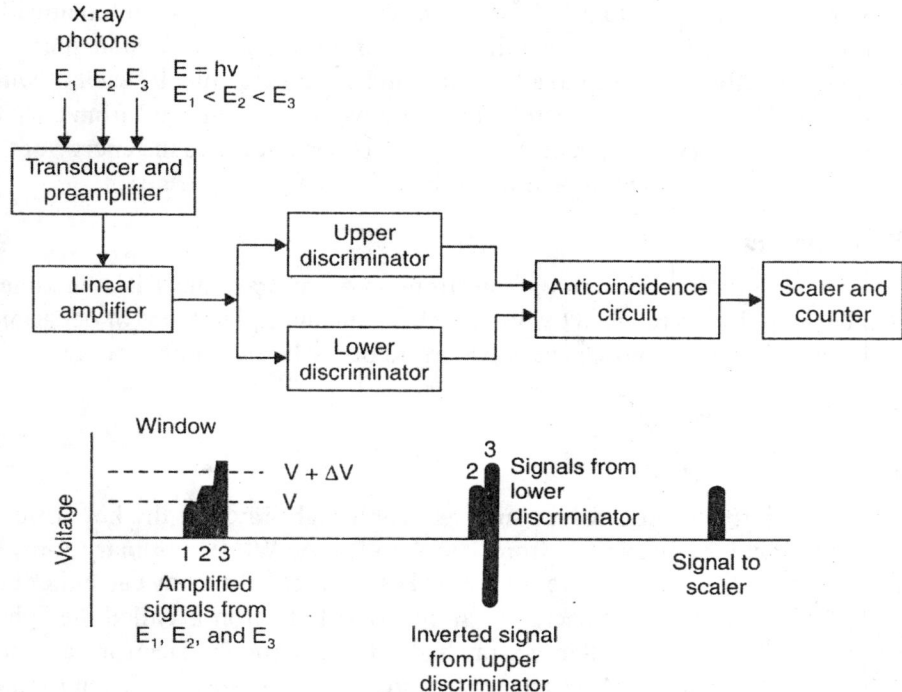

Fig. 15.15. Schematic of a signal height selector. The lower discriminator rejects pulses below V only; the upper discrimintor rejects pulses V + ΔV reaches the counter and inverts the remaining pulse. Lower plot shows the transmitted pulse at the output of anticoincidence circuit that is counted in this illustration.

pulse heights. Fig. 15.15 provides a schematic of a pulse-height sector and its method of operation. Here, the output pulses from the detector and preamplifiers are further amplified and appear as voltage signals (in the 10 voltage) as shown in the lower part of the figure. These signals are then fed into two discriminator circuits each of which can be set to reject any signal below a certain voltage. As shown in the lower part of Fig. 15.15, the lower discriminator rejects signal 1, which is smaller than V, but transmits signals 2 and 3. The upper discriminator, on the other hand, is set to V + ΔV and thus reacts all but signal 3. In addition, the lower circuit is so arranged that its output signal is reversed in polarity and pus cancels out signal 3 from the upper circuit in the anticoincidence circuit. As a consequence, only signal 2, with a voltage in the range V to V + ΔV reaches the counter.

Dispersive instruments are often equipped with pulse-height, selectors to reject noise and to supplement the monochromator in separating the analyte line from higher order, more energetic radiation that is diffracted at the same crystal setting.

Pulse-Height Analyzers

Pulse-height analyzers consist of one or more pulse-height selectors that are configured in such a way as to provide energy spectra. A single-channel analyzer typically has a voltage range of perhaps

10 V or more with a window of 0.1 to 0.5 V. The window can be manually or automatically adjusted to scan the entire voltage range, thus providing data for an energy dispersion spectrum. Multi-channel analyzers typically contain up to a few thousand separate channels, each of which acts as a single channel that corresponds to a different voltage window. The signal from each channel is then accumulated in a memory location of the analyzer corresponding to the energy of the channel thus permitting simultaneous counting and recording of an entire spectrum.

Scalers and Counters

To obtain convenient counting rates, the output from an X-ray transducer is sometimes scaled – that is, the number of pulses is reduced by dividing by some multiple of ten (of occasionally two). Counting of the scaled pulses is now generally carried out with electronic counters.

X-ray Fluorescence methods

(i) Principle

X-ray is a type of electromagnetic waves such as visible light ray, but the key difference is its extremely short wavelength, measuring from 100 A to 0.1 A. When a primary x-ray excitation source from an x-ray tube or a radioactive source strikes a sample, the x-ray can either be absorbed by the atom of transferring all of its energy to an innermost electron is called the "photoelectric effect". During this process, if the primary x-ray had sufficient energy, electrons are ejected from the inner shells, creating vacancies. These vacancies present an unstable condition for the atom. As the atom returns to its stable condition, electrons from the outer shells are transferred to the inner shells and in the process give off a characteristic x-ray whose energy is the difference between the two binding energies of the corresponding shells. Because each element has a unique set of energy levels, each element produces x-rays at a unique set of energies, allowing one to non-destructively measure the elemental composition of a sample. The process of emissions of characteristix x-rays is called "X-ray Fluorescence", or XRF. Analysis using x-ray fluorescence is called "X-ray Fluorescence Spectroscopy." In most cases the innermost K and L shells are involved in XRF detection. A typical X-ray spectrum from an irradiated sample will display multiple peaks of different intensities (Fig. 15.16).

The characteristic x-rays are labeled as K, L, M or N to denote the shells they originated from. Another designation alpha (α), beta (β) or gamma (γ) is made to mark the x-rays that originated from the transitions of electrons from higher shells. Hence, a Kα x-ray is produced from a transition of an electron from the L to the K shell, and a Kβ x-ray is produced from a transition of an electron from the M to a K shell, etc. Since within the shells there are multiple orbits of higher and lower binding energy electrons, a further designation is made as $\alpha 1$, $\alpha 2$ or $\beta 1$, $\beta 2$ etc. to denote transitions of electrons from these orbits into the same lower shell.

The XRF method is widely used to measure the elemental composition of materials. Since this method is fast and non-destructive to the sample, it is the method of choice for field applications and industrial production for control of materials. Depending on the application, XRF can be produced by using not only X-rays but also other primary excitation sources like alpha particles, protons or high energy electron beams.

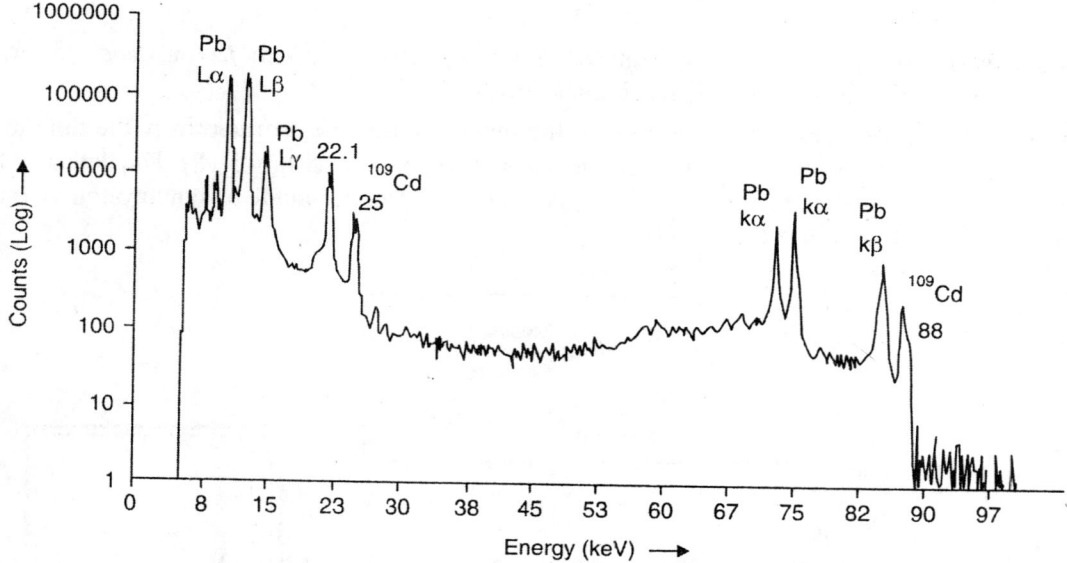

Fig. 15.16. X-ray fluorescence of lead from ^{109}Cd.

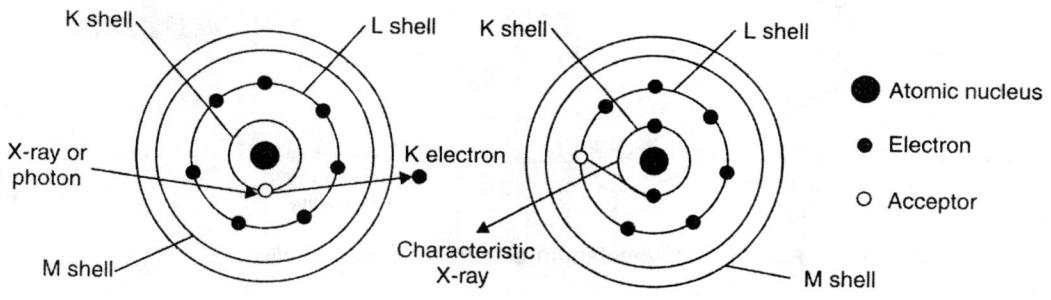

Fig. 15.17. X-ray generation.

Sometimes, as the atom returns to its stable condition, instead of emitting a characteristic x-ray it transfers the excitation energy directly to one of the outer electrons, causing it to be ejected from the atom. The ejected electron is called an "Auger" electron. This process is a competing process to XRF. Auger electrons are more probable in the low Z elements than in the high Z elements.

(ii) Instrumentation

The basic concept for all XRF spectrometers is similar to other X-ray technique. Basically it consists of a source, a device for restricting the wavelength range of incident radiation, a sample holder, and a detection system. The source irradiates the sample and a detector measures the fluorescence radiation emitted from the sample. In most cases for XRF, the source is an **X-ray tube**. Alternatives are a **radioactive source** or a **synchroton**.

(iii) Types of Instruments

There are two main types of XRF instruments: *Energy Dispersive X-ray fluorescence (EDXRF)* and *Wavelength Dispersive X-ray Fluorescence (WDXRF)*.

In **wavelength dispersive spectrometers**, the several X-ray lines emitted from the sample are dispersed spatially by crystal diffraction on the basis of wavelength (Fig. 15.18). The detector then receives only one wavelength at a time. The crystal and detector are made to synchronously rotate through angles of θ and 2θ respectively.

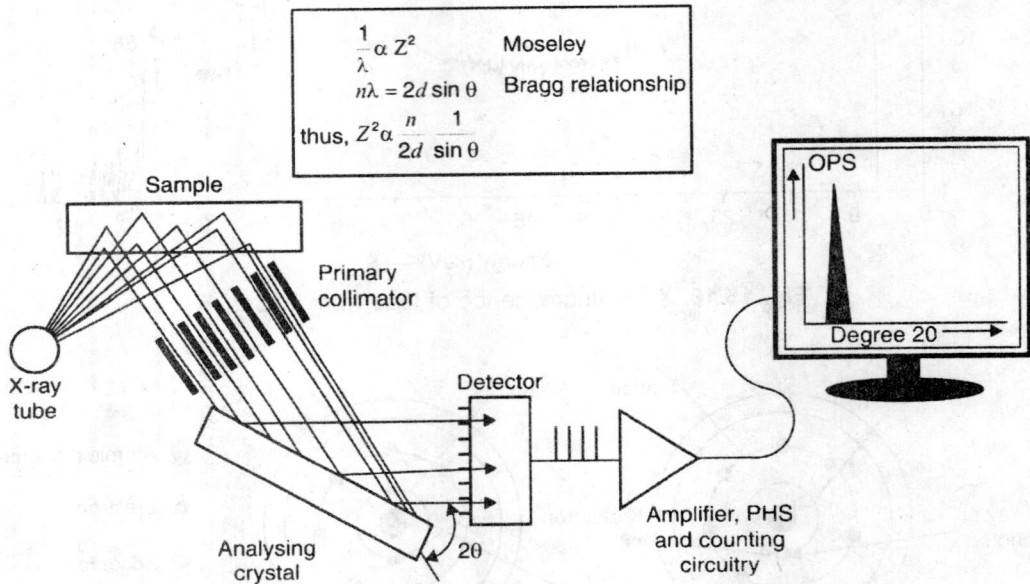

Fig. 15.18. Wavelength dispersive spectrometer.

Wavelength dispersive X-ray spectrometers function by separating the X-rays of interest using diffraction from a crystal. This follows the Bragg equation (discussed earlier);

$$n\lambda = 2d \sin \theta$$

where n is the diffraction order, d is the interplanar spacing of the atomic layer and θ is the angle of incidence.

Crystals used in WDXRF

Crystal	Primary range	Crystal	Primary range
LiF	0.025–0.272	Si	0.055–0.598
Pentaerythritol	0.076–0.834 nm	$CaSO_4.2H_2O$	0.132–1.45 nm
KAP*	0.232–2.54 nm	Lead stearate	6–15 nm

* Potassium hydrogen phthalate

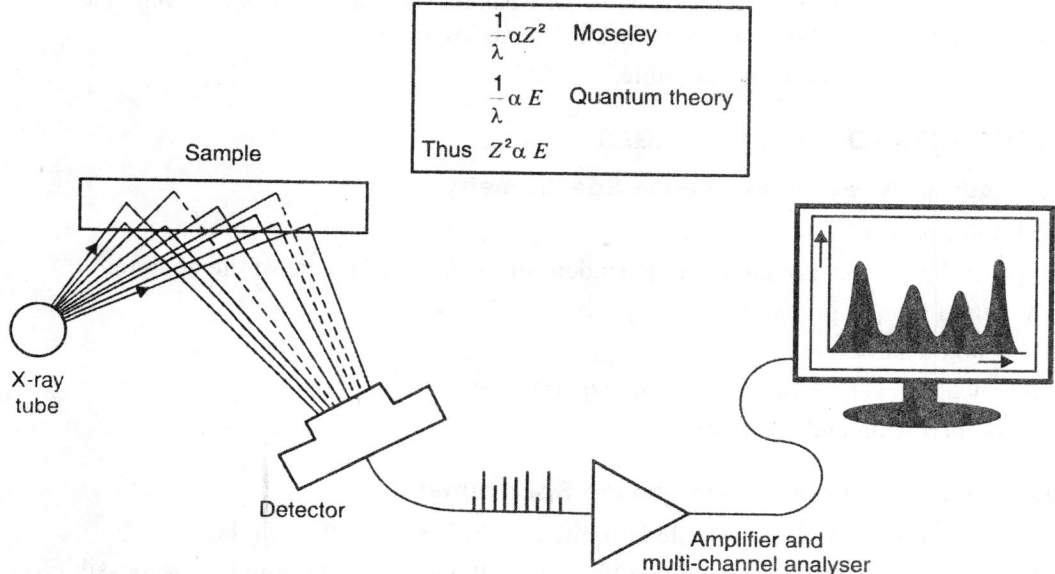

Fig. 15.19. Energy dispersive spectrometer.

On the other hand, the detector in EDX has a superior energy resolution and requires no dispersion system, which enables downsizing of the device. It is based on the detector system's capability to determine the energy of the photons (Fig. 15.19). The primary X-ray beam excites several spectral lines from the sample. In energy dispersive XRF all wavelengths enter the detector at once. The detector registers an electric current having a height proportional to the photon energy. These pulses are then separated electronically, using a pulse analyzer.

COMPARISON OF WAVELENGTH AND ENERGY DISPERSION SPECTROMETERS

Advantages of Energy Dispersion

- Simplicity of instrumentation - no moving parts.
- Simultaneously accumulation of the entire X-ray spectrum.
- Qualitative analysis can be performed in 30s, or so.
- A range of alternative excitation sources can be used in place of high-power X-ray tubes with their large, heavy, expensive and power-consuming supplies. Alternative sources include, low power x-ray tubes, secondary monochromatic radiators, radioisotopes and ion beams.

Advantages of Wavelength Dispersion

- Resolution is better at wavelengths longer than 0.08 nm.
- Higher individual intensities can be measured because only a small portion of the spectrum is admitted to the detector.

- With multichannel analysers sensitivity for weak lines in the presence of strong lines is limited because the strongest line determines the counting time.
- Lower detection limits are possible.

ADVANTAGES AND DISADVANTAGES

Advantages of X-ray Fluorescence Spectrometry

- Simple spectra.
- Spectral positions are almost independent of the chemical state of the analyte.
- Minimal sample preparation.
- It is non destructive.
- Applicable over a wide range of concentrations.
- Good precision and accuracy.

Disadvantages of X-Ray Fluorescence Spectrometry

- X-ray penetration of the sample is limited to the top 0.01–0.1 mm layer.
- Light elements (below ^{22}Ti) have very limited sensitivity although C is possible on new instruments.
- Inter element (MATRIX) effects may be substantial and require computer correction.
- Limits of detection are only modest.
- Instrumentation is fairly expensive.

Sample preparation

Reproducible sample preparation methods are essential. Samples must be in a form that are similar to available standards in terms of matrix, density and particle size.

- *Solids*, generally solids must be polished as surface roughness may give erratic results.
- *Powders and pellets*, powdered samples are often pressed into pellets, suspensions may also be analysed.
- *Fusions*, with potassium pyrophosphate ($K_2P_2O_7$) or a tetraborate ($Na_2B_4O_7$ or $Li_2B_4O_7$) present a homogenised sample which can often be analysed directly.
- *Liquids and solutions*, an X-ray transparent cover and sample cup must be provided to prevent volatility under vacuum conditions.
- *Support media*, such as filter paper, millipore filters, ion-exchange membranes.

MATRIX EFFECTS

Types of Matrix Effects

In XRF absorption-enhancement effects arise from the following phenomena:

1. The matrix absorbs primary X-rays (*primary-absorption effect*); it may have a larger or smaller absorption coefficient than the analyte for primary source x-rays.

2. The matrix absorbs the secondary analyte X-rays (*secondary-absorption effect*); it may have a larger or smaller absorption coefficient for the analyte line radiation.
3. The matrix elements emit their own characteristic lines, which may lie on the short wavelength side of the analyte absorption edge, thereby exciting the analyte to emit additional radiation to that excited by the primary source of X-rays alone (*enhancement*).

Absorption-Enhancement Effects

Absorption-enhancement effects can be *positive* or *negative* on the basis of their effect upon analyte intensity.

In the *positive absorption effect*, the matrix has a smaller absorption coefficient than the analyte for the primary and analyte line radiation, and the analyte-line radiation is higher than would be predicted.

In the *negative absorption effect*, the matrix has a larger absorption coefficient than the analyte for the primary and analyte line emission). This enhancement may take two forms: *direct enhancement* (λ_B and λ_C both excite λ_A) and the *third element enhancement* (λ_C excites λ_B which in turn excites λ_A).

Applications of X-ray Fluorescence Spectrometry

X-ray fluorescence spectrometry is a non destructive analytical technique, used to identify and determine the concentrations of elements present in solid, powdered and liquid samples. XRF is capable of measuring elements from beryllium (Be) to uranium (U) and beyond at trace levels often below one part per million and up to 100%.

Qualitative Analysis

In XRF, the sample is placed in a beam of high energy photons produced by an X-ray tube. Some of the inner-shell electrons of the sample's constituent elements absorb enough energy to be ejected from the atom. Outer-shell electrons fill the vacancies left and emit excess energies as fluorescent x-rays. With the help of characteristic peaks, identification of the elements (Fig. 15.15) can be done.

Quantitative Analysis

Following methods are adopted for quantitative analysis:
1. *Calibration-standard methods*: The analyte-line intensity from samples is compared with that from standards having the same form as the samples and, nearly as possible, the same matrix to know the concentration of particular element.
2. *Internal standardisation*: The calibration standard method is improved by quantitative addition to all samples of an internal standard element having excitation, absorption and enhancement characteristics similar to those of the analyte in the particular matrix. The calibration function involves measuring the intensity ratio of the analyte and internal standard lines.
3. *Matrix dilution methods*: The matrix of all samples is diluted to a composition such that the effect of the matrix is determined by the diluent rather than the matrix.

4. *Thin film methods*: The samples are made so thin that absorption-enhancement effects substantially disappear.
5. *Standard addition and dilution methods*: The analyte concentration is altered quantitatively in the sample itself. The sample is subjected to one or more quantitative incremental concentrations or dilutions of the analyte. The intensity of the analyte lines is measured for effectively the same matrix in each case.
6. *Mathematical corrections*: Absorption-enhancement effects are corrected mathematically by the use of *influence coefficients* for each element present (these are derived experimentally from reference samples). The basic approach is that the XRF intensity at a particular wavelength will in some way be affected by each element in the sample.

Calibration

Quantitative XRF analyses require calibration of the measuring arrangement, which may be performed by two major approaches:
- Empirical calibration
- Fundamental parameters (FP) calibration

The empirical calibration is based on the analysis of standards with known elemental compositions. To produce a reliable calibration model, the standards must be representative of the matrix and target element concentration ranges of the sample to be analyzed. Maintaining the same sample morphology (particle size distribution, heterogeneity and surface condition) and source/sample geometry for both standard and sample measurements is essential in empirical calibrations.

Alternatively, "standardless" FP techniques may be used, which rely on built-in mathematical algorithms that describe the physics of the detector's response to pure elements. In this case, the typical composition of the sample must be known, while the calibration model may be verified and optimized by one single standard sample.

Detection limits

Two types of detection limits should be considered in XRF analysis:
(a) instrument detection limits, which represent the threshold concentration of a given element that a particular instrument can resolve and
(b) method detection limits, related to sample preparation and analysis time. Depending on the element to be analyzed and the sample matrix, typically achieved detection limits vary between 10 and 100 ppm.

X-RAY ABSORPTION METHODS

In contrast to optical spectroscopy, where absorption methods are of prime importance, X-ray absorption applications are limited when compared with X-ray emission and fluorescence procedures. While absorption measurements can be made relatively free of matrix effects, the required techniques are somewhat cumbersome and time consuming when compared with fluorescence methods. Thus, most applications are confined to samples in which the effect of the matrix is minimal.

Absorption methods are analogous to optical absorption procedures in which the attenuation of a band or line of X-radiation serves as the analytical variable. Wavelength selection is accomplished with a monochromator such as that shown in Fig. 15.10 or by a filter technique similar to that illustrated in Fig. 15.9. Alternatively, the monochromatic radiation from a radioactive source is employed.

Because of the breadth of X-ray absorption peaks, direct absorption methods are generally useful only when a single element with a high atomic number is to be determined in a matrix consisting of only lighter elements. Examples of applications of this type are the determination of lead in gasoline and the determination of sulfur or the halogens in hydrocarbons.

X-RAY DIFFRACTION METHODS

Since its discovery in 1912 by Von Laue, X-ray diffractions has provided an important information to science and industry. For example, much that is known about the arrangement and the spacing of atoms in crystalline materials has been determined directly from diffraction studies. In addition, such studies have lead to a much clearer understanding of the physical properties of metals, polymeric materials, and other solids, X-ray diffraction is currently of prime importance in elucidating the structures of such complex natural product as steroids, vitamins, and antibiotic. Such applications are beyond the scope of this text.

X-ray diffraction also provides a convenient and practical means for the qualitative identification of crystalline compounds. The X-ray powder diffraction method is unique in that it is the only analytical method that is capable of providing qualitative and quantitative information about the compounds present in a solid sample. For example, the powder method can determine the percent KBr and NaCl in a solid mixture of these two compounds. Other analytical methods reveal only the percent K^+, Na^+, Br^- and Cl^- in the sample.

X-ray powder methods are based upon the text that an X-ray diffraction pattern is unique for each crystalline substance. Thus, if an exact match can be found between the pattern of an unknown and an authentic sample, chemical identify can be assumed.

IDENTIFICATION OF CRYSTALLINE COMPOUNDS

Sample Preparation

For analytical diffraction studies, the crystalline sample is ground to a fine homogeneous power. In such a form, the enormous number of small crystallites are oriented in every possible direction; thus, when an X-ray beam traverses the material, a significant number of the particles can be expected to be oriented in such ways as to fulfill the Bragg condition for reflection from every possible interlunar spacing.

Samples may be held in the beam in thin walled glass, or cellophane capillary tubes. Alternatively, a specimen may be mixed with a suitable noncrystalline binder and molded in to a appropriate shape.

Automatic Diffractometers

Diffraction patterns are generally obtained with automated instruments similar in design to that shown in Fig. 15.10. Here, the source is an X-ray tune with suitable filters. The powdered sample, however, replaces the single crystal on its mount. In some instances, the sample holder may be rotated in order to increase the randomness of the orientation of the crystals. The diffraction pattern is then obtained by automatic scanning in the same way as for an emission or absorption spectrum. Instruments of this type offer the advantage of high precision for intensity measurements and automated data reduction and report generation

Photographic Recording

The classical method for recording powder diffraction patterns, and one that still finds use, particularly when the amount of sample is small, is photographic. The most common instrument for this purpose is the *Debys Scherrer* powder camera, which is shown schematically in Fig. 15.20a. Here, the beam from a X-ray tube is filtered to produce a nearly monochromatic beam(often the copper or molybdenum k_g line) is collimated by passage through a narrow tube. The undiffracted radiation T then passes out of the camera via a arrow exit tube. The camera itself is cylindrical and equipped to hold a strip of film around its inside wall. The inside diameter of the cylinder usually is 5.73 or 11, 46 cm, so that each lineal millimeter of film is equivalent to 1.0 or 0.5 deg, respectively. The sample is held in the center of the beam by an adjustable mount.

Fig. 15.20b depicts the appearance of the exposed and developed film, each set of lines (D_1, D_2, and so forth) represents diffraction from one set of crystal planes. The Bragg angle θ, for each line is easily evaluated from the geometry of the camera.

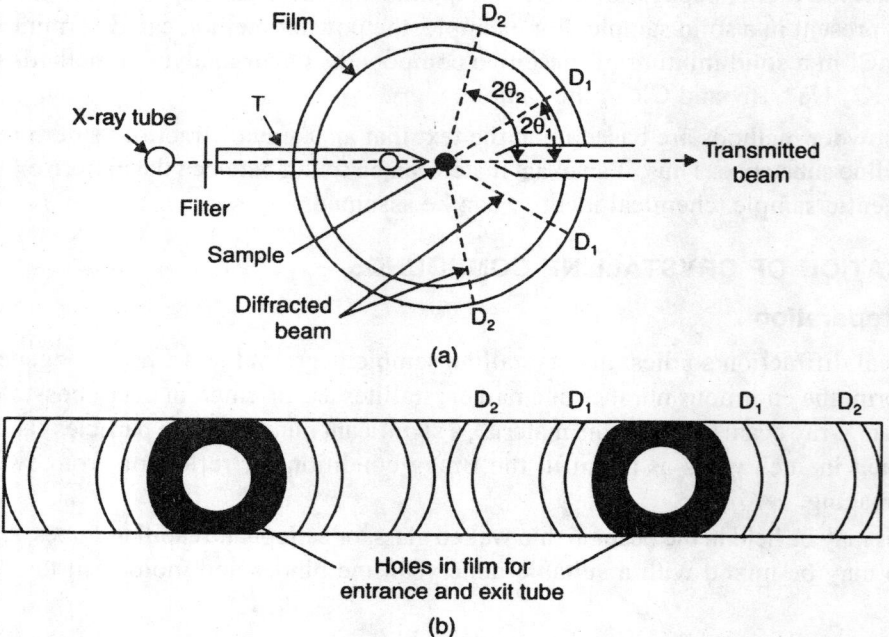

Fig. 15.20. Schematic of (a) Debye-Scherrer powder camera; (b) The film strip after development. D_2, D_1 and T indicate positions of the film in the camera.

Interpretation of Diffraction Patterns

The identification of a species from its powder diffraction pattern is based upon the position of the line (in terms of θ or 2θ) and their relative intensities. The diffraction angle 2θ is determined by the spacing between particular set of planes; with aid of the Bragg equation, this distance d is calculated from the known wavelength of the source and the measured angle. Line intensities depend upon the number and kind of atomic reflection centers in each set of planes.

Identification of crystals is empirical. A powder diffraction file is maintained by the International Center for Diffraction Data, Swarthmore, PA. In this, file contained powder diffraction patterns for over thousands of compounds. Because the file is so large as to make searching difficult and time consuming, the powder data file has been broken down into sub files that contain listings for inorganic, organic, minerals, metals, alloys, forensic materials, and others. The data in these files is in terms of d spacing and relative line intensities. The entries are arranged in order of the d spacing for the most intense line; entries are withdrawn from this file on the basis of d spacing that lies within a few hundredths of an angstrom of the d spacing of the most intense line for the analysts. Further elimination of possible compounds is accomplished by consideration of the spacing for the second most intense line, then the third, and so for the. Ordinarily, three or four spacing serve to identify the compound unambiguously. Computer search programs are now available to relive tedium of the search process.

If the sample contains two or more crystalline compounds, identification becomes more complex. Here various combinations of the more intense lines are used until a mach can be found.

By measuring the intensity of the diffraction lines and comparing with standards, a quantitative analysis of crystalline mixtures is also possible.

THE ELECTRON MICROPROBE

An important method for the determination of the elemental composition of surfaces is based upon the electron microprobe. In this technique, X-ray emission from the elements on the surface of a sample is stimulated by a narrowly focused beam of electrons. The resulting X-ray emission is detected and analyzed with either wavelength or an energy depressive spectrometer. In all the foregoing determinations, the nondestructive nature of X-ray of fluorescence is very important. This feature, coupled with the fact that sample preparation is seldom required, means that direct analysis can be performed *in situ*. Antiques and art objects can be characterized, and the original and copies of masterpieces distinguished from each other. Museums rely heavily on this method for examining works of art. In every case, the sample is unaffected physically or chemically by the analytical process. This feature is of extreme important to museums, aircraft manufacturers, and industrialists who use the technique for plant control.

Crystal Tonograpy

There are a number of experimental diffraction techniques developed in recent years, by which the micrscopial defects in a crystal can be shown. Most crystals are far from perfect crystals and exhibit regions (grains) with somewhat differing orientations, or they may contain individual defects such as dislocations or faults distributed throughout the crystal. Studies of these defects are important in understanding the nature of stress in metals, the nature and behavior of "doped" crystals used in transistors, the production of "perfect" crystals, and other phenomena.

Microradiographic methods are based on absorption and the contrast in the images is due to differences in absorption coefficients from point-to-point. X-ray diffraction topography depends for image contrast upon point-to-point changes in the direction or the intensity of beams diffracted by planes in the crystal.

One much used methods of X-ray diffraction topography is known as the Berg-Barrett method. The experimental arrangement is shown in Fig 15.21. The crystal is set so as to reflect the X-rays at the Bragg angle for some plane. Geometric resolutions of about 1 mm can be achieved and single dislocations can be resolved. The contrast on the film is due to variations of the reflecting power due to imperfections in the crystal.

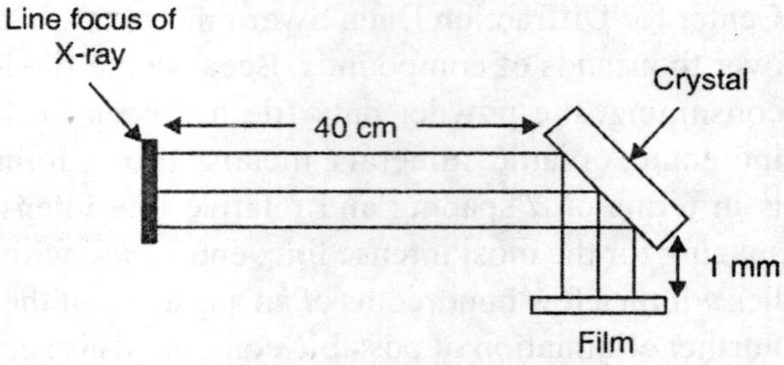

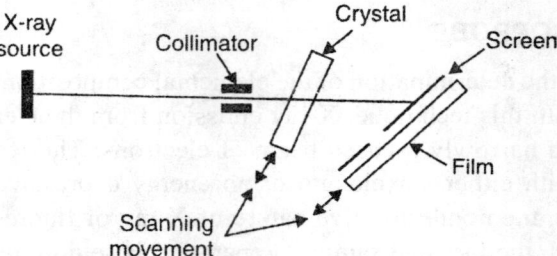

Fig. 15.21. Experimental arrangement for the Berg-Barrett method of X-ray diffraction topography.

Another method for X-ray diffraction topography is known as the Lang method. The experimental setup is shown in Fig 15.22. A ribbon X-ray beam is collimated to such a small angular divergence that only the characteristic wavelength is diffracted by the crystal. Simultaneous movement of the crystal and film allow a large area of the crystal to be investigated.

Fig. 15.22. Experimental arrangement for the Lang method of X-ray diffraction topography.

CHAPTER 16

Refractometry

The speed of light in a vacuum is always the same, but when light moves through any other medium it travels more slowly since it is constantly being absorbed and reemitted by the atoms in the material. The ratio of the speed of light in a vacuum to the speed of light in another substance is defined as the **index of refraction** (aka **refractive index** or *n*) for the substance.

$$\text{Refractive index (n) of substance} = \frac{\text{Speed of light in a vacuum}}{\text{Speed of light in a substance}} \quad \ldots(16.1)$$

Whenever light changes speed as it crosses a boundary from one medium into another, its direction of travel also changes, i.e., it is refracted (Fig. 16.1). (In the special case of the light travelling perpendicular to the boundary there is no change in direction upon entering the new medium). The relationship between light's speed in the two mediums (v_A and v_B), the angles of incidence (θ_A) and refraction (θ_B) and the refractive indexes of the two mediums (n_A and n_B) is shown below:

$$\frac{v_A}{v_B} = \frac{\sin \theta_A}{\sin \theta_B} = \frac{n_B}{n_A} \quad \ldots(16.2)$$

Thus, it is not necessary to measure the speed of light in a sample in order to determine its index of refraction. Instead, by measuring the angle of refraction, and knowing the index of refraction of the layer that is in contact with the sample, it is possible to determine the refractive index of the sample. The refractive index depends upon the temperature and the wavelength of light used. In practice usually D line sodium is used for standard measurement.

SPECIFIC AND MOLECULAR REFRACTIVITY

We know that the temperature has marked influence on refractive index and increase in temperature results in the decrease of refractive index. However, Lorentze and Lorentz (1880) introduced a term specific refraction or specific refractivity, which may be defined by the equation:

$$R = \frac{n^2 - 1}{n^2 + 2} \times \frac{1}{d}$$

where

n = refractive index

d = density of the liquid

R = specific refractivity that it is quite independent of temperature

The change of refractive index with a change in temperature is compensated by the change in density of the liquid. If the specific refractivity is multiplied by the molecular weight of the substance, the product obtained is called *molecular* or *molar refractivity*.

$$R = \frac{n^2 - 1}{n^2 + 2} \times \frac{M}{d}$$

where M is the molecular weight of the liquid.

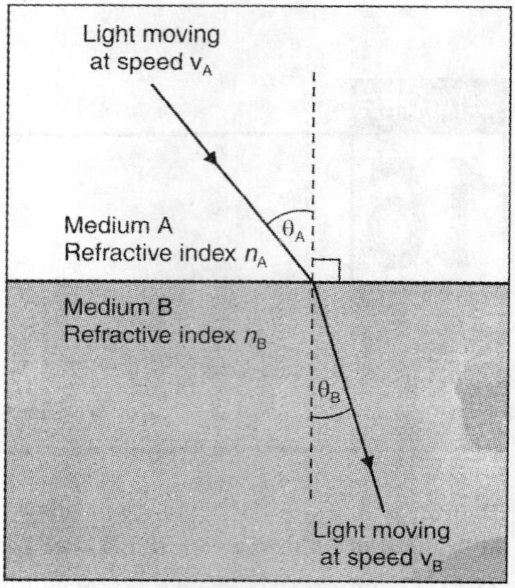

Fig. 16.1. Light crossing from any transparent medium into another in which it has different speed, is refracted.

The molecular refractivity of the solid may be determined by dissolving it first in a suitable solvent in order to get a solution of known concentration. The refractive index and the density of the solution are determined by usual methods. The molecular refractivity of the solution is then given by the following relationship:

$$R = \frac{n^2 - 1}{n^2 + 2} \times \frac{x_1 m_1 + x_2 m_2}{d}$$

where

m_1 = molecular weight of the solvent

m_2 = molecular weight of the solute

x_1 = mole fraction of solvent

x_2 = mole fraction of the solute

d = density of the solution

n = refractive index of the solution

FACTORS AFFECTING REFRACTIVE INDEX

The most important factors which affect a refractive index measurement are the temperature, pressure and wavelength.

Temperature: The refractive index of a medium is primarily affected by the temperature, because of the accompanying change in density. For most organic liquids the index of refraction decreases by approximately 0.00045 ± 0.0001 for every 1°C increase in temperature. See Table 16.2 for a few examples. Note that the index of refraction for water is much less dependent on temperature than most organic liquids, decreasing by about 0.0001 for every 1°C increase in temperature.

Table 16.1. Temperature dependence of refractive index for selected substances

Substance	n_D^{15}	n_D^{20}	n_D^{25}
Isopropanol	1.3802	1.3772	1.3749
Acetone	1.3616	1.3588	1.3560
Ethyl acetate	1.3747	1.3742	1.3700
Water	1.3334	1.3330	1.3325

Wavelength: The index of refraction is generally a decreasing function of wavelength: violet light is bent more than red light. Furthermore, the rate of change of the index of refraction also increases as the wavelength decreases. Water displays all of these characteristics. Table 16.2 shows the results of some measurements of the index of refraction of water, at various wavelength and temperature.

Table 16.2. Index of refraction of water as a function of wavelength and water temperature

Wave length (Angstrons)	$T = 10°C$	$T = 20°C$	$T = 30°C$
7065	1.3307	1.3300	1.3290
5893	1.3337	1.3330	1.3319
4047	1.3435	1.3427	1.3417

It is well evident from these dispersion phenomena that the wavelength employed should be specified in quoting a refractive index. In refractometry, D, line from sodium vapour lamp is commonly used.

Pressure

The refractive index of a substance increases with pressure because of the accompanying increase in density. The effect is more pronounced in gases than in liquids.

DETERMINATION OF REFRACTIVE INDEX

The difference between a light speed in different media results into the change of direction along which the light propagates, refraction. Refraction occurs when the light passes from one medium to a medium with a different index of refraction, except the light that approaches the boundary between the two media perpendicularly. Accordingly to the properties of an optical medium, some portion of light approaching the interface at an incident angle α is reflected back to the first medium while the rest propagates into the other medium at an angle of refraction β. The angles of incident, reflection and refraction are defined as angles between the particular ray and the interface normal (see Fig. 16.2). **Note, that the reflection angle is always equal to the incident angle.** On the other hand, the refractive angle is determined by the Snell's law:

$$n_1 \sin \alpha = n_2 \sin \beta \quad ...(16.2)$$

where n_1 is the refractive index of medium 1 and n_2 is the refractive index of medium 2. It is possible to define an optical density for the media of different refractive indices. Medium A has a higher optical density than medium B, if its refractive index is higher than that of medium B. According to the Snell's law, the light ray is "bending towards the normal" ($\beta < \alpha$), if it enters the medium with a higher optical density (Fig. 16.2). When it enters the medium with a lower optical density, it is "bending away from the normal" ($\beta > \alpha$).

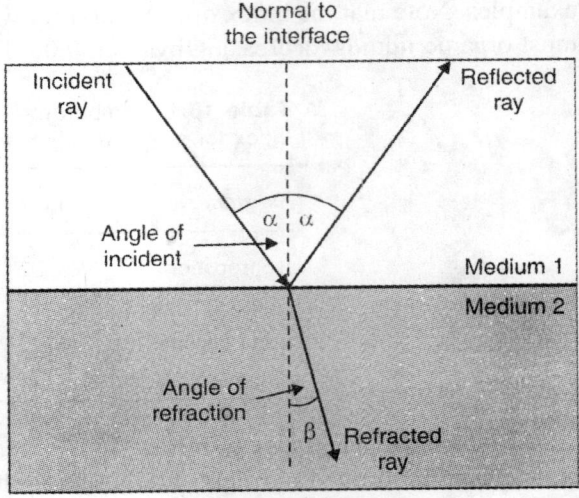

Fig. 16.2. Refraction of light.

If the angle of incidence is made so large that it becomes 90°, the angle of refraction achieves its maximum possible value. This angle of incidence is called "*grazing angle*" and maximum possible value of refraction is called "*critical angle of refraction*". In the above equation, if n_1 is known, measurement of angle of 'β' permits the estimation of n(A) because Sin 90° = 1.

Refractive index can be measured by the refractometer or inferometers.

A. Refractometers

1. Abbe's refractometer

Abbe's refractometer, shown in Fig. 16.3 is commonly used. It has mirror, to reflect light into the instrument. It consists of the two optical prisms (illuminating and refracting) with the thin layer of a liquid sample between them. The prisms are enclosed in a prism box, A. The measuring prism is made of a glass with a high refractive index ($n_2 > 1.75$), which allows this refractometer to measure refractive indices up to $n_1 < 1.75$. The light enters the refractometer from the left side of the illuminating prism at many different angles. The bottom part of this prism (AB') is rough, i.e. it consists of many small areas oriented in different directions. As such, this surface can be imagined as a source of sending incident light into all directions. Part of this light passes through the sample into the refracting prism, where the biggest possible angle of incident, α_{max}, corresponds to the ray that propagates from point A to point B (Fig. 16.4). According to Snell's law, the refraction of this ray is then described by the maximum angle of refraction β max. All other rays enter the refracting prism at smaller angles and thus end up to the left of point C. Consequently, detector located at the bottom of the refracting prism detects the illuminated region of left of point C and a dark region

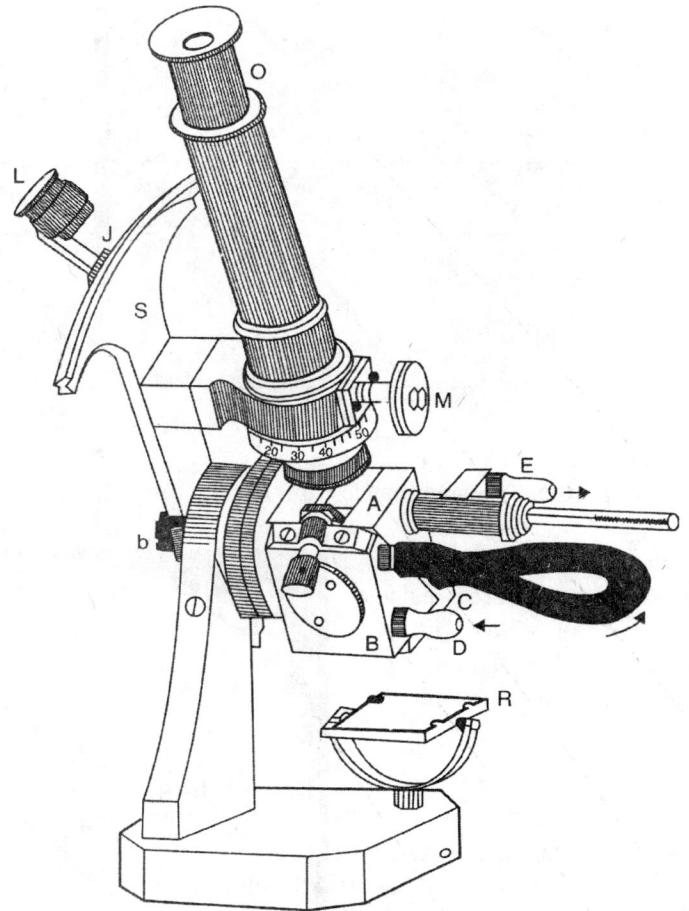

Fig. 16.3. Abbe refractometer.

of this point. Since the maximum angle, α_{max}, and the refractive index of the refracting prism, n_2, are known constants, it is straight forward to determine the refractive index of a measured liquid, n_1. The interface between an illuminated and dark region (position of point C) changes as a function of angle β_{max}, which is different for samples with different refractive indices n_1. The simple readout from the scale of refractometer then provides the refractive index directly.

Abbe refractometer is so much popular because of its convenience, its wide range (n_D = 1.3–1.7), and to the minimal sample required. The accuracy of the instrument is about $\pm$ 0.0002. The index is readout directly where the vertical cross hair intersects the scale (Fig. 16.5). The refractive index is 1.465° according to the figure.

The most serious error in the Abbe instrument is caused by the fact that the nearly grazing rays are cut off by the arrangement of the two prisms, thus the boundary is less sharp than is desirable.

The improvement in accuracy of the Abbe instrument can be obtained by replacing

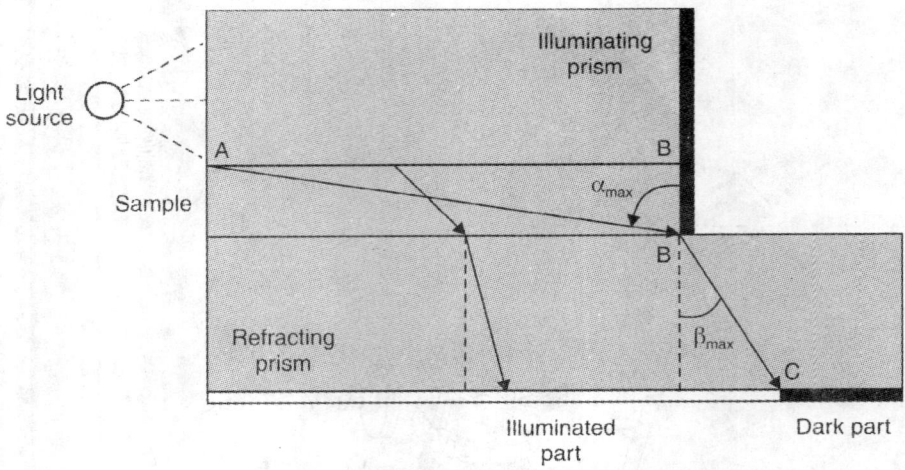

Fig. 16.4. The schematic of the Abbe's refractometer.

the compensator with a monochromatic source and by using larger and more precise prism mounts. The former provides a much sharper critical boundary, and the later permits a more accurate determination of the prism position.

2. Immersion refractometer

This instrument is very similar to the Abbe refractometer except that the refracting prism is rigidly fixed in the telescope tube and there is no diffusion prism. This instrument also contain a compensator and a scale. For liquid samples, the refracting prism is dipped completely and the sharp edge of the band of light is read off the scale.

3. Pulfrich refractometer

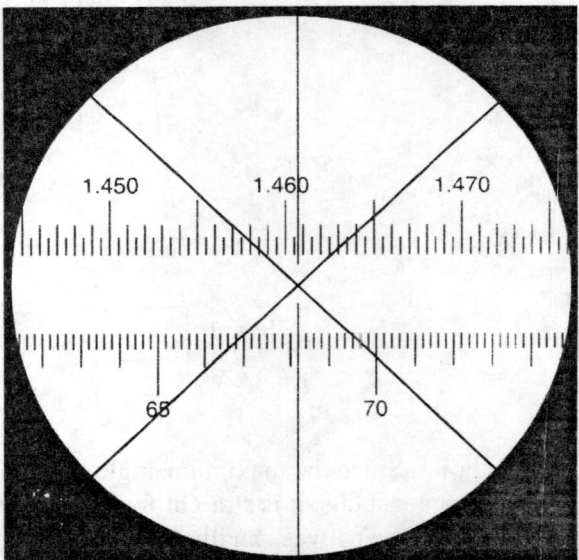

Fig. 16.5. View of internal scales in the ABBE refractometer.

This refractometer is used less frequently than the Abbe instrument. But this instrument gives great accuracy ($\pm$ 0.00002). In this refractometer, a horizontal beam of monochromatic radiation is directed along the surface of the refracting prism at the grazing angle. A sample cell is cemented on the horizontal surface of the prism, and a telescope is mounted at the side on the rotatable scale. The rays coming out of the refracting prism are reflected by a right angled prism. The telescope is turned until the sharp edge of the bend of light is centred on the cross hairs in the telescope eyepiece and the reading is taken.

B. Inferometers

These instruments utilize the interference phenomenon to obtain differential refractive indices with high precision.

APPLICATIONS OF REFRACTOMETRY

Characterization of liquid compounds

The refractive index along with melting points, boiling points and densities can be used to characterise and identify the substances. Refractometers measure the refractive index of liquids, solids or gases through which light can pass. A light ray changes direction, or bends, when it enters a material in which the velocity of light is different than in air, the extent of this refraction being directly related to the refractive index. Consequently, a refractometer is a non invasive device for the identification and characterization of substances.

Determination of Concentration of Solutions

Determining of the concentration of a solute in a solution is probably the most popular use of refractometry. For example, refractometer based methods have been developed for determining the percentage of sugar in fruits, juices, and syrups, the percentage of alcohol in beer or wine, the salinity of water, and the concentration of antifreeze in radiator fluid. Many industries use refractometer based methods in quality control applications.

In most cases the refractive index is linearly (or nearly linearly) related to the percentage of dissolved solids in a solution (Fig. 16.6). By comparing the value of refractive index of a solution to that of a standard curve the concentration of solute can be determined with good accuracy. Many refractometers contain a "Brix" scale that is calibrated to give the percentage (w/w) of sucrose dissolved in water.

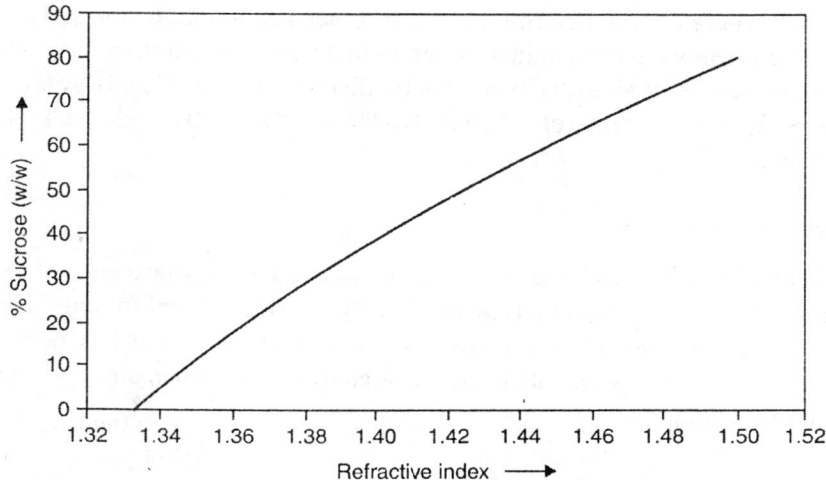

Fig. 16.6. A standard curve showing the relationship between the refractive index and the percentage (w/w) of sucrose in a solution at 20°C.

Structural Information

The refractive index does not provide detailed information about a molecule's structure, and it is not usually used for this purpose due to availability of more powerful spectroscopic techniques. One structural factor that influence the refractive index of a sample is its polarizability. Substances containing more polarizable ("soft") groups (e.g., iodine atoms or aromatic rings) will normally have higher refractive indexes than substances containing less polarizable ("hard") groups (e.g., oxygen atoms or alkyl groups). The effect of polarizibility is shown in Table 16.3.

Table 16.3. Effect of polarizable groups on refractive index

Substance	2-Iodoethanol	2-Fluoroethanol	Benzene	Cyclohexane
n_D^{20}	1.5720	1.3670	1.5010	1.4260

Determination of sulphur

Refractometeric procedures have also proved useful in determining the concentration of sulphur invulcanized rubber and the bound styrene.

Determination of composition of two liquids

The composition of a dilute solution of two liquids can be determined from the refractive index of the solution provided that the refractive indices and densities of the two liquid components are known.

Use in gem industry

For gemologists it is necessary to determine, first, whether a gem is authentic and then to determine its quality. Refractometers are used to identify gems and verifytheir authenticity. There is a unique refractive index associated with every type of gem: diamond has the highest refractive index - not only for a gem but for any substance of 2.42 whereas the topaz refractive index is 1.64. The refractive index for a vacuum is 1.

Use in veterinary medicine

Simple hand-held refractometers have been widely used by veterinarians since the early 1960s for the measurement of proteins in blood serum and density of urine of farm animals. The refractometer method enjoys the advantages of ease-of-use, rapidity of analysis and low cost. Refractometer analyses and the compare quite well with those obtained by more cumbersome and complex methods, such as the biuret method.

Use in wine making

A refractometer can be used to measure the sugar level in juice to help determine whether it is ready to be made into wine since the initial sugar level may not be sufficient to produce the desired alcohol level in the finished wine.

Use in fats and oils

RI determination can be helpful in characterize vegetable oils, animal oils, essential oils, hydrogenation.

Use in food additives

RI determination can be useful to know the conc. of citric acid, monosodium glutamate, total solids in liquid eggs.

CHAPTER 17

Thermoanalytical Methods

Thermoanalytical methods investigate the changes in a sample that take place on heating. These distinct thermoanalytical methods include thermogravimetric analysis, differential thermogravimetric analysis, differential thermal analysis, differential scanning calorimetry, thermometric titration, etc. (Table 17.1). In these techniques, physical property is measured as a function of temperature, while the sample is subjected to predetermined heating. Data are obtained in the form of continuously recorded curves, known as thermogram or thermocurve.

Table 17.1. Types of Thermoanalytical methods

Method	Property measures	Apparatus
1. Thermogravimetric analysis	Change in mass	Thermobalance
2. Differential thermogravimetric analysis	Change in mass	Thermobalance
3. Differential thermal analysis	Temperature difference	DTA apparatus
4. Differential scanning calorimetry	Heat flow	DSC apparatus
5. Thermometric titration	Change in temperature	Titration calorimeter

1. THERMOGRAVIMETRIC ANALYSIS

Thermogravimetric analysis (TGA) is the most widely used thermal method. It is based on the measurement of decrease in mass of sample material as a function of temperature. In thermogravimetry (TG), a continuous graph of mass change against temperature is obtained when a substance is heated at a uniform rate or kept at constant temperature. A plot of mass change versus temperature (T) is referred to as the thermogravimetric curve (TG curve). For the TG curve, we generally plot mass (m) decreasing downwards on the y axis (ordinate), and temperature (T) increasing to the right on the x axis (abscissa) as illustrated in Fig. 17.1.

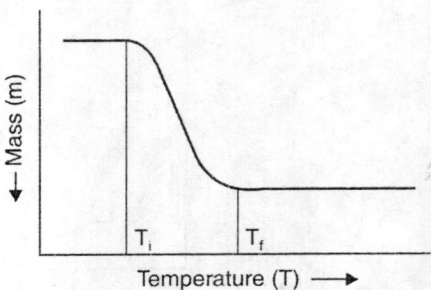

Fig. 17.1. A typical TG curve.

Sometime, we may plot time (t) in place of T. TG curve helps in revealing the extent of purity of analytical samples and in determining the mode of their transformations within specified range of temperature.

In thermogravimetry (TG) curve of a single stage decomposition, there are two characteristic temperatures; the initial T_i and the final temperature T_f (see Fig. 17.1). T_i is defined as the lowest temperature at which the onset of a mass change can be detected by thermo balance operating under particular conditions and T_f as the final temperature at which the particular decomposition process appears to be complete. Although T_i has no fundamental significance, it can still be a useful characteristic of a TG curve and so for this, the term **procedural decomposition temperature** has been suggested.

Types of thermogravimetric analysis (TGA)

It is of two types:
  (i) *Dynamic TGA*: In this type of analysis, the sample is subjected to condition of continuous increase in temperature usually linear with time.
  (ii) *Isothermal TGA*: In this type of analysis, the sample is maintained at a constant temperature for a period of time, during which any change in weight is observed.

TGA principle and method

The principle of the technique is explained by weight loss curve of a hypothetical compound, $MCO_3.2H_2O$ as shown in Fig. 17.2. As indicated from the Fig. 17.2, water evaporation started at point A. The temperature at A is called minimum weight loss temperature. At point B, the hypothetical compound is converted into $MCO_3.H_2O$. Further heating converts the hypothetical compound into anhydrous compound. It is maintained from C to D. As per the curve, the appropriate drying temperature lies somewhere between C and D for MCO_3. The values of C and D depends upon the heating rate of the furnace, a slow heating rate will shift this temperature to lower values. At point D, the compound MCO_3 starts to evolve CO_2 giving MO weight level from E to F. The thermal

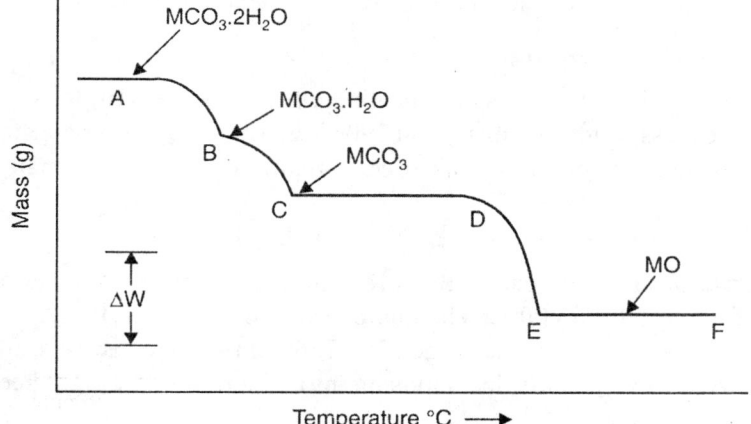

Fig. 17.2. Thermogravimetric curve of hypothetical compound, $MCO_3.2H_2O$.

stabilities of the original sample, the intermediate compound and final product can then be ascertained from the observation of the various regions in the curve. For example, MCO_3 is stable from point 'C' to 'D' and so temperature in this region can be used for drying the hypothetical compound.

The method of thermogravimetric analysis may be made more clear from the thermogravimetric curve (Fig. 17.3) of magnesium oxalate, calcium oxalate, mercurous chromate, silver chromate, etc. In the Fig. 17.3, curve 3 shows the thermogram of calcium oxalate. It is normally precipitated as calcium oxalate monohydrate. The curve exhibit several plateau corresponding to monohydrate from room temperature to 100°C, anhydrous calcium oxalate from 228 to 420°C, calcium carbonate from 420° to 660°C and calcium oxide from above 838°C. As per TG curve, the calcium carbonate is an excellent weighing form if heated in between the 420 to 660°C (generally taken 520°). The curve 4 is a thermogram for

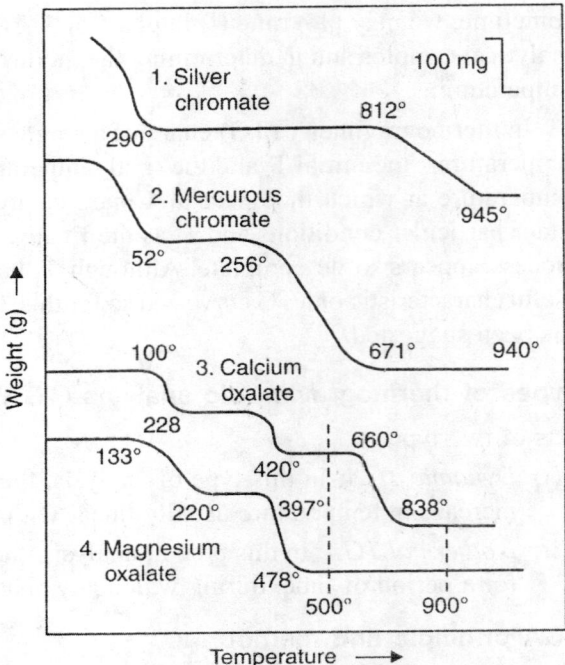

Fig. 17.3. TGA curves of precipitates of silver chromate (1), mercurous chromate (2), calcium oxalate (3), and magnesium oxalate (4).

magnesium oxalate which reveals that dihydrate is stable upto 133°C, the anhydrous compound exists between 220 to 400°C and the oxide stable from 478° to 1000°C. As per the curve, it is recommended to dry the precipitates of MgO above 500°C.

$$Hg_2CrO_4 \longrightarrow Hg_2O + CrO_3^- \longrightarrow CrO_3 + e^-$$
$$Ca(COO)_2 \longrightarrow CaCO_3 + CO\uparrow \longrightarrow CaO + CO_2\uparrow$$
$$Mg(COO)_2 \longrightarrow MgO + CO\uparrow + CO_2\uparrow$$

The curve 1 in the Fig. 17.3 represents the heating effect on silver chromate. The initial loss in weight indicates the excess water, and just about 290°C the weight becomes constant and remains so up to 812°C after which oxygen is lost. The decomposition of silver chromate can, therefore represented as:

$$2Ag_2CrO_4 \longrightarrow Ag_2Cr_2O_4 + 2Ag\downarrow + 2O_2$$

As per the observation from the curve, the silver chromate precipitates can be dried over a temperature range of about 290 to 800°C. The curve 2 is a thermogram of mercurous chromate. The mercurous chromate is stable over the range 52 to 256°C this range can be used for drying the mercurous chromate. At 256°C, it starts decomposing into Hg_2O and the weight becomes constant at about 671°C.

Another example is the analysis of copper silver alloys based on the relative stabilities of the nitrates. The TG curve of pure $AgNO_3$, $Cu(NO_3)_2$ and their mixture are given in Fig. 17.4. Curve 'a' is the curve of dry crystalline $AgNO_3$. A horizontal extends to 473°C showing its stability upto this temperature. It is followed by descent as far as 473°C. At this temperature decomposition sets in abruptly and nitrous fumes are expelled up to 608°C. After that there is much slower mass loss from 608°C to 810°C.

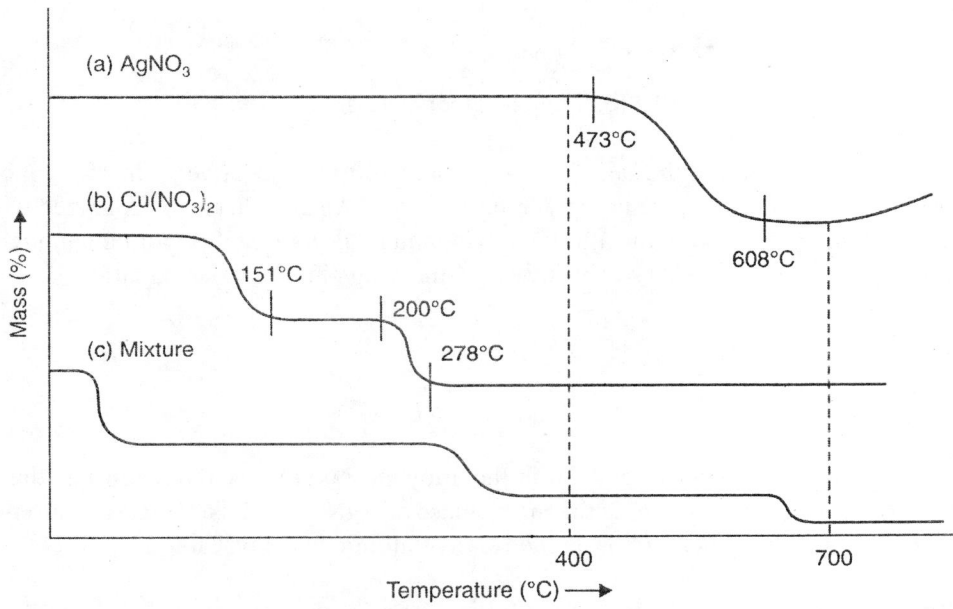

Fig. 17.4. TG curves of nitrates (a) $AgNO_3$, (b) $Cu(NO_3)_2$ and (c) $AgNO_3 + Cu(NO_3)_2$.

Decomposition of $AgNO_2$ which is not observed when CuO is present, no doubt the latter catalyses the decomposition. Above 810°C the weight is again constant due to the formation of pure Ag metal.

$$2AgNO_3(s) \longrightarrow 2AgNO_2(s) + O_2(g)$$
$$2AgNO_2(s) \longrightarrow 2Ag(s) + 2NO_2(g)$$

While the copper nitrate hexahydrate gives a quite different curve b. It decomposes into CuO in two steps. In first step, water and nitrogen oxide are driven off up to 151°C. Then a horizontal indicates the existence of zone of a new compound, which has been analysed as basic nitrate $Cu(NO_3)_2 2Cu(OH)_2$. This compound only become constant above 700°C.

$$3Cu(NO_3)_2 \cdot 6H_2O \longrightarrow Cu(NO_3)_2 \cdot 2Cu(OH)_2 + 3H_2O + 4NO_2\uparrow \longrightarrow CuO$$

If a mixture of $AgNO_3$ and $Cu(NO_3)_2$ is placed in thermobalance, the curve c is recorded. The horizontal related to the basic copper nitrate is, nevertheless, well marked. From 240°C to 400°C there is a residue keeping constant mass ($AgNO_3$ + CuO), while above 900°C a mixture of Ag + CuO is present. Thus, the weights of mixed precipitate at 400°C will permit the analysis of the Cu-Ag alloy.

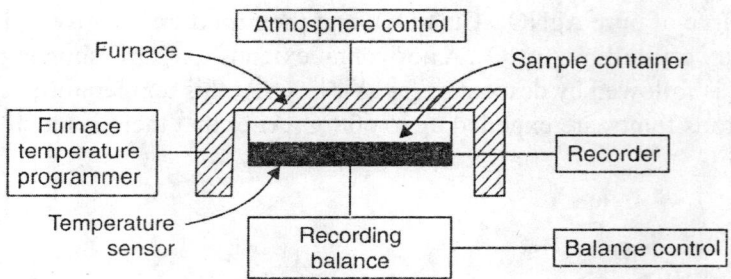

Fig. 17.5. Thermobalance.

If m_1 and m_2 are the mass of the sample at 400°C and 700°C, respectively, the amount of silver and copper in the sample can be calculated. A binary alloy of Ag and Cu can be analyzed with ±3% error by this method by dissolving the alloy in HNO_3 and then running thermogram and recording successive weight at 400°C and 700°C by solving following simultaneous equations:

$$\left(\frac{170}{108}\right)x + \left(\frac{79}{63}\right)y = m_1$$

$$x + \left(\frac{79}{63}\right)y = m_2$$

where x and y are the masses of Ag and Cu in the alloy, m_1 and m_2 are the masses of the sample at 400°C and 700°C respectively, 170 is the molar mass of $AgNO_3$, 108 is the relative atomic mass of Ag, 79 is molar mass of CuO and 63 is the relative atomic mass of Cu.

Instrumentation

In general, the thermogravimetric analytical instrument (Fig. 17.5) consists of four components:
(i) Furnace provided with control system to maintain the temperature, often to maintain the atmosphere as well.
(ii) The sample container.
(iii) The sensor for measuring temperature and sample property.
(iv) Data collection and display system.

The furnace is generally electrically operated and the furnace enclosure is purged with a suitable gas, either to provide an inert atmosphere or to provide a reactive environment in which sample may be burnt on reacted.

The analytical sample is contained in an inert crucible. It may be made of alumina, platinum or ceramic. The thermocouple is used as sensor to measure the temperature; for measuring the mass, a thermo balance is used. It is a sensitive electronic balance positioned away from the furnace to avoid the effect of heat and any corrosive gases produced by the sample and capable of detecting changes as small as 1 mg and of weighing 10–100 mg. The balance is purged with dry nitrogen for protection.

Temperature calibration cannot be carried out by the normal standards since these involve no mass change. Hence, curie-point method is used to calibrate temperature. In this, ferromagnetic material loses their magnetism on heating at an exactly reproducible temperatures or curie-points. A range of metals or alloys with curie-points between 150 to 1000°C is available.

If ferromagnetic calibration standards are placed in the sample pan of balance and a large permanent magnet is placed below the pan, the sample will experience a downward attraction heating to an apparent increase in weight (Fig. 17.6a and b) at the curie-point, the loss of ferromagnetism will be reflected by the apparent loss of weight, enabling the tempe-rature experience by the balance pan to be accurately known, for example, for nickel metal, the curie-point temperature is 354°C (Fig. 17.6c).

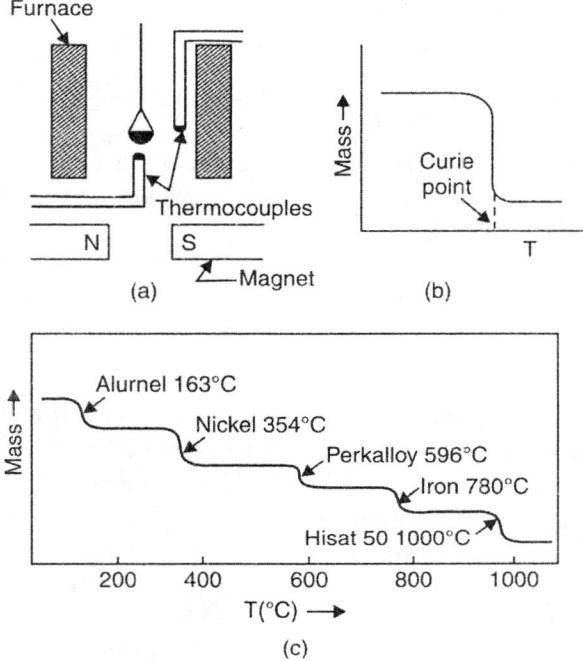

Fig. 17.6. (a) Thermobalance, (b) Curie point method of temperature calibration, (c) Curie-point temperature of various elements.

Sample containers

The geometry, size and material of the sample container or crucible have a marked influence on the shape of the TG curve. The sample holder is made of glass, quartz, aluminium, stainless steel, platinum, various alloys, etc. Generally, there are four basic designs of sample holder.

(i) Shallow pans: These are used when volatile products are produced during heating. With the use of shallow pans, there is an easy escape of gases from the surface.
(ii) Deep crucibles: These are employed in the study of industrial scale calcination or surface area measurement.
(iii) Loosely covered crucibles: These crucibles are suitable when rate of weight loss and not the exact temperature is taken into consideration, as in the case of self-generated atmospheric studies.
(iv) Retort cups: These cups are suitable in boiling point studies.

Factors Affecting Thermogravimetric Analysis

There are two important factors upon which TGA depends.
(i) Instrumental factors
(ii) Sample characteristics

Instrumental factors

Furnace heating rate, recording chart speed, furnace atmosphere, geometry of sample container,

292 Pharmaceutical Analysis

and geometry of the furnace, sensitivity of recorder and recording balance and composition of sample container are various instrumental factors.

(a) Furnace heating rate

At a given temperature, the degree of decomposition is greater at slow heating rate, and thus the shape of the TG curve can be influenced by the heating rate. For a single stage endothermic reaction it has been found that:

(i) $(T_i)_F > (T_i)_S$
(ii) $(T_f)_F > (T_f)_S$
(iii) $(T_f - T_i)_F > (T_f - T_i)_S$

where subscripts F and S indicate fast and slow heating rate respectively. For example, calcium carbonate would not show any mass loss below 600°C, when heated in a thermobalance at heating rate of 3°C per min., and yet it is known that CO_2 is evolved at 250°C (Fig. 17.7). Similarly, polytetrafluoro ethylene (PTFE) decomposition rate is illustrated in Fig. 17.8. More specifically, it is observed that the procedural decomposition temperature T_1, and also T_f (the procedural final temperature) will decrease with decrease in heating rate and the TG curve will be shifted to the left. This effect is illustrated in Fig. 17.8. The appearance of an infection in a TG curve at a fast heating rate may well be resolved into a plateau at a slower heating rate. Therefore, in TGA there is neither optimum nor standard heating rate, but a heating rate of 3°C per min gives a TG curve with maximum meaningful resolution.

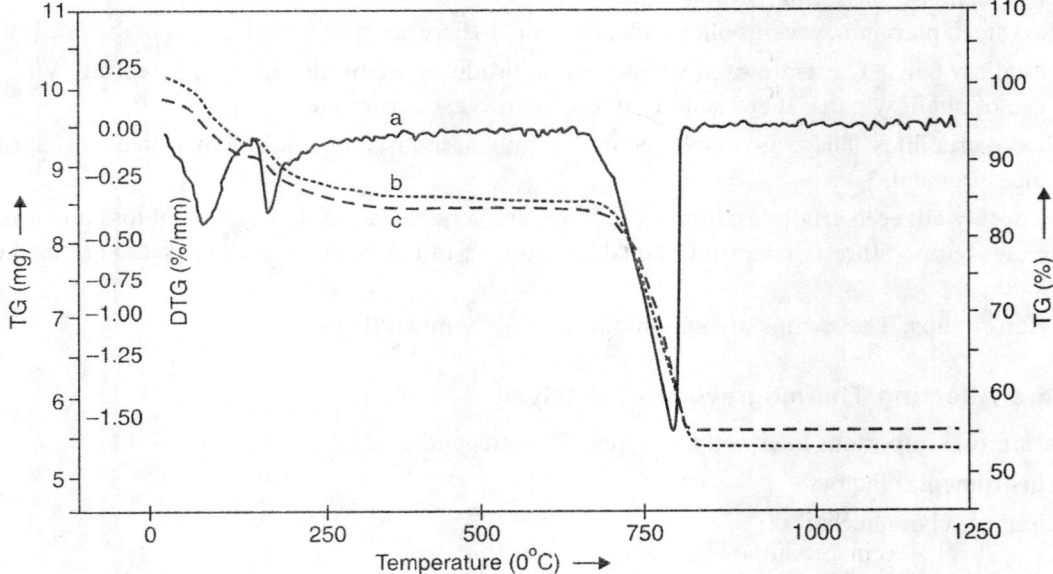

Fig. 17.7. TG and DTG curve of $CaCO_3$ at various heating rates (b = 10°C, c = 3°C) (DTG = Rate of change of mass, dm/dt) curve.

For a reversible reaction, the rate of heating has little or no effect, but it affects the position of intermediate compounds on thermogravimetric curves. For example, at a heating rate of 2.5°C per minute, the TG curves of nickel sulphate ($NiSO_4.7H_2O$) indicates one curve break corresponding to the substance $NiSO_4.H_2O$, but if nickel sulphate is heated at heating rate of 0.6°C per minute, the TG curve shows various breaks corresponding to $NiSO_4.6H_2O$, $NiSO_4.4H_2O$, $NiSO_4.2H_2O$ and $NiSO_4.H_2O$.

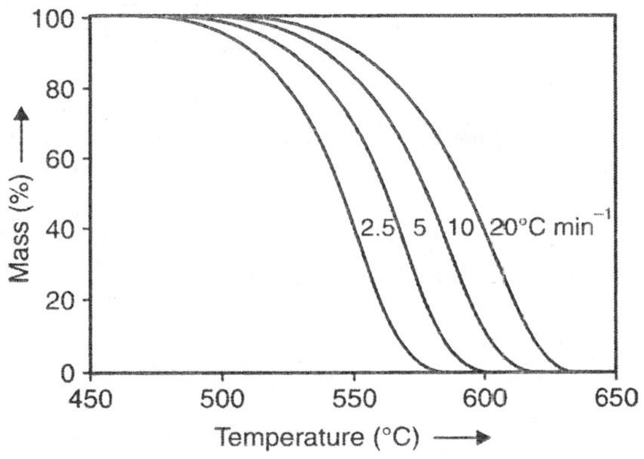

Fig. 17.8. Effect of rate of heating on 10 mg sample of PTEF 2.5, 5, 10, 20°C in nitrogen atmosphere.

(b) Recording or Chart Speed

The chart speed on the recording of the TG curve of rapid or slow reaction has pronounced effect on the shape of the TG curves. For a slow decomposition reaction, low chart speed is recommended for recording the TG curve because at high chart speed the curve will be flattened and it will not show the sharp decomposition temperature. For a slow reaction followed by a rapid one, at the lower chart speed the curve will show less separation in the two steps than the higher chart speed curve. For *fast-fast* reaction followed by slower one, similar observation is observed in shorter curve plateaus.

(c) Furnace Atmosphere

The effect of atmosphere on the TG curve depends on (i) the types of the reaction, (ii) the nature of the decomposition products and (iii) type of atmosphere employed. The effect of the atmosphere on TG curve may be illustrated by taking the example of thermodecomposition of a sample of monohydrates of calcium oxalate in dry O_2 and dry N_2 as shown in Fig. 17.9.

The first step, which is dehydration is reversible reaction.

$$CaC_2O_4.H_2O(s) \longrightarrow CaC_2O_4(s) + H_2O\uparrow$$

This is unaffected because both gases are equally effective in sweeping the evolved water vapours away from the sample surface. In the second step:

$$CaC_2O_4(s) \longrightarrow CaCO_3(s) + CO\uparrow$$

The curve diverges in O_2 atmosphere because the oxygen reacts with evolved CO, giving a second oxidation reaction which is highly exothermic and so raises the temperature of the unreacted sample. The temperature accelerates the decomposition of the compound more rapidly and completely at lower temperature as shown in the Fig. 17.9 in dry O_2 then in N_2 atmosphere.

The third step in decomposition reaction is also reversible reaction:

$$CaCO_3(s) \rightleftharpoons CaO(s) + CO_2(g)\uparrow$$

This step should not be influenced by O_2 or N_2. However there is a slight difference in curves

294 Pharmaceutical Analysis

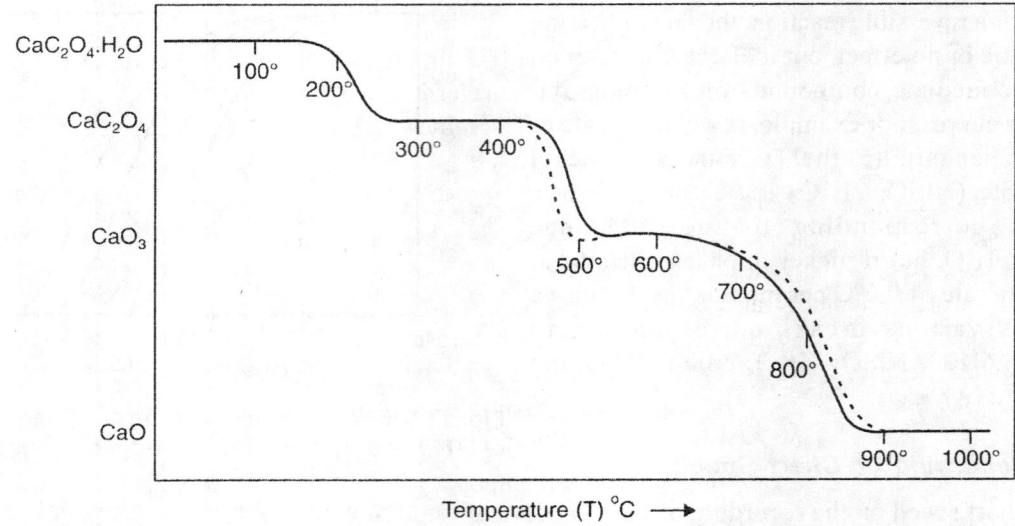

Fig. 17.9. TG curve of calcium oxalate (100 mg) in O_2 and N_2 atmosphere: [_____ N_2, ...O_2).

for the two gases as shown in Fig. 17.9. The small difference was due to the difference in the nature/composition of $CaCO_3$ formed in the two atmosphere. This is due to the particle size, surface area, lattice defects or due to the other physical characteristics of $CaCO_3$ formed.

It is however, desirable to maintain the nature of atmospheric gas as constant as possible throughout the experiment and it is achieved by heating the samples in vacuum. In thermogravimetric analysis, infact there are three common furnace atmospheres.

These are static air (air from the atmosphere is allowed to flow through the furnace), dynamic air (compressed air is allowed to flow through the furnace at a constant and measured rate of flow) and inert atmosphere (where oxygen free nitrogen gas is used as an inert atmosphere in the furnace).

Sample holder

The sample holders range from flat plates to deep crucible of various capacities. It may be made of glass, aluminium, ceramic material, metals and metallic alloys. A shallow dish is widely been used, because of rapid exchange of gaseous material between sample and surrounding atmosphere in the furnace. The slope of the TG curve is not affected by the geometry of sample holder when the furnace atmosphere is not changed. The shape of the TG curve will only vary if the sample is not be heated in identical condition. Generally, it is preconditioning that the thermocouple is placed on near the sample as possible and is not dipped into the sample because it might be spoiled due to sticking of the sample to the thermocouple on heating. So actual sample temperature is not recorded, it is the temperature at some point in the furnace near the sample. Thus, it leads to source of error due to the thermal lag and partly due to the finite time taken to cause detectable mass change. If the sensitivity of recording mechanism is not enough to record the mass change of the sample then this will also cause error in recording the weight change of the sample, or product formed or the evolved gases then this will cause error in recording the mass change of the sample.

Sample characteristics

(a) **Weight of sample**: A large sample affects the TG curve and the curve deviates from linearity as the temperature rises. Hence, small size is preferred. If 20 mg of the $CuSO_4.5H_2O$ is used, no plateau corresponding to $CuSO_4.3H_2O$ is obtained, but if only 0.5 mg of sample is used, this plateau can be observed.

(b) **Particle size**, particle size also affects the TG curve. Smaller particles decompose at lower temperature while large particle size sample take larger time and decompose at high temperature. The particle size will cause a change in the diffusion of the evolved gases which will alter the reaction rate and hence, the curve shape. The smaller the particle size, greater the extent of decomposition at any given temperature. The use of large crystals may result in apparent very rapid mass loss during heating. This may be due to the mechanical loss of part of the sample by forcible ejection from the sample container, when the accumulated evolved gases within the coarse grains are suddenly released.

(c) **Sample packing**: A compressed sample decomposes at higher in comparison to loose sample.

(d) **Nature of reaction**: The heat of reaction has affects the difference between sample temperature and furnace temperature, causing the sample temperature to lag or lead the furnace temperature depending on whether the reaction is endothermic or exothermic. When the reaction is endothermic, the effect of temperature lag is to increase furnace temperature and the differential temperature will be additive. But when the reaction is exothermic, this effect will tend to compensate each other.

(e) **Method of sample preparation**: The method of preparation may sometime affect the shape of the TG curve. For example, magnesium hydroxide is naturally occurring and can also be prepared by the precipitation method. It has been found that $Mg(OH)_2$ obtained by both these source have different temperature of decompositions when studied thermo gravimetrically.

2. DIFFERENTIAL THERMOGRAVIMETRIC ANALYSIS (DTGA)

Like TG analysis, the DTGA also involves the measurement of rate of change of weight of the sample on heating at uniform slow heating rate. Sometime it is advantageous to use DTGA because it makes the noticing of small features much easier on the curve. For example, the Fig. 17.10 indicates the comparison between TG and DTGA curves for the pyrolysis of a mixture of calcium and magnesium carbonate. It is evident from the figure that plateau in the TG curve at 700°C is quite clear but the shoulder at 870°C can only be made clear with the help of the DTGA curve. This peak at 870°C cannot be made clear from TG curve.

Application of TGA

1. *Determination of appropriate drying temperature range*: The TGA is widely used in quantitative and qualitative analysis. It indicates the appropriate drying temperature range for the drying the precipitates for conventional gravimetric analysis. The Fig. 17.3 indicates the appropriate drying temperature for calcium oxalate, silver chromate, magnesium oxalate and mercurous chromate as discussed earlier.

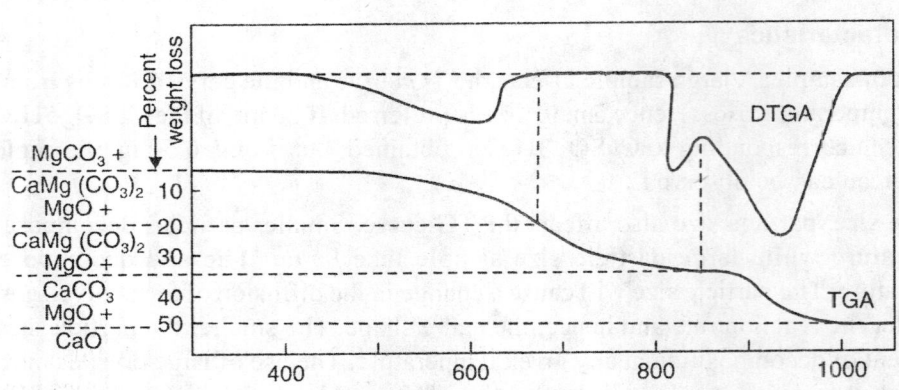

Fig. 17.10. TG/DTG curve for the pyrolysis of $CaCO_3$ and $MgCO_3$.

2. *Characterization of sample compound*: TG may be used to identify and compare samples using TG curve as a fingerprint.
3. *Analysis of inorganic and organic mixtures*: The pure single compound gives characteristic TG curves. On this basis, TGA can be used in predicting relative quantities of the components of a mixture.

For example, consider a mixture of two compounds AB and CD having characteristic TG curves which are different from each other as shown in Fig. 17.11.

The decomposition of pure compound AB and CD occur at T_1, labelled as bc and temperature T_2, and labeled as fg respectively, as illustrated in Fig. 17.1(a). The TG curve of mixture of AB nd CD together is shown in Fig. 17.1 (b). You can see in this figure, the plateaus (corresponding to the regions of constant mass) commence at about the same temperature as they do in the TG curves for the pure compounds AB and CD. You can also noticd that the

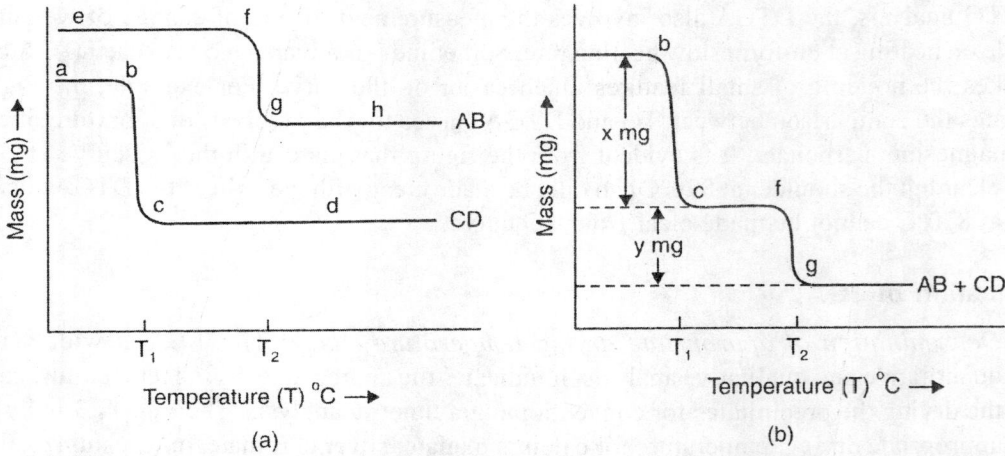

Fig. 17.11. (a) Thermogravimetric curves of two pure compounds AB and CD and (b) Mixture.

mass loss overall up to T_1 is x mg and from T_1 to T_2 it is an additional y mg. By measuring these two quantities of x and y from the TG curves of Fig. 17.11b, the relative quantities of of AB and CD can be determined present in the original binary mixture.

4. *Miscellaneous*: It includes the use of TGA in kinetic studies and surface area measurement.

3. DIFFERENTIAL THERMAL ANALYSIS

Differential thermal analysis (DTA) is a technique in which the temperature of the substance under investigation is compared with the temperature of a thermally inert material such as α-alumina and is recorded with furnace temperature as the substance is heated or cooled at a predetermined uniform rate. The range of temperature measurable in the course of DTA is much larger than TG determination. Thus, during thermogravimetric analysis, pure fusion reactions, crystalline transition, glass transition and crystallization and solid

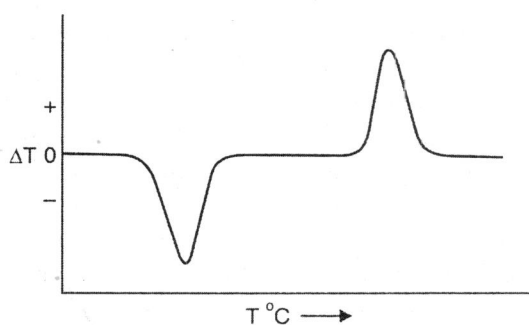

Fig. 17.12. Typical DTA curve.

state reactions without evolution of volatile product are not indicated because they provide no change in mass of the specimen. However, these changes are indicated during DTA by endothermal or exothermal departure from the base line (Fig. 17.12). Since DTA is a dynamic method, it is essential that all aspects of the technique be standardized in order to obtain reproducible results. These include pretreatment of specimen, particle size and packing specimen, dilution of the specimen and nature of the inert diluent.

The principle of method consists of measuring the change in temperature associated with physical or chemical changes during the gradual heating of the substance. Thermal changes due to fusion, crystalline structure inversions, boiling, dissociation or decomposition reactions, oxidation and reduction reactions, destruction of crystalline lattice structure and other chemical reactions are generally accompanied by an appreciable rise or fall in temperature. Hence, all these are accounted in DTA. Generally speaking, phase transitions, dehydration, reduction and some decomposition reactions produce endothermic effects whereas crystallization, oxidation and some decomposition reactions produce exothermic effects.

Characteristics of DTA Curves

An idealized representation of the two major processes observable in DTA is illustrated in Fig. 17.13, where ΔT is plotted on y-axis and T on x-axis. Endotherms are plotted downwards and

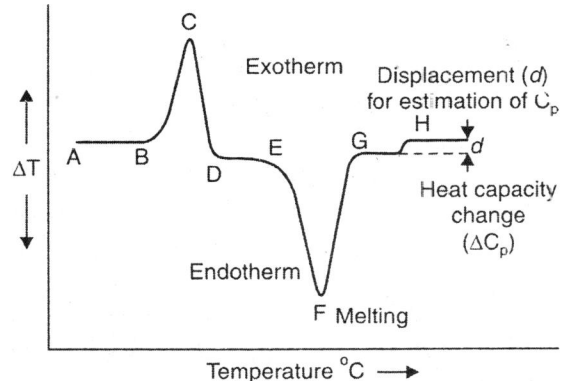

Fig. 17.13. DTA curve showing exotherm, endotherm and base line changes.

exotherms upwards. Similarly, the temperature of the sample is greater for an exothermic reaction, than that of the reference, for endotherms the sample temperature lags behind that of the reference.

When no reaction occurs in the sample material, the temperature of the sample remains similar to that of reference substance. This is because both are being heated exactly under identical condition i.e. temperature difference ΔT ($T_s - T_r$) will be zero for no reaction. But as soon as reaction starts, the sample becomes either hot or cool depending upon whether the reaction is exothermic or endothermic. A peak develops on the curve for the temperature difference ΔT against temperature of furnace or time. Let us consider the DTA curve in Fig. 17.13 again, where ΔT along the line AB is zero indicating no reaction but at B where the curve begins to deviate from the base line corresponds to the onset temperature at which the exothermic reaction starts and give rise to a peak BCD with a maximum at point C. Where rate of heat evolution by the reaction is equal to the difference between the rate of evolution of heat and inert reference material. The peak temperature C corresponds to the maximum rate of heat of evolution. It does not represent the maximum rate of reaction nor the completion of the exothermic process. Thus, the position of C does not have much significance in DTA experiments.

At some determinant point, the heat of evaluation process is completed and after this point heat evaluation goes on decreasing up to D. The usefulness of the method arises from the fact that peak temperature is normally characteristic of the material in the sample. Area of the peak BCD is proportional to the amount of reacting material. For endothermic reaction the peak EFG will be obtained as shown in the idealised curve. The peak shows that the ΔT i.e. ($T_s - T_r$) will be negative because heat is absorbed and consequently T_s will be smaller than T_r. Note the levels of base lines of exotherm curve, AB and DE. Both are at different levels above x-axis. This is due to the fact that heat capacity of sample has changed as a result of the exothermic process. Similar explanation can be given for the difference in levels of base lines of endotherm curve i.e. DE and GH. DTA curves are not only help in the identification of materials but their peak areas provide quantitative information regarding mass of sample (m), heat of reactions (enthalpy change, ΔH) and factors such as sample geometry and thermal conductivity. If latter two factors are expressed by a factor K called calibration factor, then peak area can be expressed as follows.

$$\text{Peak area (A)} = \pm \Delta H \, m \, K \qquad \ldots(17.1)$$

There is positive (+ve) sign for endothermic reaction ($\Delta H > 0$) i.e. when the temperature of the sample will lag behind that of the reference, and negative sign for exothermic reaction ($\Delta H < 0$) the temperature of the sample will exceed that of reference, factor K is called calibration constant which is **temperature dependent**. It can be determined by calibrating DTA with some standard. Once we know the value of K at a particular temperature, the peak area can be used for quantitative analysis to determine the mass of sample of energy (enthalpy changes) of a reaction.

The Fig. 17.14 shows a thermogram for the DTA of calcium oxalate monohydrate indicating also the effect of changing the atmosphere from nitrogen to air. The DTA of the same compound in an atmosphere of air and nitrogen gives three points of weight loss corresponding to the three endothermic processes.

$$CaC_2O_4H_2O \longrightarrow CaC_2O_4 + H_2O$$

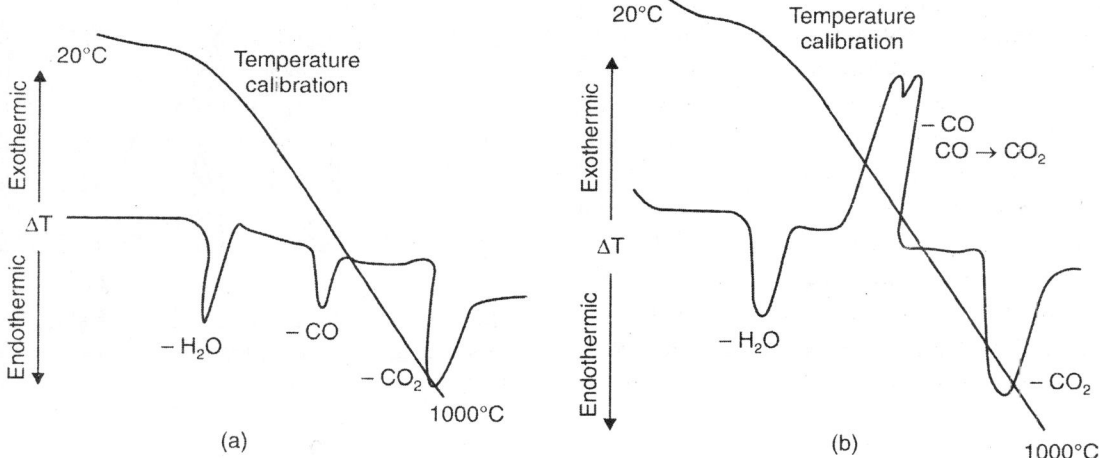

Fig. 17.14. DTA curves of $CaC_2O_4 \cdot H_2O$ showing the effect of changing the atmosphere from (a) nitrogen, (b) air.

$$CaC_2O_4 \longrightarrow CaCO_3 + CO$$
$$CaCO_3 \longrightarrow CaO + CO_2$$

First and third DTA maxima are similar but the second maximum corresponds to the elimination of carbon monoxide at 500°C is sharply exothermic when the atmosphere is air. But both the peaks correspond to same weight loss. The reason for the difference in DTA behaviour is the exothermic burning CO in air at the temperature of the furnace.

Instrumentation

The typical DTA apparatus is shown in Fig. 17.15. It consists of following components:

(i) Furnace or heating device.
(ii) Sample holder.
(iii) Microvolt or millivolt amplifier.
(iv) Furnace temperature control system.
(v) Furnace atmosphere control system.

Furnace contains both the sample and reference which are heated at the same rate. The temperature of the sample and reference are measured respectively by individual thermocouples. A thermogram is then plotted between the difference in temperature of sample and reference versus overall furnace temperature.

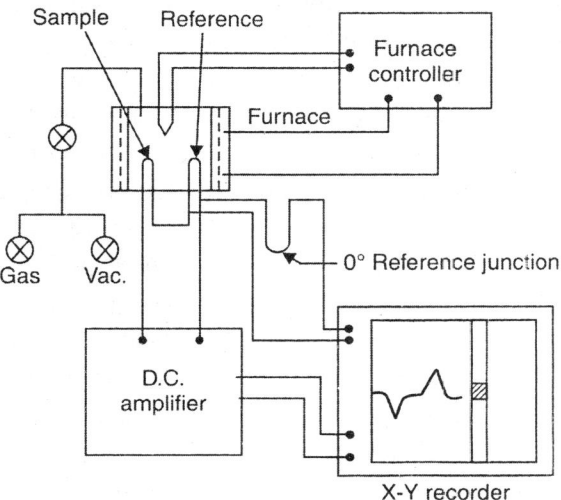

Fig. 17.15. Typical DTA apparatus (schematic).

There are two types of system for keeping the sample and reference in furnace. In the first, the sample and reference substance are heated in the same heating block, Fig. 17.16(a). In the second type of arrangement, the sample and reference pans are separate heating blocks or heat sinks. In this, temperature of block is measured rather than sample itself, Fig. 17.16(b). This type of arrangement is present in calorimeter or buersma DTA instrument. The two variations provide the same data but the latter type is less dependent. On the thermal properties of the sample and has a slower response to thermal change.

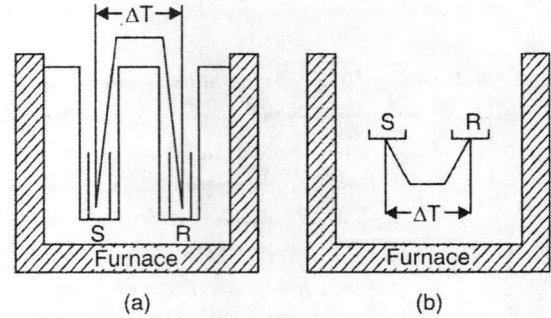

Fig. 17.16. Differential thermal analysis (a) classical apparatus (S sample; R = reference); (b) Calorimetric.

Factors affecting DTA data

DTA is a dynamic temperature technique. Therefore, a large number of factors can affect the resulting experimental curves. Similar to TGA curves, these factors can be divided into the two groups:

(i) Sample factors, and
(ii) Instrumental factors.

The *instrumental factors* includes various factors like size and shape of sample holder, sample holder material, heating rate of the sample, sensitivity of recording system, location of thermocouple in the sample and atmosphere around sample. Most of these factors are associated with instrumental desgn. We have very little control on these factors.

Sample characteristics includes amount of sample, particle size, packing density, heat capacity and thermal conductivity, degree of crystallinity, dilutes of diluents, swelling and shrinkage of the sample. Some of the important factors are given here.

1. **Amount of sample:** In DTA analysis, peak area of DTA curve is proportional to the mass of the sample. Certainly this assumption is valid only over a certain range of amount of the sample. Generally in DTA experiments, a few mg of powdered solid sample is used.

2. **Particle size:** In DTA experiments, samples in the form of fine powers are generally preferred except polymers, in which case we might have to use plastic fragments or chopped fibers. The sample should have similar particle size for comparison purpose.

3. **Sample packing:** Packing density of sample influences the shape of DTA curve. Tight packing influences the escape of volatiles and interaction of sample with atmosphere of furnace due to thermal experiments. Therefore, a reproducible method of packing the sample is desirable.

4. **Heating rate:** It is observed that an increase in heating rate increases, the procedural peak temperature, and some time it also increases peak area. Often high heating rate results in poor resolution of fine peak in DTA curve. Therefore slower heating rate is preferred for DTA experiments. Heating rate of 10°C min^{-1} and 5°C min^{-1} are commonly preferred.

5. **Atmosphere around sample:** Similar to DTG, a flowing gas is preferable to a static atmosphere as in static atmosphere. There is a possibility of change of atmosphere around sample on its degradation or decomposition especially in case of a volatile sample. In such a case we generally use flowing gas technique. Flowing gas sweeps away volatile by products and keeps homogenous atmosphere around sample. In Table 17.2, we have summarized the major factor which can affect the DTA curve.

Table 17.2. Factors that influence DTA curve

Factor	Effect	Suggestions
1. Heating rate	Change in peak size and position	Use a low heating rate
2. Location of thermocouple location	Irreproducible curve	Standardise thermocouple
3. Atmosphere around sample	Change in the curve	Inert gas should be allowed to flow
4. Amount of sample	Change in peak size and position	Standardise sample mass
5. Particle size of sample	Irreproducible curves	Use small, uniform particle size
6. Packing density	Irreproducible curves	Standardise packing technique
7. Sample container	Change in peak	Standardise container

Application of DTA

The Fig. 17.13 illustrate the DTA curves, provided with exotherms and endotherms. These endotherm and exotherms are unique to particular sample composition. Thus, pattern of thermogram can be used a fingerprint for qualitative analysis while area under the curve may be used for quantitative analysis. This principle can be applied for the analysis of mineral, inorganic compounds, foodstuff and biological specimen.

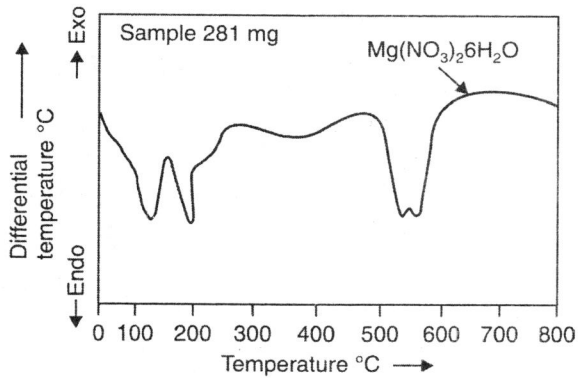

Fig. 17.17. DTA curve of $Mg(NO_3)_2.6H_2O$.

DTA curve can be used to identify the polymer, fats, oil, amino acid, carbohydrates, etc. by studying the melting characteristic of a specimen. The Fig. 17.17 illustrates a complex behaviour for an inorganic compound and Fig. 17.18, the characterization of starch in foodstuff. Application in polymer analysis is illustrated in Fig. 17.19 and 17.20. The first one shows schematically the typical thermal processes which occur on heating a polymer. The latter an analysis of a seven components mixture based upon melting point. The Fig. 17.20 is differential thermal curve of seven components polymeric mixture for their melting points: Polytetrafloroethylene (PTFE), High Pressure (high density) Polypropylene (HPPE), Low Density Polypropylene (LPPE), Polypropylene (PP), Polypropylene POM, Nylon 6, Nylon 66. It shows characteristics peaks of all the polymers and hence confirm the presence of individual polymers in the analyzed sample. The

302 Pharmaceutical Analysis

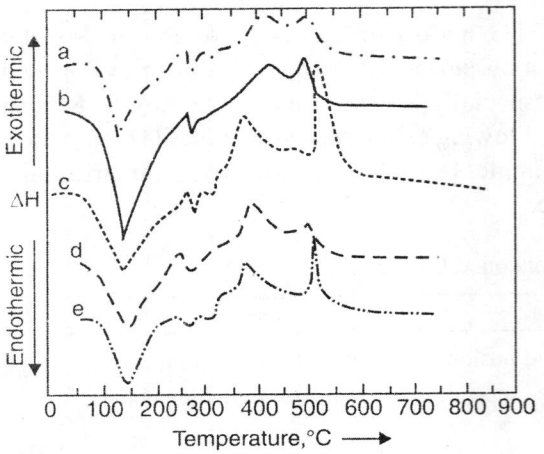

Fig. 17.18. DTA curves of potato and corn starch (a) potato starch, (b) potato starch duplicate run, (c) corn starch, (d) methanol extracted corn starch, (e) ammonia pregelatinized corn starch.

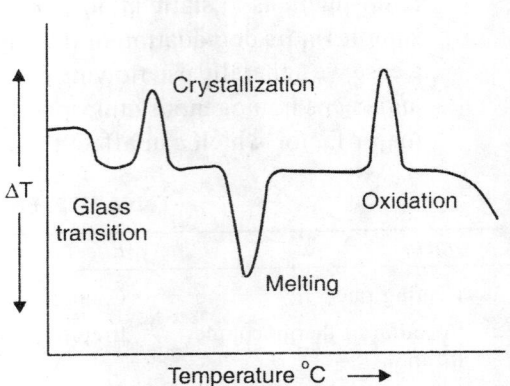

Fig. 17.19. DTA curve of a typical polymeric sample.

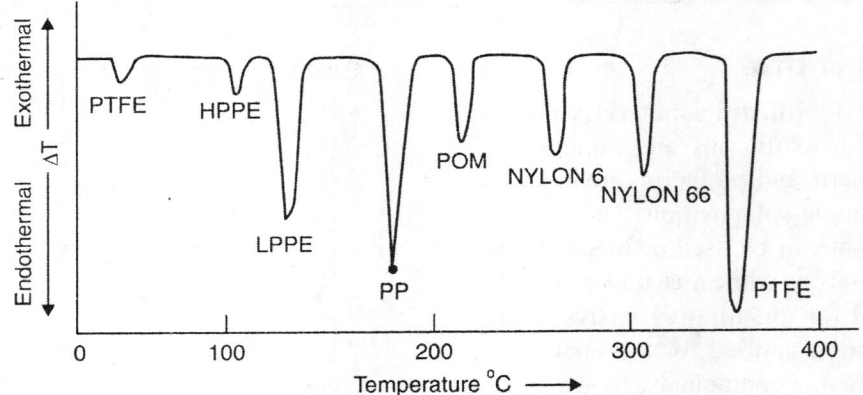

Fig. 17.20. DTA curve of a typical polymeric mixture.

area under the peak is related to the heat of reaction and related to the quantity of material present in the mixture.

4. DIFFERENTIAL SCANNING'S CALORIMETRY

Differential scanning calorimetry (DSC) is a similar technique like DTA but work on different principle. The data obtained in both the technique is similar in nature. In principle like DTA, DSC involves the heating of sample and inert reference in parallel with the help of separate heating device. The heaters are programmed to ensure that the temperatures of both sample and reference advance at exactly the same rate. On heating, when endotherms or exotherm occurs in the sample, the power of the heater is varied in order to maintain the temperatures difference (ΔT) = 0 (Fig.

Thermoanalytical Methods 303

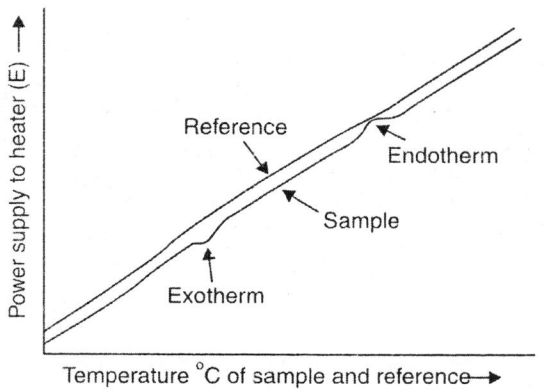

Fig. 17.21. Schematic representation of the variation of power supply to the sample and reference in DSC.

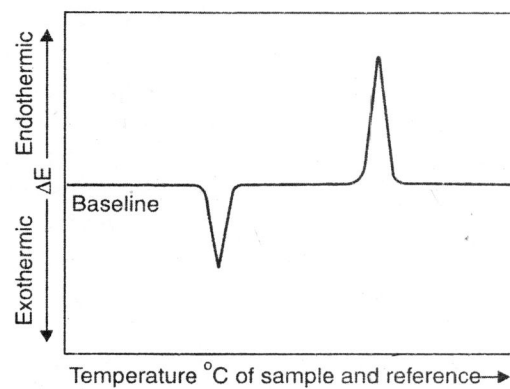

Fig. 17.22. A typical DSC curve.

17.21). Thus by monitoring the difference in power supplied to the heaters (ΔE), the thermal change in the sample may be followed. The Fig. 17.22 illustrates a typical DSC curve which indicates that measurement of ΔE is effectively a direct measurement of energy change in the sample.

Instrumentation

The instrument for power compensated DSC consists of two parallel temperature measurement systems. Sample (about 50 mg) and reference in small pans are placed on the separates heating blocks (Fig. 17.23). Each heating block is provided with separates heater and thermocouple connected

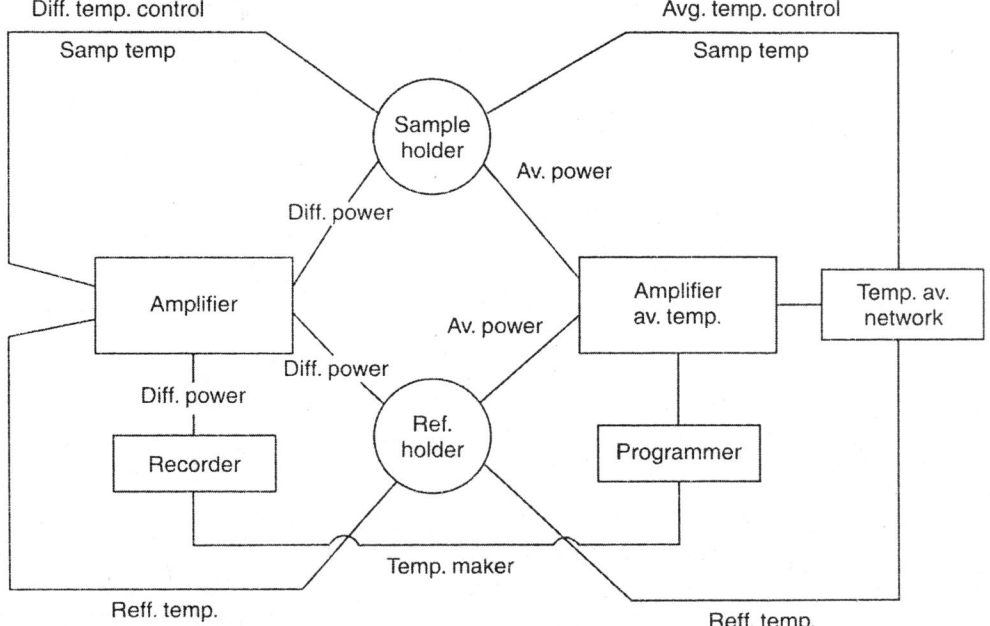

Fig. 17.23. Block diagram of a DSC instrument.

to heater so that power supply can be varied to ensure the temperature difference $\Delta T = 0$ at all times on increasing the temperature. A DSC curve is than generated by monitoring the difference in power supplied to the two heaters (ΔE) and plotting this against the overall temperature (Fig. 17.24). Analytical data is presented in a sample form on a chart recorder but microcomputers or microprocessors are used to provide flexibility in data presentation. There is in built system to control the atmosphere of the sample. For heat flux, the sample and reference are placed in a separate sample container on separate platforms, kept on heated metal (Cu/Ni alloy) disc. Thermocouples are placed to monitor the heat flow from the disc to the sample and standard. The differential heat flow will then reflect the different thermal behaviour of the sample and standard. A plot of this against overall temperature produces a graph analogous to those from power compensated DSC. Calibration is done with the use of standard (like indium) with known thermal characterization.

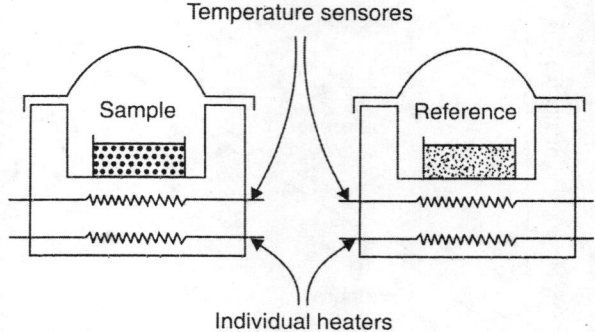

Fig. 17.24. Heating arrangement in DSC instrument.

Factors affecting DSC curve

There are many factors which influence a DSC curve. These factors may be due to instrumentation or nature of sample. We have listed the main factors which affect the shape, precision and accuracy of the experimental results:

1. *Instrumental factors*:
    (a) Furnace heating rate
    (b) Recording or chart speed
    (c) Furnace atmosphere
    (d) Geometry of sample holder/location of sensors
    (e) Sensitivity of recording mechanism
    (f) Composition of sample container
2. *Sample characteristics*:
    (a) Amount of sample
    (b) Solubility of evolved gases in sample
    (c) Particle size
    (d) Heat of reaction
    (e) Sample packing
    (f) Nature of sample
    (g) Thermal conductivity

Some of these factors, we have are already described above under DTA technique.

Advantages of DSC

1. Small sample size 1 to 10 mg.
2. Simple and rapid procedure of analysis, typically 15 to 30 min per determination.
3. Ideal for comparison of sample purity for example in quality control.
4. Does not require high absolute temperature accuracy (in contrast with melting point depression method).
5. Does not require calibration with known impurity levels, cryoscopic constant is obtained simultaneously.

Application of DSC

The DTA and DSC provide similar in applications but DSC generally has better resolution. The example DTA/DSC of $CuSO_4.5H_2O$ shows the superiority of DSC (Fig. 17.25). Peak areas are more accurate and temperature ramp is less disturbed by thermal events in the sample (e.g. difference in specific heats and thermal conductivities between the sample and reference). In the curve below, the peaks correspond to loss of two, two and finally one molecule of water.

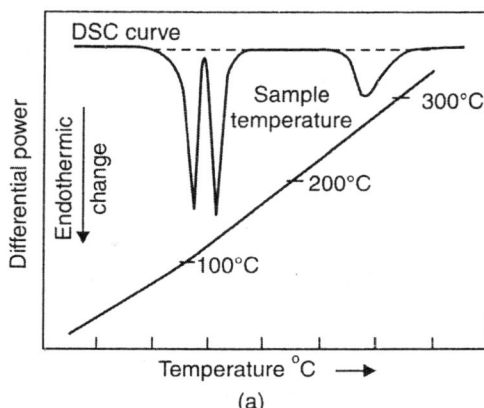

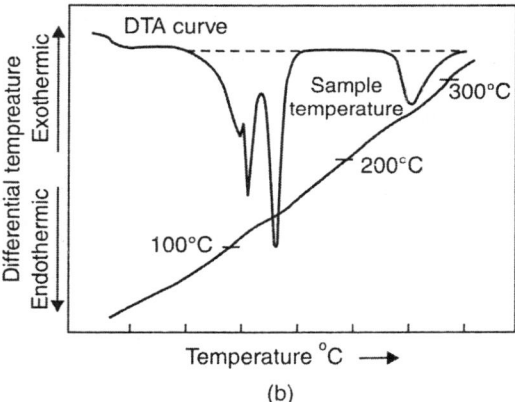

Fig. 17.25. DTA and DSC curve of $CuSO_4.5H_2O$.

Some of the prominent uses of DSC are given here.

1. DSC is commonly used to measure melting temperature of crystalline solid.
2. DSC is commonly used to measure the heat of fusion of a crystalline solid. Heat of fusion is an integrated area under melting curve.
3. DSC is used to determine solubility of crystalline small molecule in polymer.
4. DSC is used to identify the polymorphs as different polymorphs usually have different **melting temperatures** and **heat of fusions**.
5. DSC can be used to determine percent purity. The melting of a pure material takes place over an infinitely narrow temperature range. The result is a sharp melting spike on a DSC curve at a temperature characteristic of that material. For a material that only has a small amount of impurity (that dissolves in the melt, but not in the solid) the melting point is depressed and the melting range is broadened. This is the basis of the calorimetric purity determination by observed melting point depression. The Fig. 17.26 shows the melting endotherms of phenacetin (p-acetophenetidide) at three levels of impurity (99.97, 99.5 and

99.0%). The Fig. 17.26 indicates the broadening of peak due to increase in impurity level. The thermodynamic relationship for determination of percent purity is described by simplified van't Hoff law.

$$T_m = T_0 - \frac{RT_0^2}{\Delta H_0} X^2$$

where T_0 is the melting point of the pure substance, T_m is the sample temperature at equilibrium, X^2 is the mole fraction of impurity in the liquid base. ΔH_0 is the heat of fusion of pure substance and R is gas constant (1.9872 cal mol^{-1} deg^{-1}. The DSC technique can determine the extent of impurity to within 5 to 10 percent.

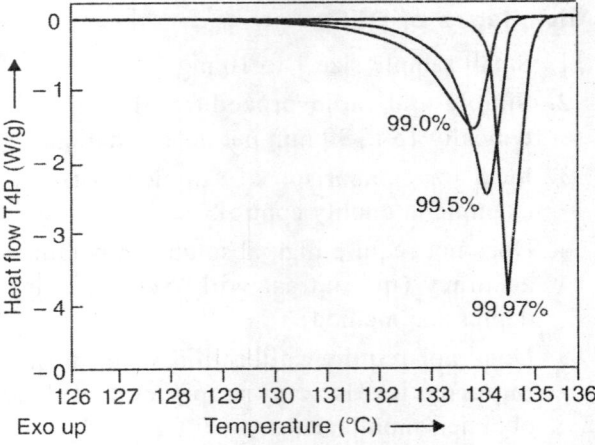

Fig. 17.26. DSC melting curves of phenacetin at three purity level.

5. THERMOMETRIC TITRATIONS

Thermochemistry is a branch of physical chemistry that deals with the heat changes during the chemical reactions. All the reactants possess certain amount of energy. The total energy content of reaction products therefore will be different from total sum energy of the reactants. The difference in energy is either evolved (exothermic reaction) or absorbed (endothermic reaction) as heat. In thermometric titration heat changes is measured during the course of titration. For example, when a solution of hydrochloric acid is added from a burette in thermostatic condition into a solution of NaOH present in thermostatically controlled flask, the neutralization reaction takes place.

$$HCl(aq) + NaOH(aq) \longrightarrow NaCl(aq) + H_2O$$

During neutralization, heat of neutralization is liberated (also called heat of reaction, $-\Delta H$). This liberated heat is measured with the help of calibrated thermocouple. Then graph of solution temperature versus volume of HCl added is plotted as shown in Fig. 17.27. The sharp break in the curve indicates the end points. Dielectric constant of the solvents does not affect the thermometric titration. It can therefore be performed in non-aqueous solvents as well.

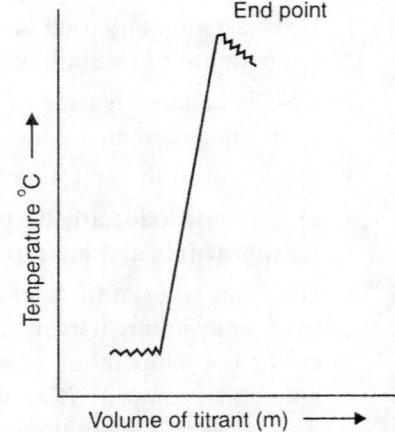

Fig. 17.27. Typical thermometric curve.

Apparatus for thermometric titrations

The essential parts of the apparatus (Fig. 17.28) are:
1. Motor driven burette.
2. Thermally insulated beaker or Dewar flask.

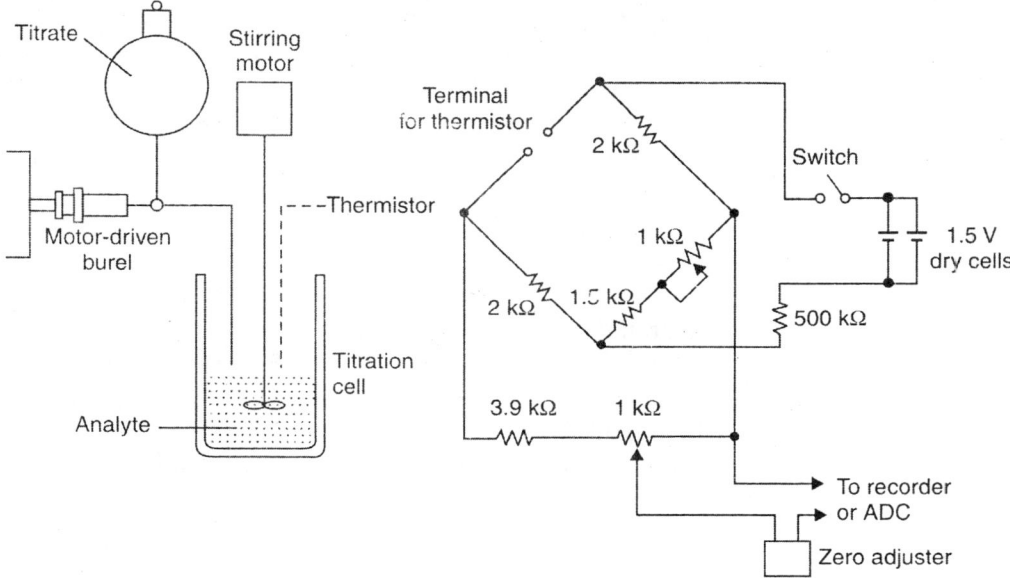

Fig. 17.28. Schematic layout for thermometric titration assembly and bridge circuit.

3. Thermister bridge assembly for measuring the temperature changes.
4. Recorder.

Technique of thermometric titration

The technique is simple in operation. It is illustrated with the titration of hydrochloric acid solution with standard NaOH solution.

1. Transfer 50 ml of sodium hydroxide solution to a polystyrene cup. Allow it to stand for a few minutes, then record the temperature of the solution.
2. Add 5.0 ml of hydrochloric acid from a burette to the cup. Immediately stir the mixture with the thermometer and record its temperature. Repeat until a total of 50.0 ml of acid is added. Record the result in data table.

Note: The concentration of HCl is maintained higher in comparison to NaOH in order to minimise the error due to change in volume.

Data table. Titration of acid with NaOH solution

Volume added ($\pm$ 0.01 ml)	0	5	10	15	20	25	30	35	40	45	50
Temperature ($\pm$ 0.5°C)	–	–	–	–	–	–	–	–	–	–	–

3. Plot a graph of temperature (vertical axis) against total volume of acid added (horizontal axis).
4. Draw straight lines of best fit and extend them until they cross (Fig. 17.29). The point at

which the two lines meet corresponds to the volume of acid needed for neutralisation and to the maximum temperature.

Application of thermometric titration

Thermometric titration is suitable for such titration where the end point is obscured due to presence of coloured solution or poisoning of electrodes. A large number of volumetric titrations e.g. neutralization, precipitation, redox, and complexation, etc. can be carried out by thermometric method. Determination of the end point in this method depends upon the free energy change ΔG, hence at equilibrium constant of reaction, the quantity measured is ΔH, not ΔG as in the familiar thermodynamic equation:

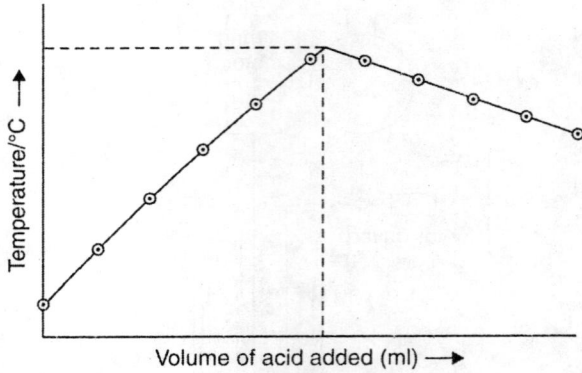

Fig. 17.29. Titration of HCl with NaOH solution.

$$\Delta H = \Delta G + T\Delta S$$

Hence, it is possible that thermometric may give useful result even if DG is zero or positive.

(a) **Acid base titration:** A large number of acid and base can be titrated by using this technique some of which are given below:

| NaOH vs. HCl, | H_3PO_4 vs. NaOH, | Alanine vs. NaOH |
| NH_3 vs. HCl | C_6H_5N vs. HCl, | Glutaric acid vs. NaOH |

The most important limitations of thermometric titration are due to the fact that level of neutralization of various acids differs by only 50% or less.

(b) **Precipitation:** Thermometric titration can also be done successfully with the formation of slightly soluble substance, XY as given here.

$$X^+ \text{ (aq.)} + Y^- \text{ (aq.)} \longrightarrow XY \text{ (s)} \pm \Delta H$$

The heat of reaction, ΔH evolved or absorbed in the above reaction is of enough magnitude to give a suitable curve. Some of the compounds which can be determined are given below.

$$Ca^{2+} + (NH_4)C_2O_4 \longrightarrow CaC_2O_4\downarrow + 2NH_4^+$$
$$Ag^+ + HCl \longrightarrow AgCl\downarrow + H^+$$
$$Hg^+ + 2KI \longrightarrow HgI_2\downarrow + 2K^+$$
$$Ni + 2KCN \longrightarrow Ni(CN)_2\downarrow + 2K^+$$

(c) **Complexometric titrations:** Thermometric titration can be done to form the complex, for example, $Pb^+, Cd^+, Ni^{2+}, Ca^{2+}, Zn^{2+}, Co^{2+}$ and Mg^{2+}, can be titrated separately against standard EDTA solution, where by a complex of the form $M(EDTA)^{2-}$ is formed where M = Pb, Cd, Cu, Ni, Ca, Zn, Co, Mg etc.

Analysis of mixtures is possible when the two species have different equilibrium constants and heats of reactions with the titrant. For example, in the titration of mixture of calcium and magnesium with EDTA. Calcium ($Kf = 10^{11}$) reacts first and exothermally ($\Delta H = -5.7$ kcal/mole) and then magnesium ($Kf = 10^{9.1}$) reacts endothermally ($\Delta H = 5.5$ kcal/mole) as illustrated in Fig. 17.30.

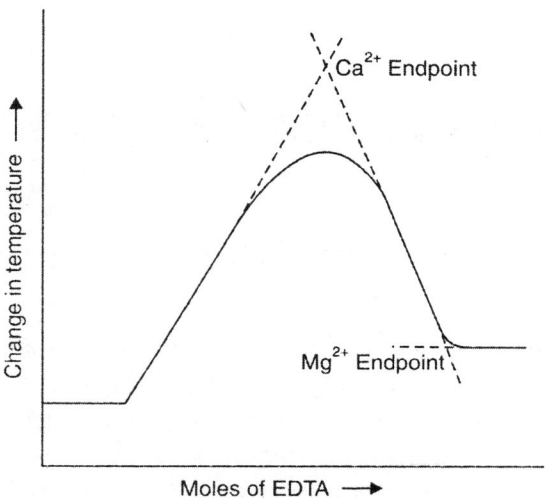

Fig. 17.30. Typical curve for thermometric titration of a mixture of Ca^{2+} and Mg^{2+} with EDTA.

(D) **Redox titration:** Very little work has been done on redox titration. Some of the redox reactions e.g. oxidation of Fe^{2+} ion, potassium ferro cyanide ion, titanium (III) ion, and H_2O_2 by ceric (Ce^{4+}) ion, the oxidation of oxalic acid and Ferro cyanide ion by permangnate ion has been studied.

CHAPTER 18

Electron Spin Resonance (ESR) Spectroscopy

Introduction

Electron Spin Resonance (ESR) spectroscopy, invented by Zavoiskii in 1944, is similar to NMR spectroscopy, ESR spectroscopy is an absorption spectroscopy which involves the study of spin changes at the electron level when a microwave frequency (10^4–10^6 MHz) is absorbed in the presence of a magnetic field. The substance with one or more unpaired electrons are paramagnetic and exhibit ESR. Thus ESR spectroscopy is also called by other names such as **electron paramagnetic resonance (EPR) spectroscopy** and **electron magnetic resonance (EMR) spectroscopy**.

The systems which can be investigated by ESR spectroscopy are organic or inorganic free radicals and ions of transition metals which contain unpaired d and f orbital electrons. One of the most important uses of ESR technique is detection of extremely short-lived (transient) free radical intermediates in chemical reactions.

Substances containing unpaired electrons, i.e. paramagnetic are of two types:

(i) **Stable paramagnetic substances:** These include simple molecules like NO, O_2, NO_2 and the ions of transition metals and their complexes, e.g. Fe^{3+}, $[Fe(CN)_6]^{3-}$ etc.

(ii) **Unstable paramagnetic substances:** These are generally called free radical ions and are formed either as intermediates in chemical reactions or by irradiation of a stable molecule with UV or X-ray radiation or with a beam of nuclear particles. If the life times of such radicals are greater than 10^{-6} s, they may be studied by ESR spectroscopy. Paramagnetic substances with life time shorter than 10^{-6} s may also be studied by ESR spectroscopy if they are produced at low temperatures in the solid state, called matrix technique, as this increases their life times.

Theory of ESR Spectroscopy

The theory of ESR is similar to NMR, except that electron spin is involved in ESR instead of nuclear spin which is involved in NMR. In ESR, the energy levels are produced by the interaction of the magnetic moment of an unpaired electron in a molecular ion with an applied magnetic field.

The ESR spectrum results due to the transitions between these energy levels by absorbing radiations of microwave frequency.

An unpaired electron has a spin and this spin has an associated magnetic moment. An electron of spin S = 1/2 can have the spin angular momentum quantum number values of Ms = ± 1/2. In the absence of applied magnetic field, the two values of Ms, i.e. +1/2 and −1/2 will give rise to a doubly degeneracy spin energy state (two spin energy states with same energy).

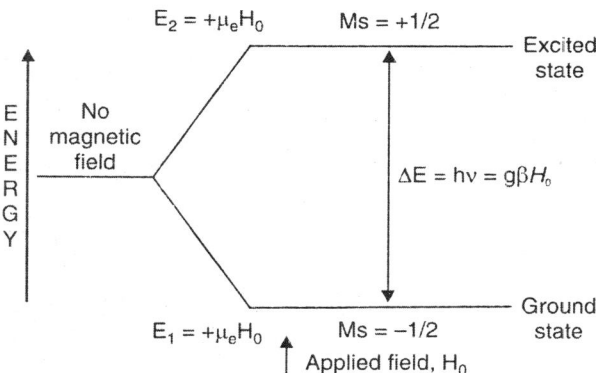

Fig. 18.1. Energy states.

When a magnetic field is applied, this degeneracy disappears and two non-degenerate spin energy states result. The low energy state (more stable) has the spin magnetic moment aligned with the applied magnetic field and corresponds to the quantum number Ms = −1/2. On the other hand the high energy state (less stable) will have the spin magnetic moment opposed to the field and correspond to the quantum number, Ms = +1/2. These energy states are illustrated in Fig. 18.1.

These two states will possess energies that are split up from the original state with no applied magnetic field by the amount $-\mu_e H_0$ and $+\mu_e H_0$ for the low energy and high energy states, respectively; here μ_e is the magnetic moment of the spinning electron and H_0 is the applied field acting on the unpaired electrons.

In ESR, a transition between the two different energy levels takes place by absorption of a quantum of radiation of appropriate frequency in the microwave region. When the absorption takes place the following relation holds good.

$$2\mu_e H_0 = h\nu = \Delta E$$

where $2\mu_e H_0$ is the difference between the two electron spin energy states (Fig. 18.1).

$$\mu_e H_0 - (-\mu_e H_0) = 2\mu_e H_0$$

The energy of transition ΔE in substances containing and unpaired electron is more accurately given by the relation.

$$\Delta E = h\nu = g\beta H_0 \qquad \qquad ...(18.1)$$

where h is the Plank's constant, ν is the frequency in cycles per sec., β the Bohr's magneton which is a factor for converting angular momentum into magnetic moment and spectroscopy splitting factor or lande splitting factor.

The value of β is defined as

$$\beta = \frac{eh}{4\pi mc} = 0.9723 \times 10^{-20} \text{ erg/gauss} \qquad \qquad ...(18.2)$$

where e is the electronic charge, m is mass of electron and c the velocity of light.

The value of g is not constant but it is a tensor quantity. For a free electron its value is 2.0023. All free radicals and some ionic crystals have almost the same g value, i.e. 2.0023 with a variation of ± 0.003 from this value.

The value of g depends on the orientation of the molecule containing the unpaired electron with respect to the applied magnetic field. It also depends upon the physical state of the sample i.e. gas, liquid or solid.

In gas and liquid states, the value of g is averaged over all orientation. However, in case of a paramagnetic ion or radical situated in a perfectly cubic crystal site the value of g does not depend upon the orientation of the crystal. But a paramagnetic ion or radical situated in a crystal of low symmetry depends upon the orientation of the crystal.

In case of a tetragonal site, the values of g_x and g_y are equal and referred to as g-perpendicular, when the external magnetic field is perpendicular to z-axis. The value of g_z is obtained when the magnetic field is parallel to z-axis. The value of g_z is denoted by g-parallel.

ESR Absorption Positions: the g factor

Equation 18.1 shows that an ESR absorption will occur at a Frequency $\nu = \Delta E/h$ Hz. Thus the position of ESR absorption may be expressed in terms of absorption frequency. The absorption position varies with the applied field H_0.

Thus the ESR absorption position can be expressed in terms of the observed g values.

$$G = \Delta E/\beta H_0 = h\nu/\beta H_0$$

For measuring the g values of free radical it is convenient to measure the field separation between the center of the spectrum of the unknown sample and that of a reference substance whose g value is accurately known.

The most widely used reference is 1,1-diphenyl-2-picryl hydrazyl free radical (DPPH) which is completely in free radical state and its g value is 2.0036. The reference substance is placed along with the unknown in the same dual resonant cavity.

DPPH

The g factor for unknown sample is given by:

$$G = g_{ref}(1 - \Delta H_0/H)$$

where g_{ref} is the g factor for the reference, H is the resonance frequency. ΔH_0 is positive if the unknown has its center at a higher field than the reference.

Instrumentation

The description of various components of the ESR spectroscopy instrument is given as follows.

(i) Microwave radiation source

(a) **Klystron valve** is a powerful source of microwave radiation of a small frequency range. For free radical study Klystron 3 cm wavelength is normally operated in the microwave region

(b) **Isolator** is a strip of ferrite material. It minimizes variations in the frequency of microwaves produced by Klystron. The variations in frequency are caused by the back-ward reflections in the regions between the klystron and the circulator.

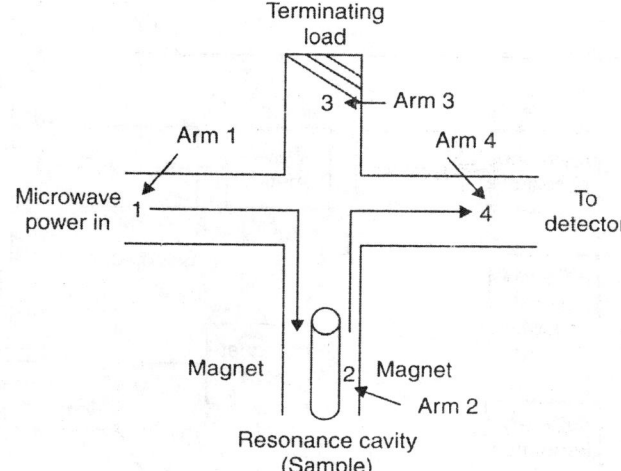

Fig. 18.2. A four port microwave circulator.

(c) **Wavemeter** is put in-between the isolator and attenuator to know the frequency of microwave produced by the klystron.

(d) **Attenuator** is put in between the wave meter and circulator. It is similar to a filter in a spectrophoto-meter. It adjusts the level of the microwave power incident upon the sample.

(ii) Microwave bridge (Circular-T or Magic-T)

From the attenuator, the microwave radiations enter the microwave circulator. Fig. 18.2 indicates the operation of a four-port circulator which works as a balanced bridge with all the advantages of null method in electrical circuits. The microwave radiations enter through arm 1, then enter into arm 2, attached to resonant cavity which contains the sample. Arm 3, which has a balancing load, absorbs any power reflected from the detector arm 4 which is connected to the detector. The microwave circulator does not allow the microwave power to pass in a straight line from one arm to the opposite arm.

(iii) The resonant cavity (sample cavity)

The resonant cavity containing the sample is the heart of an ESR spectrometer. The cavity system is constructed in such a way to maximize the applied magnetic field along the sample dimension. A sample volume of 0.15 to 0.5 ml can be used which do not possess high dielectric constant. Flat cells with a thickness of 0.25 mm and sample volume of 0.05 ml are generally used for samples having high dielectric constant. For studying anisotropic effects in single crystal and in solid samples, rotatable cavities are generally used.

(iv) Magnet system

It consists of an electromagnet which provides a homogeneous magnetic field. The strength of

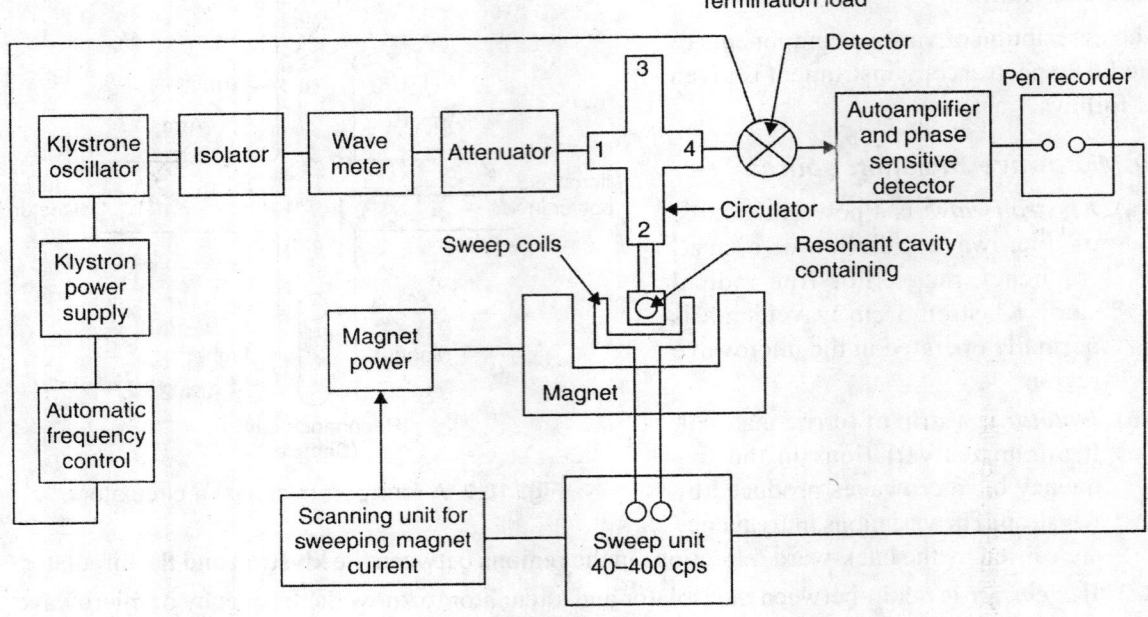

Fig. 18.3.

magnetic field can be varied (swept) over a small range (zero to 500) by varying the current in a pair of sweep coils. The resonant cavity is placed between the pole pieces of electromagnet. The stability of field is achieved by energizing the magnet with a highly regulated power supply. The stability of 1 part in 10^6 is satisfactory for samples whose g-factor ranges from 1.5 to 6.

(v) Crystal detectors

The most commonly used detector is a semiconducting silicone-tungsten crystal which acts as a microwave rectifier and converts the microwave power into a direct current output.

(vi) Autoamplifier and phase sensitive detector

The signal received from the detector undergoes narrow-band amplification by the operation of autoamplifier. This amplified signal contains a lot of noise. The operation of the phase sensitive detector reduces noise by rejecting all the noise components except those in a very narrow band.

(vii) Recorder

Finally, the signal from phase sensitive detector and sweep unit is recorded by the oscilloscope or pen-recorder.

Working

(i) The sample is placed in the resonant cavity. The cavity serves as a long path-length cell in which the waves are reflected to and fro for thousands of times.

(ii) The microwaves produced by the Klystron oscillator pass through the isolator, wavemeter and attenuator, and then they are received by the circular through arm 1.

(iii) The microwave power entering arm 1 is divided between arms 2 and 3.

(iv) If the impedance of arms 2 and 3 are the same, then the circulator is balanced and no power will be received by detector through arm 4.

(v) If the impedance of arm 2 changes because of some ESR absorption by a sample, then bridge becomes unbalanced and some microwave power will enter into the detector.

(vi) The detector acts as rectifier and converts microwave power into direct current.

Presentation of the ESR spectrum

Derivative curve is used instead of an absorption curve, to get more information. The results represented by derivative curves in ESR can be readily interpreted. Each negative slope in the derivative curve represents a peak or shoulder in the absorption spectrum. Every crossing of the derivative axis with a negative slope indicates a true maximum whereas a crossing with positive slope indicates a minimum.

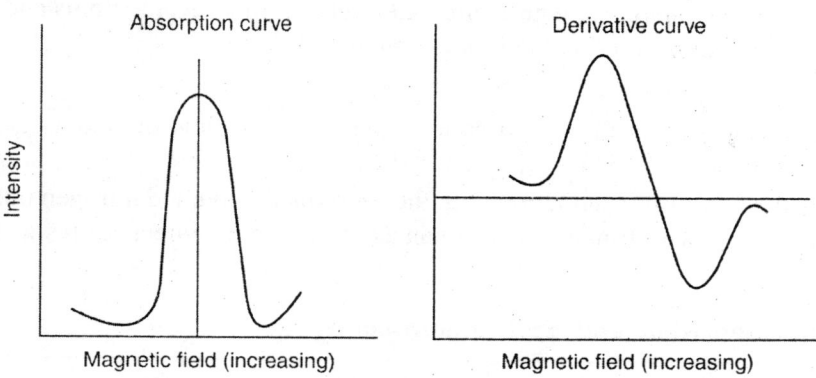

Fig. 18.4.

Choice of solvents

Water, alcohol and other high dielectric constant solvents are not used because they strongly absorbs microwave radiation. However these solvents can be used for a sample which has strong absorbance.

Hyperfine splitting (H_{hfs})

The ESR spectrum exhibits hyperfine splitting which is caused by the interaction between the spinning electrons and adjacent spinning magnetic nuclei. When a single electron interacts with one nucleus, the number of splitting will be equal to $2I + 1$, where I is the spin quantum number of the nucleus. In general, if a single electron interacts magnetically with n equivalent nuclei, the electron signal is split up in to a $(2nI + 1)$ multiplet.

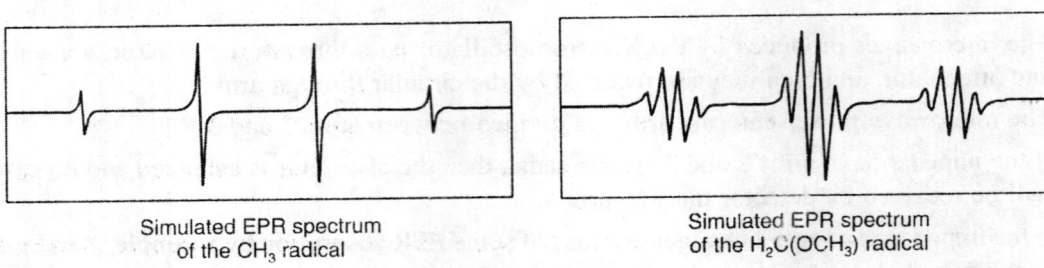

Simulated EPR spectrum of the CH₃ radical   Simulated EPR spectrum of the H₂C(OCH₃) radical

Fig. 18.5.

For example, when the electronic spin of a transition metal or a free radical interacts with its own nuclear spin (S) the hyperfine interaction is described by the Hamiltonian term:

$$H_{hfs} = A\text{I.S} \qquad \ldots 18.1$$

A is the coupling constant.

The hyperfine coupling constant varies with the nuclear species, and it is a measure of the strength of the interaction between the nuclear and electronic spins. The Fig. 18.5 illustrates well the phenomenon: the hyperfine interaction between the electronic spins.

In the molecules, the unpaired electron circulates between the several atoms and the resulting hyperfine structure is the result of a Hamiltonian term of the form:

$$H_{hfs} = \Sigma A_i m_i \qquad = 18.2$$

where the projection m_i of the ith nuclear spin on the magnetic field direction may take on the following $2Ii + 1$ values: $Ii, I_i -1, I_i - 2, \ldots, 1 - Ii, - Ii$.

For example, the hyperfine interaction with the two equally coupled nitrogen nuclei (I = 1) in DPPH molecule leads to a splitting of the resonance into five components of respective intensity 1:2:3:2:1.

Comparison between NMR and ESR spectroscopy

NMR spectroscopy	*ESR spectroscopy*
1. Different energy states are produced relative to the applied magnetic field and a transition between these energy states occurs on the application of an appropriate frequency in the radiofrequency region	1. Different energy states are produced relative to the applied magnetic field and a transition between these energy states occurs on the application of an appropriate frequency in the microwave region
2. NMR absorption positions are expressed in terms of chemical shifts	2. ESR absorption position are expressed in terms of g values
3. Nuclear spin-spin coupling causes the splitting of NMR signals	3. Coupling of the electronic spin with nuclear spins (hyperfine coupling) causes the splitting of ESR signals

Application of ESR Spectroscopy

ESR spectroscopy is useful in the study of chemical, photochemical and electrochemical reaction which proceeds through free radical mechanism.

(i) Study of free radicals

ESR spectroscopy is used to detect the presence of the radicals and to determine their concentration. The method is very sensitive than NMR.

For example, in the oxidation of Hydroquinone in alkaline solution by oxygen, the formation of semiquinone free radical has been proved by ESR.

(ii) Effect of ionizing radiations on matter

ESR spectroscopy is used for the study of the effects of radiation on polymers. For example, polyethylene, on irradiation with γ-rays, exhibits a seven line pattern in its ESR spectrum indicating the formation of the following free radical:

$$—H_2C—\overset{\bullet}{\underset{\underset{|}{CH_2}}{C}}—CH_2—$$

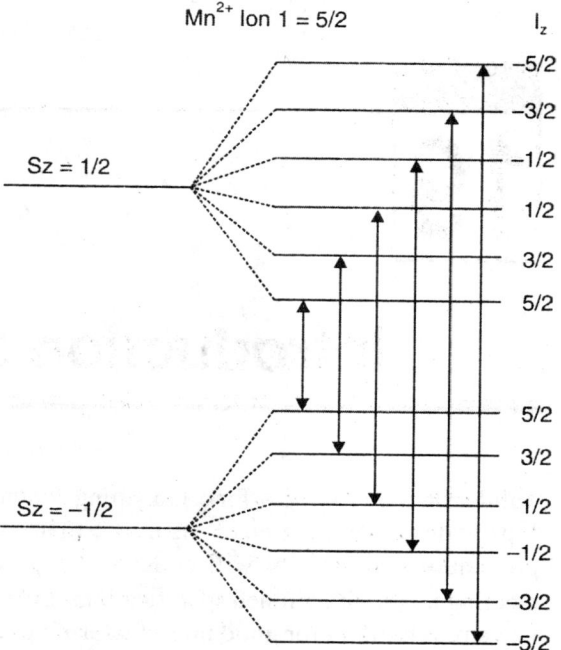

Fig. 18.6. Splitting of the ESR line in Mn^{2+} ion due to hyperfine interaction.

(iii) Analytical applications

ESR spectroscopy is used for the determination of various transition metal ions like Mn^{2+}, V^{4+}, Cu^{2+}, Cr^{3+}, Fe^{3+}, Ti^{3+} etc. For example, the ESR spectrum of a solution of Mn^{2+} ions exhibits six lines. The multiplicity is given by $2I + 1$, i.e. $2 \times 5/2 + 1 = 6$, where I for Mn^{2+} ions is $5/2$.

ESR technique is also used for the estimation of polynuclear hydrocarbons.

(iv) Biological applications

Some examples of biological applications of ESR spectroscopy:
1. ESR spectroscopy has demonstrated the presence of free radicals in healthy and diseased tissue.
2. ESR studies of leaves, seeds and tissue preparations revealed that there is correlation between the concentration of free radicals and the metabolic activity of the material.
3. ESR studies have shown that most of the enzymes function via one-electron redox reactions involving the production of enzyme-bound free radical.
4. ESR studies on photosynthesis can be performed with photosynthesis bacteria.

(v) Miscellaneous application

ESR spectroscopy confirms that electrons in impurities (donor) are responsible for conducting properties of semiconductor.

It has been also used to detect conduction electrons in solution of alkali metals in liquid ammonia, alkaline earth metals, alloys etc.

CHAPTER 19

Introduction to Validation Process

Validation is a procedure for establishing documented evidence. It provides a high degree of assurance that a specific process, procedure and activity will consistently produce a product, meeting its pre-determined specifications and quality attributes. It is a requirement for good manufacturing practices and other regulatory requirements.

Reasons for Validation

Validation is *"Establishment of documented evidence that provides a high degree of assurance that a specific process will consistently produce a product meeting its pre-determined specifications and quality attributes"*. A properly designed system will provide a high degree of assurance that every step, process, and change has been properly evaluated before its implementation. Testing a sample of a final product is not considered sufficient evidence that every product within a batch meets the required specification.

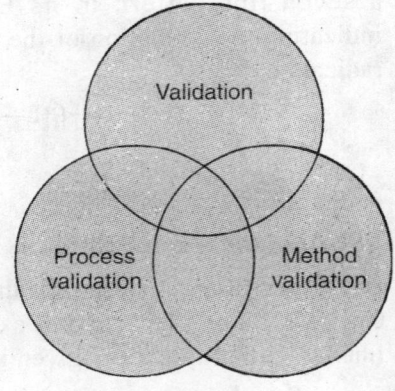

Fig. 19.1.

1. PROCESS VALIDATION

Process validation is defined as the collection and evaluation of data, from the process design stage through commercial production, which establishes scientific evidence that a process is capable of consistently delivering quality product.

WHY VALIDATE PROCESSES?

First, and certainly foremost, among the reasons for validation is that it is a regulatory requirement for virtually every process in the global health care industry for pharmaceuticals, biological, and medical devices. Regulatory agencies across the world except firms to validate their processes.

The containing trend toward harmonization of requirements will eventually result in a common level of expectation for validations worldwide. Utility for validation beyond compliance is certainly available. The rationale compliance has reduced our visibility towards other advantages of validation process, thereby preventing us from developing an inuing complete validation process. Some years ago, identified a number of tangible and intangible benefits of validation realized at his employer at the time. In the intervening years, there has been repeated affirmation of those expectations at other firms, large and small. Regrettably, there has been little quantification of these benefits. The predominance of compliance-based validation initiatives generally restricts objective discussion of cost implications for any initiative. But once a process/product is properly validated, it would seem that reduced sample size and intervals could be easily justified, and thus provide a measurable return on the validation effort. Aside from utility systems, this is hardly ever realized and represents one of the major failings relative to the implementation of validation in our industry. Validation and validation-like activities are found in a number of industries, regulated and unregulated. Banking, aviation, software, microelectronics, nuclear power, among others all incorporate practices closely resembling validation of health care product production. That such verification activities for products, processes, and systems have utility in other areas should not be surprising. The health care industries fixation on compliance has perhaps blinded us to the real value of validation practices.

PROCESS VALIDATION: ORDER OF PRIORITY

Because of resource limitation, it is not always possible to validate an entire company's product line at once. With the obvious exception that a company's most profitable product should be given a higher priority, it is advisable to draw up a list of product categories to be validated. The following order of importance or priority with respect to validation is suggested.

A. Sterile Products and their Processes
1. Large-volume parenterals (LVPs)
2. Small-volume parenterals (SVPs)
3. Ophthalmics, other sterile products, and medical devices

B. Nonsterile Products and their Processes
1. Low-dose/high-potency tablets and capsules/transdermal delivery system (TDDs)
2. Drugs with stability problems
3. Other tablets and capsules
4. Oral liquids, topicals, and diagnostic aids

TYPES OF PROCESS VALIDATION
1. Prospective process validation (also called premarket validation),
2. Retrospective process validation,
3. Concurrent validation, and
4. Revalidation

1. Prospective Process Validation

In prospective process validation, an experimental plan called the validation protocol is executed (following completion of the qualification trials) before the process is put into commercial use. Most validation efforts require some degree of prospective experimentation to generate validation support data. This particular type of process validation is normally carried out in connection with the introduction of new drug products and their manufacturing processes.

The formalized process validation program should never be undertaken unless and until the following operations and procedures have been completed satisfactorily:

1. The facilities and equipment in which the process validation is to be conducted meet CGMP requirements (completion of *installation qualification*).
2. The operators and supervising personnel who will be "running" the validation batch(es) have an understanding of the process and its requirements.
3. The design, selection, and optimization of the formula have been completed.
4. The qualification trials using (10 × size) pilot-laboratory batches have been completed, in which the critical processing steps and process variables have been identified, and the provisional operational control limits for each critical test parameter have been provided.
5. Detailed technical information on the product and their manufacturing process have been provided, including documented evidence of product stability.
6. Finally, at least one qualification trial of a pilot-production (100 × size) batch has been made and shows, upon scale-up, that there were no significant deviation from the expected performance of the process.

2. Restrospective Validation

Retrospective validation is the validation of a process based on accumulated historical production, testing, control, and other information for a product already in production and distribution. This type of validation makes use of historical data and information which may be found in batch records, production log books, lot records, control charts, test and inspection results, customer complaints or lack of complaints, field failure reports, service reports, and audit reports. Historical data must contain enough information to provide an in-depth picture of how the process has been operating and whether the product has consistently met its specifications. Retrospective validation may not be feasible if all the appropriate data was not collected, or appropriate data was not collected in a manner which allows adequate analysis.

Retrospective validation may be conducted in the following manner:

1. Gather the numerical data from the completed batch record and include assay values, end-product test results, and in-process data.
2. Organize these data in a chronological sequence according to batch manufacturing data, using a spreadsheet format.
3. Include data from at least the last 20–30 manufactured batches for analysis. If the number of batches is less than 20, then include all manufactured batches and commit to obtain the required number for analysis.

4. Trim the data by eliminating test results from noncritical processing steps and delete all gratuitous numerical information.
5. Subject the resultant data to statistical analysis and evaluation.
6. Draw conclusions as to the state of control of the manufacturing process based on the analysis of retrospective validation data.
7. Issue a report of your findings (documented evidence).

3. Concurrent Validation

In-process monitoring of critical processing steps and end-product testing of current production can provide documented evidence to show that the manufacturing process is in a state of control.

4. Revalidation

Almost all GMP texts recommend that whenever there are significant changes in the facility, equipment or process, revalidation should be carried out.

The FDA process validation guidelines refer to a quality assurance system in place that requires revalidation whenever there are changes in packaging (assumed to be the primary container-closure system), formulation, equipment or processes (meaning not clear) which could impact on product effectiveness or product characteristics and whenever there are changes in product characteristics.

Conditions requiring revalidation study and documentation are listed as follows:
1. Change in a critical component (usually refers to raw materials).
2. Change or replacement in a critical piece of modular (capital) equipment.
3. Change in a facility and/or plant (usually location or site).
4. Significant (usually order of magnitude) increase or decrease in batch size.
5. Sequential batches that fail to meet product and process specifications.

BENEFITS OF PROCESS VALIDATION

- Increased throughput.
- Reduction in rejections and reworks.
- Reduction in utility costs.
- Avoidance of capital expenditures.
- Fewer complaints about process related failures.
- Reduced testing in process and finished goods.
- More rapid and accurate investigations into process deviations.
- More rapid and accurate investigations into process deviation.
- More rapid and reliable start-up of new equipment.
- Easier scale-up from development work.
- Easier maintenance of the equipment.

- Improved employee awareness of processes.
- More rapid automation.

2. METHOD VALIDATION

Method validation is the process used to confirm that the analytical procedure employed for a specific test is suitable for its intended use. Results from method validation can be used to judge the quality, reliability and consistency of analytical results; it is an integral part of any good analytical practice.

Strategy for the Validation of Methods

The validity of a specific method should be demonstrated in laboratory experiments using samples or standards that are similar to unknown samples analyzed routinely. The preparation and execution should follow a validation protocol, preferably written in a step-by-step instruction format. Possible steps for a complete method validation are listed in Table 19.1. This proposed procedure assumes that the instrument has been selected and the method has been developed. It meets criteria such as case of use; ability to be automated and to be controlled by computer systems; costs per analysis; sample throughput; turnaround time; and environmental, health and safety requirements.

Table 19.1. The range of different analytical procedures

Analytical procedure	Range
Assay of a drug substance	80%–120% of test concentration
Impurity determination	50%–120% of specification
Content uniformity	70%–130% of test concentration
Dissolution testing	$\pm$ 20% over the specified range

1. Develop a validation protocol, an operating procedure or a validation master plan for the validation.
2. For a specific validation project define owners and responsibilities.
3. Develop a validation project plan.
4. Define the application, purpose and scope of the method.
5. Define the performance parameters and acceptance criteria.
6. Define validation experiments.
7. Verify relevant performance characteristics of equipment.
8. Qualify materials, e.g. standards and reagents for purity, accurate amounts and sufficient stability.
9. Perform pre-validation experiments.
10. Adjust method parameters or/and acceptance criteria if necessary.
11. Perform full internal (and external) validation experiments.
12. Develop SPOs for executing the method in the routine.

13. Define criteria for revalidation.
14. Define type and frequency of system suitability tests and/or analytical quality control (AQC) checks for the routine.
15. Document validation experiments and results in the validation report.

PARAMETERS FOR METHOD VALIDATION

- Accuracy
- Precision
- Specificity
- Limit of detection
- Limit of quantitation
- Linearity
- Range
- Robustness

Accuracy

The accuracy of an analytical method is the closeness of test results obtained by that method to the true value. The accuracy of an analytical method should be established across its range.

In assay of a drug substance, accuracy may be determined by application of the analytical method to an analyte of known purity (e.g. a reference standard) or by comparison of the results of the method of a second, well characterized method, the accuracy of which has been stated or defined. The ICH documents recommended that accuracy be assessed using a minimum of nine determinations over a minimum of three concentration levels, covering the specified range (i.e., three concentrations and three replicates of each concentration).

Precision

The precision of analytical method is the degree of agreement among individual test results when the method is applied repeatedly to multiple sampling of a homogeneous sample. The precision of an analytical method is usually expressed as the standard deviation or relative standard deviation of a series of measurements. Precision may be measure of either the degree of reproducibility or repeatability of the analytical method under normal operating conditions. In this context, reproducibility refers to the use of analytical procedure in different laboratories, as in a collaborative study. Intermediate precision expresses within laboratory variation, as on different days, or with different analysts or equipment with the same laboratory. Repeatability refers to the use of analytical procedure within a laboratory over a short period of time using the same analysts with the same equipment.

The precision of an analytical method is determined by assaying a sufficient number of aliquots of a homogeneous sample to be able to calculate statistically valid estimates of standard deviation or relative standard deviation. Assay in this context are independent analyses of samples that have been carried through the complete analytical procedure from sample preparation to final test result.

ICH documents recommend that repeatability should be assessed using a minimum of nine determinations covering the specified range for the procedure (i.e., three concentrations and three replicates of each concentration, or a minimum of six determinations at 100% of the test concentration).

Specificity

The specificity of an analytical method is defined as the ability to assess unequivocally the analyte in the presence of components that may be expected to present, such as impurities, degradation products, and matrix components. Lack of specificity of an analytical procedure may be compensated for by other supporting analytical procedures.

In qualitative analyses, the ability to select between the compounds of closely related structure that are likely to be present should be demonstrated. This ability should be confirmed by obtaining positive results from the samples containing the analyte, coupled with negative results from samples that do not contain the analyte, and by conforming that a positive response is not obtained from materials structurally similar to or closely related to the analyte.

In an analytical procedure for impurities, specificity may be established by spiking the drug substance or product with appropriate levels of impurities and demonstrating that these impurities are determined with appropriate accuracy and precision.

The ICH documents state that when chromatographic procedures areused, representative chromatograms should be presented to demonstrate the degree of selectivity, and peaks should be appropriately labeled. Peak purity tests may be useful to show that the analyte chromatographic peak is not attributable to more than one component.

Limit of detection

Limit of detection is a characteristic of limit tests. It is the lowest amount of analyte in a sample that can be detected but not necessarily quantitated, under the stated experimental conditions. Thus, limit tests merely substantiate that the amount of analyte is above or below a certain level. The detection limit is usually expressed as the concentration of analyte in the sample.

For non-instrumental methods, the detection limit is generally determined by the analysis of samples with known concentrations of analyte and by establishing the minimum level at which the analyte can be reliably detected. For instrumental procedures, the same method may be used as for non-instrumental. In the case of methods submitted for consideration as official compendia methods, it is almost never necessary to determine the actual detection limit. Rather, the detection limit is shown to be sufficiently low by the analysis of samples with known concentrations of analyte above and below the required detection level.

In case of instrumental analytical procedures that exhibit background noise, the ICH documents describe a common approach, which is to compare measured signals from samples with known low concentration of analyte with those of blank samples. The minimum concentration at which the analyte can reliably be detected is established. Typically acceptable signal-to-noise ratios are 2:1 or 3:1. Other approaches depend on the determination of the slope of the calibration curve and the standard deviation of responses. Whatever method is used, the detection limit should be subsequently validated by the analysis of a suitable number of samples known to be near, or prepared at, the detection limit.

Limit of quantitation

The limit of quantitation is a characteristic of quantitative assays for low levels of compounds in sample matrices, such as impurities in bulk drug substances and degradation produced in finished pharmaceuticals. It is the lowest amount of analyte in a sample that can be determined with acceptable precision and accuracy under the stated experimental conditions. The quantitation limit is expressed as the concentration of analyte (e.g. percentage, parts per billion) in the sample.

For non-instrumental methods, the detection limit is generally determined by the analysis of samples with known concentrations of analyte and by establishing the minimum level at which the analyte can be determined with acceptable accuracy and precision. For instrumental procedures, the same method may be used as for non-instrumental. In the case of methods submitted for consideration as official compendia methods, it is almost never necessary to determine the actual quantitation limit. Rather, the quantitation limit is shown to be sufficiently low by the analysis of samples with known concentrations of analyte above and below the required quantitation level.

In case of instrumental analytical procedures that exhibit background noise, the ICH documents describe a common approach, which is to compare measured signals from samples with known low concentration of analyte with those of blank samples. The minimum concentration at which the analyte can reliably be quantified is established. A typically acceptable signal-to-noise ratio is 10:1. Other approaches depend on the determination of the slope of the calibration curve and the standard deviation of responses. Whatever method is used, the quantitation limit should be subsequently validated by the analysis of a suitable number of samples known to be near, or prepared at the quantitation limit.

Linearity and range

Linearity of an analytical method is its ability to elicit test results that are directly, or by a well-defined mathematical transformation, proportional to the concentration of analyte in samples within a given range.

Range: The range of an analytical method is the interval between the upper and lower levels of analyte that has been demonstrated to be determined with a suitable level of precision, accuracy, and linearity using the method as written. The range is normally expressed in the same units as test results (e.g. percent, parts per million) obtained by the analytical method.

Linearity should be expressed across the range of the analytical procedure. It should be established initially by visual examination of a plot of signals as a function of analyte concentration of content. If there appears to be a linear relationship, test results should be established by appropriate statistical methods.

The range of the method is validated by verifying that the analytical method provides acceptable precision, accuracy, and linearity when applied to samples containing analyte at the extremes of the range as well as within the range.

ICH recommends that, for the establishment of linearity, a minimum of five concentrations normally be used. It is also recommended that the following minimum specified ranges should be considered.

Robustness: The robustness of the analytical method is a measure of its capacity to remain unaffected by small but deliberate variations in method parameters and provide an indication of its reliability during normal usage.

One consequence of evaluation of robustness should be that a series of system suitability parameters is established to ensure that the validity of the analytical method is maintained whenever used. Typical variations are the stability of analytical solutions, equipments and analysts. In liquid chromatography, typical variations are the pH of the mobile phase, the mobile phase composition, different lots or suppliers of columns, the temperature and the flow rate. In the case of gas chromatography, typical variations are different lots or suppliers of columns, the temperature, and flow rate.

Question Bank

Chapter 1

1. (a) Define the terms qualitative and quantitative analysis.
   (b) Differentiate between micro and semi-micro analytical methods.
   (c) What are advantages and limitations of chemical methods?
2. Classify the various instrumental methods. Discuss their advantages and disadvantages.
3. Give a brief account on methods for repoorting analytical data?

Chapter 2

1. What is the principle of mass spectrometry?
2. Discuss the various components of mass spectrometer.
3. Clarify the various ionization sources. Discuss them in view of their advantages and disadvantages.
4. What do you meant by low resolution and high resolution mass spectrometer? How the resolution power is calculated?
5. How the ions of different mass value are separated in mass spectrometer? Discuss in detail.
6. What is nitrogen rule?
7. How the index of hydrogen deficiency is calculated? What is index of hydrogen deficiency of benzaldehyde and cyclohexane?
8. Discuss the various types of positive ions, formed during ionization/fragmentation in mass spectrometry along with their importance.
9. How the molecular formula is determined with the help of mass spectrometry?
10. Discuss the importance of mass spectrometry.
11. Discuss the role of molecular ion and isotopic ion peaks to determine the molecular formula.

12. Discuss the chemical ionization method, using methane, isobutane and ammonia gases.
13. Write short notes on following:
    (a) Maclafferty rearrangement
    (b) Diel-alder rearrangement
    (c) Importance of mass spectrometry in structural elucidation of organic compounds
    (d) Stevenson rule
    (e) Metastable ion peak
    (f) Quadrupole
14. Discuss the rules governing the fragmentation pattern in mass spectrometry.
15. Give the fragmentation pattern of following:
    (a) Acetophenone
    (b) Hexanone
    (c) Toluene
    (d) Benzyl alcohol
    (e) Isopentane
    (f) o-Methyl ethyl benzoate
16. Discuss the qualitative and quantitative applications of mass spectrometry.
17. The mass spectrum of a compound contain only C, H and O, have the following intensity pattern for molecular and isotopic ion peaks.

m/e	Intensity of peak
100 (M+)	100
101 (M + 1)	6.67
102 (M + 2)	0.41

    Due to structure of the compound.
18. (a) Distinguish the 3-methyl cyclohexene and 4-methyl cyclohexene on the basis of their mass spectrum
    (b) Show the fragmentation peaks of cyclohexane at m/e 69, m/e 56, m/e 55, and m/e 41
    (c) A compound whose molecular ion peak was observed at m/e 122 has an equally intense (M + 2) peak. Give the molecular formula of the compound.
19. In the mass spectrum of methyl butylate peaks at m/e 102, 74, 59 and 53 are observed. Explain the formation of these ions.
20. (a) (i) Write a brief note on application of mass spectrum in the analysis of halogen compounds.
        (ii) Explain about meta stable ion peaks in mass spectrometry.
    (b) (i) Write a note on β-cleavage in mass spectrometry.
        (ii) Determine the molecular formula and structure of organic compound by the following mass spectral data.

m/e	109	108	93	78	77	66	65	51	39	30
Relative abundance:	(7)	(100)	(18)	(50)	(30)	(3)	(46)	(12)	(18)	(40).

Chapter 3

1. State Beers and Lamberts law.
2. What are the differences between the single beam and double beam UV visible spectrophotometers?
3. Explain the relationship between wavelength, wave number and frequency of electromagnetic radiations.
4. Enumerate the different types of monochromators used in spectrophotometers and mention advantages of each.
5. Define and explain chromophore and auxochrome.
6. State and explain Beers and Lamberts law. Give its mathematical expression.
7. Define molar extinction coefficient.
8. Bring out differences between grating and prism monochromator.
9. Explain the construction and working of any two detectors used in colorimeters.
10. Define the terms of bathochromic shift and hypochromic shift.
11. Why is the absorption maximum of the compound preferred for the quantitative determination?
12. Enumerate the applications of UV spectrometry.
13. What is wave number? What unit is used to express it.
14. Define wave number and how is it related to energy.
15. Define hypsochromic shift and hyperchromic shift.
16. Describe the construction and working of prism monochromators and interference monochromators in UV spectrophotometers.
17. With a Beat diagram, explain the construction and working of a barrier layer cell. Compare the merits and demerits of barrier layer cell with that of phototube.
18. What are the type of electronic transitions observed, when the organic molecule absorbs ultra violet radiations? Give examples.
19. Mention the detectors used in UV spectrophotometers and explain the working of any one of them.
20. Explain with the help of a neat diagram, the construction and working of a UV visible spectrophotometer with special emphasis on the monochromators and detectors present in them.
21. Define and explain the Beers Lamberts law. Explain the factors affecting this above law and discuss its applications.
22. Write a note on following:
    (a) Woodward-Feiser rule

330 Pharmaceutical Analysis

(b) Effect on hydrogen bonding on absorption maxima in UV spectroscopy

(c) Effect of solvent on absorption maxima in UV spectroscopy

23. What are the effects of solvent and pH upon the UV spectra of an organic compound? Show with examples.
24. What are the requirements of a molecule for absorption of ultraviolet radiations?
25. Calculate the absorption maxima of following compounds.

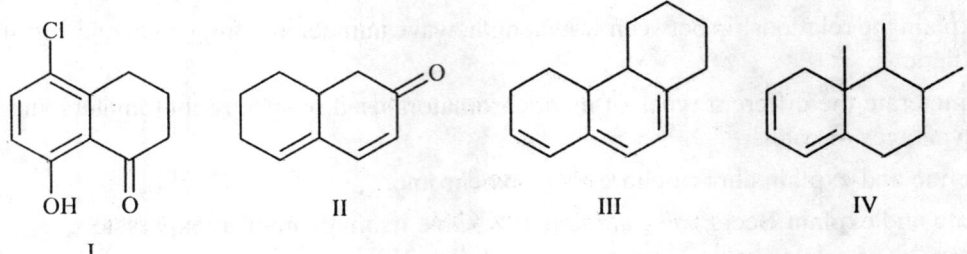

I   II   III   IV

26. Distinguish between cis-trans isomers and keto-enol tautomers using UV spectroscopy.
27. Discuss the different types of radiation sources used in UV visible spectrometric method.

Chapter 4

1. Explain why water cannot be used as a solvent in IR spectrophotometry? Explain why IR spectrophotometer should be used in humid free conditions.
2. Explain sample handling in IR spectroscopy.
3. How are the following organic compounds, distinguished by IR spectra?

    (a) Aldehydes and ketones

    (b) Alcohol and ether

4. What is fingerprint region? What is its importance?
5. What are the means of handling samples in IR spectroscopy? Describe suitable methods to obtain IR spectra for solid samples.
6. Write a note on the different sources of light used in IR spectrophotometers.
7. Discuss the various types of detectors used in IR spectrophotometer.
8. How the IR technique differs from the UV spectroscopical technique.
9. What are the factors causing deviation from Beers law.
10. Describe the instrumentation of IR spectroscopy with the help of neat diagram.
11. Explain the working of Golay cell.
12. With the help of a neat diagram, explain the various parts and working of IR spectrophotometer.
13. Explain Beers Lamberts law and its applications and limitations.
14. Discuss the theory of IR spectroscopy and give its applications.

15. Write short notes on the following:
    (a) Types of fundamental vibrational changes in IR spectroscopy
    (b) Selection rule
    (c) Non-fundamental vibrational changes in IR spectroscopy
    (d) Effect of hydrogen bonding in IR spectroscopy
    (e) Strokes law and its importance
16. Using IR how can you differentiate between:
    (i) Primary, secondary and tertiary amine
    (ii) Alcohol and phenol
    (iii) Cyclic and acyclic anhydride
17. Predict the frequency shift of carbonyl in the benzaldehyde and o-hydroxy benzaldehyde.
18. Calculate the frequency (in Hz and cm^{-1}) of O–H band, if the force constant and reduced mass of the atom pair are 770 Nm^{-1} and 1.563×10^{-27} kg respectively.
19. Discuss the application of IR spectroscopy in the structural elucidation of organic compounds.
20. Discuss the effect of hydrogen bonding on IR absorption bands. Differentiate the intermolecular and intramolecular hydrogen bonding.
21. Discuss the different types of radiation sources used in IR spectrometric methods and mention the different types of detectors used in IR spectrometer.
22. What are the different regions of the IR spectrum? Explain various types of stretching and bending vibrations.
23. Which of the following molecules are IR active and why?
    (i) CO_2
    (ii) HCN
    (iii) N_2O
    (iv) CH_4
24. Define Fourier transform? Describe IR instrumentation.
25. Define cut-off wavelength and Beer-Lambert law in detail.

Chapter 5

1. What is the principle behind NMR spectroscopy?
2. What is the reference standard used in NMR? What is the reaction behind its selection? What is chemical shift?
3. Name one reference standard each used in NMR and ESR spectroscopy.
4. Explain the shielding and deshielding effects.
5. Write a note on spin-spin splitting. How it differs from chemical shift?
6. Define chemical shift and mention its application.

7. Explain in detail about chemical shift and spin-spin coupling.
8. Discuss the factors affecting the chemical shift.
9. Write a note on following:
   (a) Equivalent and non-equivalent protons
   (b) NMR instrumentation
   (c) Use of deuterated solvents in NMR spectroscopy
10. Discuss the NMR spectrum of following:
    (a) ortho-Aminoacetophenone
    (b) Ethyl acetate
    (c) p-Hydroxy toluene
    (d) Ethyl acetoacetate
11. Discuss the effect on hydrogen bonding on NMR spectra with example.
12. What is principle of ^{13}C-NMR spectroscopy?
13. What is advantages of ^{13}C-NMR spectroscopy over ^{1}H-NMR spectroscopy.
14. Compare the ^{1}H-NMR and ^{13}C-NMR spectroscopy with example.
15. What is 2D-dimensional NMR spectroscopy? Classifythem.
16. Discuss the NMR spectrum of acetylene and benzene.
17. A compound having molecular formula $C_4H_8O_2$ shows three peaks in proton NMR at delta 1.2 (triplet), 2.1 (singlet) and 4.4 (quartet). Identify the compound.
18. What are the magnetically active and inactive nuclei? Explain with examples.
19. Why TMS is used as reference standard in NMR technique?
20. Explain the relaxation process as a taking place in NMR technique.
    1. (a) Discuss about ^{13}C-NMR and simplification of ^{13}C-spectra by process of decoupling.
       (b) What are the main differences between ^{1}H^{13}C-NMR and ^{13}CNMR.
    2. (a) Describe the ^{1}H-NMR of neat ethanol.
       (b) Assign the ^{13}CNMR chemical shifts for the following compounds.
           (i) $C_6H_5-CH_2-CH_3$
           (ii) $C_6H_5-CH=CH_2$
       (c) Sketch the off resonance decoupled ^{13}C-NMR spectra of n-propylchloride and acetaldehyde.
    3. (a) Write short notes on off resonance decoupling.
       (b) Suggest structure based on the given ^{1}HNMR data and molecular formula
           Molecular formula C_9H_{12}.
           0.95 (t, 3H), 1.70 (sexhet: 2H), 2.6 (t, 2H), and 7.25 (s, 5H)
       (c) Predict the CMR values of the following compound
           ph–CO–CH_2–CH_3

(d) Deduct the structure of the organic compound with following data, having Molecular formula C_9H_{10} × 7.30 (m, 5H), 5.34 (d, 1H), 5.05 (m, 1H), 2.11 (d, 3H).
21. (a) Explain the principle involved in CMR spectra.
    (b) Why it is not possible to determine relative ratio of carbon atoms in a compound by integration of peak area in ^{13}C NMR as in PMR?
22. What are the basic principles and advantages of FT-NMR?

Chapter 6

1. Explain in brief the light source used in atomic absorption spectroscopy.
2. Under what circumstances N_2O acetylene flame would be preferred over oxyacetylene flame in atomic absorption spectroscopy. Explain with example.
3. Give an account of various interferences that may affect atomic absorption analysis.
4. What is the principle of atomic absorption spectroscopy? How the sample preparation is done in this technique.
5. Discuss the instrumentation of atomic absorption spectroscopy.
6. (a) What is atomic absorption? What are its advantages and disadvantages?
   (b) Give some of its limitations.

Chapter 7

1. (a) Distinguish fluorescence and phosphorescence in terms of their mechanism by which an excited molecule is deactivated.
   (b) How would you distinguish the two experimentally?
2. Compare absorption and fluorescence procedures as to (a) sensitivity and (b) selectivity.
3. What are the two basic differences in the construction of a fluorimeter as compared to an absorption spectrophotometer?
4. Define singlet and triplet states.
5. What is the relation between phosphorescence intensity and concentration?
6. What are the fluorescent indicators?
7. How will you determine vitamin B_1 by fluorimetry?
8. Describe the double beam fluorimeter with neat diagram.
9. Explain how a spectrofluorimetric method is more sensitive and selective than spectrophotometric method.
10. Explain the term quenching. Discuss the different types of quenching.
11. Enumerate and discuss the different factors that affect the intensity of fluorescence.
12. Whay is quenching? Explain various types of quenching with suitable examples.
13. Explain the relationship between fluorescence and chemical structure of organic compound.

14. Outline the procedure by which thiamine is estimated by fluorimetry.
15. Show the relationship between fluorescence intensity and concentration. Describe any four factors that influence the efficiency of fluorescence.
16. Write the difference between fluorescence and phosphorescence.
17. Add a note on fluorescent indicators and explain the estimation of quinine sulphate or riboflavin by fluorescence spectroscopy.
18. Why do the fluorescence measured at right angles with respect to incident activation beam?
19. List four examples of drugs that are assayed by measuring their inherent fluorescence.
20. Explain the necessity of using 2 filters in fluorimetry.
21. Explain the advantages of fluorimeter over colorimeter. How can non-fluorescent drugs can be assayed by fluorimetry.
22. Explain the theory, instrumentation and applications of spectrofluorimetry.

Chapter 8

1. Outline the principle of flame photometry.
2. Explain the principle and applications of flame photometry.
3. Discuss the instrumentation and working of flame photometry.
4. Write a note on atomizers used in flame photometry.
5. Explain in detail about photoluminescence? What are the relationship between the concentration and fluorescence, and mention the structural features required to give fluorescence with the help of a neat label diagram.
6. How you estimate the sodium by using flame photometry? What criteria were considered in selecting the method and designing the experimental procedure?

Chapter 9

1. Compare the relative sensitivities of the nephelometer and turbidimeter.
2. Compare the nephelometer, turbidimeter and spectrophotometer, as to the type of samples.
3. Compare the three instruments as to the geometrical arrangements of the samples and detectors.
4. What is the main criterion for deciding whether turbidimetry or nephelometry should be used in the analysis of a medium containing suspended particles?
5. Write applications of turbidimetry and nephelometry.
6. Discuss the theory of nephelometry and turbidimetry.

Chapter 10

1. Write short notes on:
    (a) Liquid membrane electrode
    (b) Solid state membrane electrode

(c) Precipitate membrane electrode
   (d) Double membrane electrode
2. Discuss the applications of ion selective electrode.
3. Write advantages of potentiometric titration over other indicator method.
4. Show how following titrations are carried out by potential measurement.
   (a) Acid-base titration
   (b) Redox titration
   (c) Complexometric titration
   (d) Precipitation titration
5. Explain graphical method and differential method for the determination of end point in the potentiometric titration.
6. Derive the Nernst equation.
7. What are the different types of electrodes used in potentiometric titration?
8. Write short note of glass electride with diagram.
9. Enumerate any two reference electrodes and two indicator electrodes used in potentiometry.
10. What is null point potentiometry? Under what circumstances it is applied?
11. Explain any two methods to locate the equivalence point by potentiometry.
12. Define indicator and reference electrodes.
13. Explain the significance of dead stop end point technique.
14. Name the indicator electrodes that can be used in acid base titrations using a potentiometer.
15. Explain the principle underlying dead stop end point technique and null-point potentiometry.

Chapter 11

1. Definethe terms, conductance, specific resistance, cell constant, molar conductance.
2. Give the relation between specific conductance and equivalent conductance and discuss the effect of dilution on various conductances.
3. Show how following titration are carried out by conductance measurements.
   (a) Acid-base titration
   (b) Complexometric titration
   (c) Precipitation titration
   (d) Replacement titration
   (e) Redox titration
4. Describe the principle of conductometric titration of a strong acid with a weak base.
5. What is the effect of temperature on conductivity of a solution.
6. What is the principle of conductometric titrations?

7. Explain with graph, the conductometric titration of a mixture of weak and strong acid with strong alkali.
8. Draw and explain the conductometric titration curve of a strong base against a strong acid.
9. Explain the conductometric titration curve of a strong acid against a weak base.
10. Explain the principle underlying conductometric titration? Explain how the presence of mineral acid in vinegar be determined by a conductometric titration.
11. Show how solubility of sparingly soluble salt and basicity of organic acid are determined by conductance measurement.
12. Show how solubility of ionic product of water and hydrolysis constants/dissociation constants is determined by conductance measurement.
13. What is cell constant? Discuss the method to determine conductance and hence the cell constant by conductance measurement.
14. Discuss the applications of conductometry in detail.
15. Discuss the effect of dilution on various conductances. Write short note on conductivity cell.
16. Write about the general concept and basis of conductometric titrations.

Chapter 12

1. Explain polarographic maxima and mention how this can be prevented.
2. Why is it necessary to remove dissolved oxygen from the electrolyte solutions before polarographic analysis? How is oxygen removed? Add a note on polarographic maxima.
3. Describe the construction and working of saturated calomel electrode.
4. Describe the construction and working of glass electrode.
5. Explain the role of supporting electrolyte in polarography.
6. Mention the importance of half wave potential.
7. Explain the experimental arrangement of polarography and construction of current voltage curve with diagram.
8. Explain the basic principle involved in polarography and discuss the factors affecting diffusion current.
9. What is diffusion current and discuss the factors affecting diffusion current.
10. Justify the statement – "Half wave potential is a characteristic constant for a reversible oxidation-reduction system. Add a note on Ilkovic equation and polarographic maxima.
11. Describe the construction and working, advantages, disadvantages and applications of a standard hydrogen electrode.
12. Explain the principle involved in polarography. Explain the half wave potential and applications of polarography.
13. Define electrochemical cell.
14. What is a Nernst equation?
15. Draw and explain the various features of polarographic curve.

Chapter 13

1. Explain amperometric titrations of curves with example.
2. Write short notes on amperometric titrations and discuss its importance in analysis of metallic ions.
3. Write about the technique of amperometric titrations with the dropping mercury electrode.

Chapter 14

1. What is polarized light? How it can be obtained?
2. Explain the function of each part of polarimeter with the help of neat diagram.
3. Define the term specific rotation. Explain the factors affecting the specific rotation.
4. Explain what the following term mean (i) $[\alpha]^{25} = +4.21$; (ii) $[\alpha] = -10°$; (iii) optically inactive.
5. Discuss the applications of polarimetry.

Chapter 15

1. What is Bragg's law?
2. Discuss the some applications of XRF technique.
3. Discuss some of applications of X-ray diffraction techniques.
4. Explain the applications of X-ray diffraction in pharmaceutical application.
5. Explain the concept of reciprocal lattice concept. Add a note on different X-ray diffraction patterns.
6. What is principle of X-ray fluorescence spectroscopy? Discuss its applications.

Chapter 16

1. Define the terms index of refraction, angle of incidence, and critical angle of refraction.
2. What is effect of temperature on refractive index? How it is measured?
3. Discuss the applications of refractometry.
4. What is molecular refraction? Discuss the application of refractometry and Abbe type of refractometer.

Chapter 17

1. What are common source of errors in thermogravimetric analysis?
2. What are the common instrumental factors affecting TG curves.
3. Explain different types of thermal balances.
4. Explain thermometric titrations. Give a detailed account on applications of thermometric titrations.

5. Write a note on differential thermal analysis 10 M.
6. What is principle of DSC technique. How the purity of sample can be determined by this technique.
7. Explain briefly differential thermal analyses and differential scanning calorimetry.
8. Explain the principle of DSC analysis? How is it different from DTA?
9. (i) Give the principle of TGA and DTA? Discuss the DTA and TGA curve of calcium oxalate monohydrate.
   (ii) List out the information obtained from a DTA curve.

Chapter 18
1. (a) What is the principle of ESR. Discuss some important applications of ESR.
   (b) What are the limitations of ESR.
2. Why ESR spectroscopy is widely used in the study of chemical, photochemical and electrochemical reactions? Justify your answer.
3. What is 'g' value and shift in 'g' values in ESR spectra.

Chapter 19
1. What is validation? Why validation is performed?
2. Discuss the various parameters for validation process.

Index

A

Abbe's refractometer, 280, 281
Absorption spectroscopy, 49
Absorption frequencies, 85
    factors affecting, 85, 87
Absorption-enhancement effects, 271
Aliphatic ether, 42
Amides, 46
Amines, 45
Amperometric titrations, 232, 233
    advantages of, 235
    applications of, 236
    concept of, 233
    curves of, 234
        common types of, 234
    disadvantages of, 236
    examples of, 236
Analytical techniques, 1, 6
    characterization of, 6
Apparatus for thermometric titrations, 306
Application of DTA, 301
Application of TGA, 295
Applications of IR spectroscopy, 95
Aromatic ether, 43

Asymmetrical stretching, 81
Atomic absorption spectrometer, 145, 153
    source modulation in, 153
    types of, 154
Atomic absorption spectrophotometer, 144, 154
Atomic absorption spectroscopy, 141, 142, 143, 156, 161
    applications of, 161
    basic principle of, 143
    interferences in, 156
Atomic emission spectroscopy, 142
Atomic fluorescence spectroscopy, 143
Atomizers, 148
Automatic diffractometers, 273
Auxochrome, 54

B

Bathochromic shift, 54
Beer-Lambert's law, 66
    deviation from, 68
    validation of, 75
Bending vibrations, 84
Biamperometry end point method, 238
Biot's law, 241

Blue effect, 54
Blue shift, 54
Bolometer, 90
Bonds, 31
    energy profile of, 31
    relative strength of, 31
Bragg's law, 252
Broadband decoupling, 133

C

C-13 NMR spectroscopy, 132
Calomel electrode, 202
Carbon rod analyser, 152
Carbonyl compounds, 43
Carboxylic acid, 44
Cast film technique, 93
Cation-anion interference, 156
Cation-cation interference, 157
Cell constant, 213
Characteristic IR absorption frequencies, 109
Characteristics of DTA curves, 297
Charge-transfer complex, 52
Chemical interferences, 156, 184
Chemical shift, 118, 120
    factors affecting, 120
Chromophores, 53, 54
    types of, 54

Classical polarographic setup, 220
Classical techniques, 2
Classical vs instrumental techniques, 2
Combination tones, 84
Components of instruments, 253
Concentration polarization, 221
Concentric tube nebulizer, 149
Conductance measurements, 217
    applications of, 217
Conductometer, 212
Conductometric titrations, 208, 214
Conjugation, 70
    detection of, 70
Continuous and characteristic x-ray spectra, 248
Continuous wave NMR instruments, 114
COSY - correlation spectroscopy, 136
COSY spectra, 136
Coupled interactions, 86
Coupling constant, 127
Critical angle of refraction, 280
Crystal tonograpy, 275
Crystals used in WDXRF, 268

D

Daniel cell, 194
Deactivation process, 164
Dead stop end point technique, 205
Dead-stop end point method, 238
DEPT, 134
Deshielding effect, 118
Detection limits for selected elements, 161
Determination of vitamin B_1 (thiamine), 172
Deuterium exchange, 128
Deviation from Beer-Lambert's law, 68

Dextrose solution by polarimetric method, 245
    quantitative analysis of, 245
Differential scanning's calorimetry, 302
Differential thermal analysis, 297
Differential Thermo Gravimetric Analysis (DTGA), 295
Diffuse reflectance technique, 93
Diode array detector, 64
Dispersive infrared spectophotometers, 88
Doppler effect, 159
Double beam atomic absorption spectrophotometer, 154
Double beam UV-visible spectrometers, 65
DSC, 305
    advantages of, 305
    application of, 305
DSC instrument, 303
Dynamic quenching, 168

E

EMF of cell and its measurement, 195
Effect of hydrogen bonding on IR absorption, 87
Effect of polarizable groups on refractive index, 284
Effective line width, 158
Elastic scattering, 186
Electrochemical cell, 192, 194
Electrodeless discharge lamp, 148
Electromagnetic radiation, 49
Electromagnetic spectrum, 51
Electrometric determination of pH, 198
Electron microprobe, 275
Electron multiplier, 19
Electron spin, 163
Electron spin resonance spectroscopy, 310
Electronegativity effect on chemical shift, 120
    effect of, 120

Electronic transition, 52
    energy levels of, 52
Electrothermal atomizers, 151
Elemental mass spectrometry, 21
Elimination reaction, 34
Emission spectra, 177
Energy dispersive X-ray fluorescence (EDXRF), 268
Energy level diagram for a hypothetical atom, 248
Equivalent conductance, 210
ESR absorption positions, 312
ESR spectroscopy, 310, 316
    application of, 316
    theory of, 310
ESR spectroscopy instrument, 313
ESR spectrum, 315
    presentation of, 315
Esters, 45
Ethers, 42

F

Factors affecting absorption frequencies, 85, 87
Factors affecting chemical shift, 120
Factors affecting conductance, 210
Factors affecting DSC curve, 304
Factors affecting DTA data, 300
Factors affecting fluorescence, 166
Factors affecting refractive index, 278
Factors affecting thermogravimetric analysis, 291
Factors that influence DTA curve, 301
Fermi resonance, 84
Filter or monochromator, 60
Filters, 60
Fingerprint region, 79
Flame absorbance profiles, 150

Flame atomic absorption spectroscopy, 149
   fuels and oxidants used in, 149
Flame atomizers, 148, 151
   advantages of, 151
   disadvantages of, 151
Flame photometry, 175, 178
   application of, 182
Flame structure, 150
Fluorescence, 162
Fluorescence/Phosphorescence, 163
   theory of, 163
Fluorescent indicators, 173
Fluorimetry, 162, 171, 172
   applications of, 172
Fluorimetry in inorganic analysis, 173
   application of, 173
Fluorimetry or spectrofluorometry, 172
   advantages of, 172
Formazin, 187
Fourier transform IR spectrometers, 90
Fourier transform NMR instruments, 116
Fourier-transform spectrometers, 91
Fragment ions, 24
Fragmentation, 31, 37
   factors influencing, 31
   general rules of, 37
Functional group region, 79
Fundamental vibrations, 81

G

Gas filled transducers, 259
GC-MS, 29
Geiger tube, 261
Glass electrode, 199
   determination by, 199
Globar source, 89
Golay cell, 90

Graphite tube furnance, 151
Grazing angle, 280

H

Half shadow prism, 243
Half wave potential, 223
Heteronuclear correlation spectroscopy, 138
HMBC, 140
HMQC, 139
Hollow cathode lamp, 144, 147
Homonuclear correlation spectroscopy, 136
Hook's law, 82
HSQC, 139
Hydrocarbons, 40
Hydrogen bonding, 121
Hydrogen bonding on IR absorption, 87
   effect of, 87
Hydrogen electrode, 199
   pH determination, 199
Hydroxylated compounds, 40
Hyper chromic effect, 54
Hyperfine splitting, 315
Hyphenated techniques, 29
Hypochromic or blue effect, 54

I

Ilkovic equation, 223
Immersion refractometer, 282
Incandescent wire source, 89
Index of refraction, 277
Inferometers, 283
Infrared absorption, 80
   theory of, 80
Infrared spectroscopy, 78
Instrumental factors, 291
Instrumental methods, 6
   principle of, 6
Instrumental techniques, 2
Interference due to oxide formation, 157

Interpretation of diffraction patterns, 275
Ion-molecule interaction, 26
   ions formed by, 26
Ionisation interferences, 183
Ionisation potential, 10
Ionisation source, 10
   desorption sources, 13
      Electron Spray Ionisation (ESI), 15
      Fast Atom Bombardment (FAB), 14
      field desorption, 13
      laser desorption, 14
      Matrix Assisted Laser Desorption Ionisation (MALDI), 14
      photoionisation, 14
      thermal ionisation (surface ionisation), 13
   Gaseous sources, 10
      chemical ionisation, 12
      electron impact ionisation, 10
      field ionisation, 13
Ionization chambers, 262
Ionization interference, 157
Ions, 21
   types of, 21
IR instrumentation, 88
   detectors used in, 89
IR instrumentation, 89
IR region, 78
IR sources, 88
IR spectral analysis of organic compounds, 98
IR spectroscopy, 92, 95
   applications of, 95
   sample preparations in, 92
IR spectrum, 78
Isotope effects, 96
   study of, 96
Isotope ratio mass spectrometry, 21

Isotopes, 22
    natural abundance of, 22
Isotopic ions, 22

J

Jablonski diagram, 165
Jet separator, 30

K

Karl Fischer method, 205
KBr press method, 93

L

Larmor frequency, 113
Limiting current, 221
Line width, 158
Lithium-drifted silicon detector, 263
Lorentz effect, 159

M

Maclafferty Rearrangement (MR), 35
Magnetic anisotropy, 121
Magnetic quantum number, 111
Magnetogyric ratio, 112
Mass absorption coefficient, 251
Mass analyser, 15
    high resolution and low resolution, 16
        double focussing mass spectrometer, 17
        ion trap analysers, 19
        quadrupole mass analyser, 18
        single focussing mass spectrometer, 17
        time of flight (ToF) analyser, 18
        single focussing mass spectrometer, 17
Mass spectrometry, 8, 9, 19, 26
    application of, 26
    detectors used in, 19

Matrix effects, 270
    types of, 270
Matrix interference, 158
Maxima suppressors, 224
Metastable ions, 25
Michelson interferometer, 91
Migration current, 222
Minimum wavelength, 249
Miscellaneous atomization method, 153
Molar conductivity, 209
Molecular formula by mass spectrometer, 22
    determination of, 22
Molecular ions, 21
Molecular or molar refractivity, 278
Molecular refractivity, 278
Molecular vibrations, 81
    types of, 81
Molecular weight, 76
    determination of, 76
Monochromators, 60, 89
Multicenter fragmentations and steric factors, 34
Multiple charged ions, 25
Multiple ion detection, 28

N

Negative ions, 26
Nephelometer, 188
Nephelometric titrations, 186
Nephelometric Turbidity Unit (NTU), 187
Nephelometry, 191
    applications of, 191
Nernst glower, 88
NMR and ESR spectroscopy, 316
    comparison between, 316
2D NMR 136
    types of 136
^{13}C-NMR chemical shifts 134
NMR coupling constant, 127
NMR instrumentation, 114

NMR spectroscopy, 111, 129
    applications of, 129
2D-NMR spectroscopy 135
NMR spectrum, 116
NMR to quantitative analysis, 130
    application of, 130
NOESY, 137
Non-fundamental vibrations, 84
Nuclear Overhauser Enhancement (NOE), 135
Nuclear spin, 111
Nujol mull methods, 93

O

Organic compounds, 98
    IR spectral analysis of, 98
Organic compounds, 40, 230
    classes of, 40
        Common fragmentation pattern of, 40
    Polarographic analysis of, 230
Organic functional groups, 109
    IR absorption frequencies of, 109
Ortho effect, 35
Output devices, 64
Overtones, 84

P

Pascal's triangle, 125
pH determination by using hydrogen electrode, 199
Phosphorescence, 163
Photodiode array spectrometer, 65
Photoelectric detectors, 90
Photographic recording, 274
Photoluminescence, 162
Photomultiplier tube, 63
Phototube, 63
Polarimeter, 242
    components of, 243
Polarimeter, 243
Polarimetry, 240
    applications of, 244

Polarizer, 240
Polarogram, 222, 232
Polarographic apparatus, 228
Polarographic determination of ascorbic acid, 231
Polarographic maxima, 224
Polarography, 220, 229
　applications of, 229
　principle of, 220
Polymorphs, 96
　identification of, 96
Potentiometer, 195, 196
Potentiometric titration, 192, 202
Potentiometric titrations with conductometric titration, 206
　comparison of, 206
Presentation of the ESR spectrum, 315
Proportional counters, 261
Proton chemical shifts, 119
Pulfrich refractometer, 282
Pulse-height analyzers, 265
Pulse-height selectors, 264
Pyroelectric detectors, 90

Q

Qualitative and quantitative polarographic analysis, 225
Qualitative flame photometry, 181
　interferences in determinations of, 183
Qualitative UV-visible spectroscopy, 73
Quantitative atomic absorption spectroscopy, 159
Quantitative determination methodology, 74
Quantitative flame photometry, 181, 183
Quantitative fluorescence analysis, 169
Quantitative infrared spectroscopy, 94

Quantitative mass spectrometry, 29
Quantitative nephelometry, 189
Quantitative polarographic analysis, 227
Quantitative turbidimetry, 189
Quantitative UV-visible spectroscopy, 74
Quenching, 168
　dynamic, 168
　static, 168
Question Bank, 327
Quinhydrone electrode, 200
　determination by, 200
Quinine sulphate solution, 174
　assay of, 174

R

Radiant energy, 50
　absorption of, 50
Radiation sources (UV and visible), 59
Radioisotopes, 254
Rayleigh scattering, 186
Rearrangement ions, 24
Red shift, 54
Redox reaction in electrochemical cells, 193
Refractive index, 279
　determination of, 279
Refractometers, 280
Refractometry, 277, 283
　applications of, 283
Relative tendencies of electrodes, 195
Relative vs absolute techniques, 5
Relaxation processes, 114
Residual current, 224
Retro Diels-Alder reaction, 36
ROESY, 137

S

Salt bridges, 202
Sample handling system, 19

Scattering, 186
　origin of, 186
Scattering and diffraction, 252
Scheibe-Lomakin equation, 181
Scintillation counters, 262
Scintillation type detector, 19
Secondary fluorescent sources, 255
Selection rule, 80
Semiconductor transducers, 263
Sheilding effect, 118
Signal processing, 64
Signal processors, 259, 264
Silver bromide emulsion, 19
Silver-silver chloride electrode, 202
Single beam atomic absorption spectrophotometer, 154
Single beam UV-visible spectrometers, 64
Single electrode potential, 198
Single ion detection, 27
Single-channel vs multi-channel techniques, 3
Singlet/triplet excited states, 163
Snell's law, 280
Sodium ions in NaCl solution by flame photometry, 185
　determination of concentration of, 185
Specific and molecular refractivity, 277
Specific conductance, 209
Spectral interferences, 156, 183
Spectral line, 158
　broadening of, 158
Spectroscopy, 49
　absorption spectroscopy, 49
　emission spectroscopy, 49
Spin-lattice relaxation, 114
Spin-spin relaxation, 114
Stable neutral molecule, 37
　expulsion of, 37
Stable paramagnetic substances, 310

Standard addition method, 76
Static quenching, 168
Stevenson's rule, 38
Stokes' shift, 166
Stretching vibrations, 82
Symmetrical stretching, 81
Synchroton, 255

T

Tandem or multistage mass spectrometry, 20
Tantalum boat analyser, 152
Technique of thermometric titration, 307
Tetramethylsilane (TMS), 118
TGA, 295
    application of, 295
TGA principle and method, 287
Thermal detectors, 89
Thermoanalytical methods, 286
    types of, 286
Thermobalance, 290
Thermocouples, 90
Thermogravimetric analysis, 286
    types of, 287
Thermogravimetric analytical instrument, 290
Thermometric titration, 308
    application of, 308
Thermometric titration assembly and bridge circuit, 307
Thermometric titrations, 306
TMS, 118
TOCSY, 137
Transition, 51
$n \to \pi^*$ Transitions 58
$p \to \pi^*$ Transitions, 58
Turbidimeter, 188
Turbidimetric determination of sulphate in water, 191

Turbidimetric titrations, 186
Turbidimetry, 191
    applications of, 191
Turbidimetry versus nephelometry, 188
Typical DTA apparatus, 298

U

Ultraviolet spectroscopy, 70
    applications of, 70
Unstable paramagnetic substances, 310
Uranium, 173
    determination of, 173
UV absorption, 55
    effect of solvent on, 58
    importance of conjugation in, 55
UV and visible radiation, 51
    absorption of, 51
UV radiation source, 59
UV spectrum, 53, 59
    effect of hydrogen bonding on, 59
UV-visible spectrophotometer, 59, 63
    detectors used in, 63
    types of, 64
        double Beam, 65
        photodiode Array, 65
        single Beam, 64
UV-visible spectroscopy, 49
    detection of impurities by, 74

V

Vacuum system, 20
vacuum ultraviolet region, 52
Visible radiation sources, 60
Vitamin B_1 (thiamine), 172
    determination of, 172

Vitamin B_2 (riboflavin), 172
    determination of, 172

W

Wavelength and energy dispersion spectrometers, 269
    comparison of, 269
Wavelength dispersive spectrometers, 268
Wavelength Dispersive X-Ray Fluorescence (WDXRF), 268
Wavelength on specific rotation, 241
    effect of, 241
Wavelength selector, 60
Woodward rules, 70

X

X-ray absorption methods, 246, 272
X-ray diffraction methods, 246, 273
X-ray fluorescence methods, 246, 266
X-ray fluorescence spectrometry, 271
    applications of, 271
X-ray monochromators, 256
X-ray spectrum of a copper tangent, 249
X-ray transducers, 259
X-ray tube, 254
X-ray with matter, 250
    interaction of, 250
X-rays, 247, 256
    filters for, 256
    origin of, 247